The Orbit and the Visual Pathway

The Orbit and the Visual Pathway

Anatomical and Pathological Aspects and Detailed Clinical Accounts

Editors

Dieter Voth
Paul Glees

W DE G

Walter de Gruyter
Berlin · New York 1994

Editors

Professor Dr. Dr. h. c. med.
Dieter Voth
Neurochirurgische Universitätsklinik
Langenbeckstr. 1
55131 Mainz am Rhein

Professor Dr. med. Paul Glees
In der Russbreite 26
37077 Göttingen

This book contains 175 illustrations and 53 tables.

Library of Congress Cataloging-in-Publication Data

The Orbit and the visual pathway : anatomical and pathological aspects and detailed clinical accounts / editors, Dieter Voth, Paul Glees.
p. cm.
Includes indexes.
ISBN 3-11-012803-9 (pbk. : alk. paper)
1. Eye-sockets—Diseases. 2. Visual pathways—Diseases. I. Voth, D. (Dieter), 1935– . II. Glees, Paul.
[DNLM: 1. Orbit—physiology. 2. Orbit—pathology. 3. Orbital Diseases—pathology. 4. Visual Pathways—pathology. 5. Graves' Disease—pathology. WW 202 0635 1993]
RE71.068 1993
617.7'8—dc20
DNLM/DLC
for Library of Congress 93-34354
CIP

Die Deutsche Bibliothek — Cataloging-in-Publication Data

The **orbit and the visual pathway** : anatomical and pathological aspects and detailed clinical accounts / eds. Dieter Voth ; Paul Glees. – Berlin ; New York : de Gruyter, 1993
ISBN 3-11-012803-9
NE: Voth, Dieter [Hrsg.]

Medical science is constantly developing. Research and clinical experience expand our knowledge, especially with regard to treatment and medication. For dosages and applications mentioned in this work, the reader may rely on the authors, editors and publisher having taken great paints to ensure that these indications reflect the standard of knowledge at the time this work was completed.
Nevertheless, all users are requested to check the package leaflet of the medication, in order to determine for themselves whether the recommentations given for the dosages or the likely contraindications differ from those given in this book. This is especially true for medication which is seldom used or has recently been put on the market and for medication whose application has been restricted by the German Ministry of Health.
The quotation of registered names, trade names, trade marks, etc. in this copy does not imply, even in the absence of a specific statement that such names are exempt from laws and regulations protecting trade marks, etc. and therefore free for general use.
Printing: Gerike GmbH. — Binding: Lüderitz & Bauer, Berlin. — Printed in Germany.

CONTENTS

I INTRODUCTION

II BASIC RESEARCH AND DIAGNOSTIC METHODS

III TUMORS OF THE ORBIT AND THE VISUAL PATHWAY

IV GRAVE'S OPHTHALMOPATHY

V CAROTID CAVERNOUS FISTULA - DISTURBANCES OF CIRCULATION

I

INTRODUCTION

Preface and overview

D. Voth, P. Glees

The treatment of diseases of the orbit and the visual pathway has been a challenge to both the ophthalmologists and the neurosurgeons. Space occupying lesions within the orbital cavity were originally dealt with and the domain of ophthalmic surgeons, while all intracranially localised diseases, such as space occupying lesions involving the intracranial space were and are treated by neurosurgeons. This is certainly valid for tumors and inflammatory diseases.

A variable border line between the ranges of the two competitors in this field arose in the surgical treatment of orbital tumors. The 'invasion' by neurosurgery into territory of orbital surgery started with the publications of DANDY (1922), GRINKER (1930), MARTIN and CUSHING (1923). In addition the contributions of RETTELBACH and SCHUTZBACH (1943) concerning gliomas of the optic nerve should be noted as well as the relevant publication of LÖHLEIN and TÖNNIS (1949).

In consequences of these investigations the treatment procedures followed a two pronged course for disease processes transgressing the orbit and entering the intracranial space. The first step was the removal of the eye ball (exenteratio orbitae) and the second step the resection of the intracranial portion of the optic glioma. SCHÜRMANN (1960) however proposed a single approach via a transfrontal orbitotomy, which he performed on a number of patients. Following this procedure, techniques are developed to allow neurosurgeons to operate on space occupying lesions in the retrobulbar area. The results of the transfrontal approach in a number of cases have been reported by K. SCHÜRMANN and D. VOTH (1968, 1972). For this reason the legitimate and scientific claim of the Neurosurgical Clinic of Mainz University devoting a special meeting on orbital lesions is well founded and a full report of the contributions justified.

The present report deals with the criteria of the operational procedures and the diseases demanding surgical intervention. Special emphasis has been given to diagnostic problems, dealt with extensively in the first part of this publications. The basis of all diagnostic considerations is the erudition and the detailed knowledge of the anatomical structures refered to by J. LANG on account of extensive personal studies.

Computerised tomography and magnetic resonance imaging have greatly facilitated diagnostic considerations and promoted a better understanding of the topography confronting the neurosurgeon. The informative range of both new methods is extensively accounted for by several groups of investigators, emphasizing their importance for disease processes transgressing the border of the orbit and stressing the greater usefulness of high resolving power computer tomography with multiplanar reconstructions.

When following the proceedings of the meeting it became evident that the methods of sonography, the videoangiography as well as SPECT allow important diagnostic insight of intra-orbital pathology. A similar diagnostic progress was brought about by the systematic studies of evoked visual potentials, proving that the last ten years have seen a considerable progress in diagnostics.

As present volume of the published Mainz series of the annual neurosurgical meeting essentially deals with the treatment of tumors of the orbit and the visual pathway, and explains the numerous contributions by neuropathologists. They support the observations of neurosurgeons, ophthalmic surgeons and oro-pharyngeal surgeons, proving at the same time that no single speciality can claim priority in the field of orbital surgery. A further conclusion can be reached that the most satisfactory can only be achieved when interdisciplinary co-operation is available. This view is specially demonstrated when an operational intervention is necessary in diseases involving the optic chiasm due to pituitary adenoma directly or intraglandular haemorrhage, craniopharyngoma, or disease processes of cortical tissue close to the visual pathway.

Few contributions have been devoted to endocrine aspects of ophthalmic pathology, discussing the diagnostic problems ranging from the results of conservative treatment to those of operative decompression. In any case it is apparent, that a systematic conservative therapy can prevent operative intervention in many cases.

A further range of clinical indications stem from circulatory disturbances within the orbit, e.g. the carotis-cavernous sinus fistula and other arterio-venous fistulas. The clinical pictures of retinal stroke and chronic ocular ischemia have been discussed including arterial and venous circulatory disturbances affecting the retina including amaurosis fugax. The relevant diagnostic procedures and the therapeutic conclusions have been fully discussed.

A final chapter embraces traumatic lesions related to orbital structures or close to the orbit. The combined cranio-facial injuries, fractures of the skull base, disturbances of eye ball mobility due to fractures of the orbital floor including trans-ethmoidal decompression of the optic nerve after cranio-cerebral injuries have been evaluated.

We learn from these communications that every orbital involvement in head injuries is a further important clinical indication when dealing with the treatment by demanding special experience and skill from members of the team.

Thus by stressing the interdisciplinary approach and cooperation in treating the patient it is obvious that no single medical speciality should claim priority for the therapeutic course to be taken.

D. Voth P. Glees

Mainz und Göttingen 1993

Introduction

D. Voth

In Berlin, on August 3, 1881, at around 6 p.m. the surgeon HAHN performed a small craniotomy on a 45-year-old patient and removed a tuberculous abscess. This was the beginning of neurosurgery as a new branch of surgery in Germany. This first neurosurgical operation was also the result of a new and direction setting neurological diagnosis, that is, a homonymous hemianopsia towards the right. The report of this case impressively shows how the diagnosis of a neurologist, WERNICKE, and that of an ophthalmologist, SCHILLING, together provided the decisive topical suggestion of the disease. It is certain, in any case, that a dysfunction in the optical system brought about the beginning of the development of neurosurgery in Germany.

Today operations in the region of the orbit and the intracranial parts of the optical canal still require the special knowledge and techniques of the neurosurgeon. Even space-occupying processes of the eye socket, which are sometimes considered to be in the domain of the opthalmological surgeon, are operated on by the neurosurgeon in many clinics. Of course, opthalmologists remain, with good reason, responsible for operations on the eyeball itself and for corrections of dysfunctions such as crossed eyes. Because of this early division of responsibility, the treatment of diseases of the orbit, have required an interdisciplinary strategy. When process of the orbita walls are involved, specialists in otorhnolaryngoly and dental, oral, and jaw surgery have been consulted.

If we look back to the time before August 3, 1881, it is obvious that vision and the phaenomenology of the process of vision has interested and fascinated people long before the scientific epoch. In the fragments of the pre-Socratic thinkers, in the writings of the Hippokratic School, in the relicts of the Alexandrinic School, in the knowledge theories of Plato - and one could continue this list without end - we find curiosity about the world of pictures and their nature.

This should not surprise us when we remember the enormous importance of vision for the aquisition of knowledge. We know, for example, as is shown by nature's experiment of the congenital blind, that although tactile feeling is partly able to substitute for vision, the experience of color cannot be described verbally, and, in the last consequence, is not teachable.

Even when we add our knowledge about the physical nature of light and of the physiology of the senses to a (fragmentary and sometimes questionable) whole, there remain great deficits in our knowledge about optical experience and the psychology of color. Here, on the borderline of our knowledge, we see that the conflict between NEWTON, the representative of the dispassionate and presently dominating natural sciences and GOETHE, the antagonist of "the Papism of the one-sided natural science", is not at all obsolete, but rather still exemplary.

Even today, there is great enmity between those who believe in the refraction indices, virtual images and, therefore, "one-sided natural science" and those who believe that "Colors are the deeds of light, acts, and suffering". As GOTTFRIED BENN once wrote so pertinently, GOETHE and NEWTON could have existed together without destroying each other; that each had standpoint on which he stood, from which he attacked, is clearer to us today than it was then.

When one finds, for example, the 6th Section in "The Theory of Color" entitled "Sensual-traditional effect of color", it becomes immediately clear that the adversaries have no common language, even though CARL FRIEDRICH VON WEIZSÄCKER, as a physicist, thinks: "But we know that this science does not represent absolute truth, but is rather a certain methodological procedure. It is necessary to think about the dangers and limits of this procedure. Thus, we must ask what is in GOETHE's science which is different from the prevailing natural science. And acutally we find that it is the procedure that is different: in GOETHE's science the experiment does not require the destruction of the form, but rather viewing becomes thinking and thinking becomes viewing.

And we, who usually regard NEWTON more highly than GOETHE, should, sometimes, at least, take the opportunity and the time to be convinced of the existence of this other, certainly fascinating, view of the world.

Returning to the medical and surgical aspects, we find two viewpoints which were important for the publication of the proceedings of this meeting. On the one side, the development of the perfection of diagnostic procedures with computed tomography and magnetic resonance imaging has made the early detection of even small processes possible. The demonstration of space occupation in the area of the orbits presents a challenge to the surgeon to remove these processes without affecting function. The development of microsurgical techniques has brought enormous improvements in the last two decades. Here we will just mention the systematic construction of the pterional approach for, for example, processes in the dorsal region of the orbit, the optical nerve canal, and in the region of the chiasma itself. The new techniques for operating through the smallest approaches has greatly reduced the burden for the patient from the operation itself, and, at the same time, allowed preservation of functions and reduced secondary damage to a minimum.

On the other side, surgical procedures have also been greatly improved. Quite early in the history of the Neurosurgical Department of the University Hospital in Mainz, neurosurgeons took responsibility for surgery of the orbit, and consequently developed and expanded procedures in this area. This is certainly to the credit of the past Director of the Clinic, Prof. Kurt Schürmann. It is a special pleasure and satisfaction to me that during our many years of cooperation two large publications on intraorbital space-occupying processes and their neurosurgical treatment could be published.

The editors hope that this book describes new developments in this field and can, therefore, serve as a foundation for further improvements in surgical techniques for the benefit of our patients.

I would like to acknowledge the assistance of my daughter Imogen and my son Malte, who worked long hours helping me in the editorial work related to this book.

II

BASIC RESEARCH AND DIAGNOSTIC METHODS

The orbit, some anatomical details

J. Lang

The term "orbit" was used for the first time by Gerardus Cremonesis. This man translated the papers of AVICENNA (980 - 1037) who already learnt by heart the Koran in his 10th year of life, studied drama, dialectics, astronomy and geometry as well as medicine and lived then in Bagdad and finally in Isphahan. His name was ABU ALI el HOSSEIN ben Abdallah ibn SINA: The translation "orbita" was loaded onto the Anatomical speech - according to HYRTL (1880) - by GERARDUS and is barbarous - as a term for our eye socket - because of neither being used during the blossom nor during the decline of the Latin speech. Orbita means "wheel, circle or line". A hollow four-sided lying pyramid should get another name [14].

Aditus Orbitae

The aditus of the orbit is the orbital margin. The supraorbital margin is a part of the frontal bone which is laterally connected with the zygomatic bone. The lateral rim of the orbit is the strongest, and built up by the zygomatic bone and its frontal process. The zygomatic bone is also situated on the lower part of the orbital rim and extends medially to the sutura zygomaticomaxillaris. At this suture is palpable a small tubercle in most of the cases: Tuberculum infraorbitale marginale. In the most cases the foramen infraorbitale is situated below this tubercle. The medial part of the orbital rim belongs to the processus frontalis maxillae which extends upwards to the sutura frontomaxillaris and dorsally to the fossa sacci lacrimalis and the lacrimal bone. The maxillofrontal point is located superior to the anterior lacrimal crest at the frontomaxillary suture. Between this maxillofrontale and the ectoconchion (this is the midzone of the lateral orbital rim) was measured the width of the orbit. In adults this orbital width was found to be 41.3 (35 - 45) mm. The height of the orbit is formed right-angled to the transverse diameter and is in our material 34.4 (31.8 - 38.5) mm. According to BARTELS (1897) the superior orbital rim is situated in male 5.9, in female 7.8 mm above the nasion. The nasion is the suture zone between os nasale and os frontale. At Figure 1 is also seen that the orbital width line which sinks sidewards and downwards by an angle of 11.9 (7 - 17)°. Visible is also the axis of the nasolacrimal canal to the median sagittal plane. In most of the cases we found this axis to run downwards and medially but in about 12 % it was found to be orientated downwards and laterally.

During the postnatal life the growth of the orbital rims and of the parietes orbitae respectively is interesting, too. At Figure 2 there is to be seen that the segment of the orbital roof grows to the front for 50 % of its original length, the side wall of the orbit (and the lateral orbital rim) for 58 %, the medial for 60.6 %, and the lower wall and rim for 67.4 %. Additionally the lengths of the orbital walls (measured from the side wall of the intraorbital aperture of the optic canal) to the respective rim zones are indicated. Accordingly, the roof of the orbit is on an average something more than 50 mm long in adults, the side wall of the orbit something more than 47 mm, the medial wall 46.5 mm, and the lower 48.4 mm. The limits of these measurements of length are given in brackets [30]. Actually the sagittal entry angle of the orbit is on average 69.2° in newborns, and 83.3° in adults. Thus the lower orbital rim relatively grows more to the front than the upper in postnatal period - or that the part of the calvarium is more developed than the part of the facial bones before birth [24]. It may be emphasized that the right orbital rim in the region of the frontozygomatic suture lies on an average for about 1 mm more dorsally than the left. We found such an asymmetry in 63.6 % of our material. Also the length of the tendons of the eye muscles is on an average for about 1 mm shorter on the right side than on the left [27]. Additionally we examined the extraorbital prominence of the cornea in 430 cases.

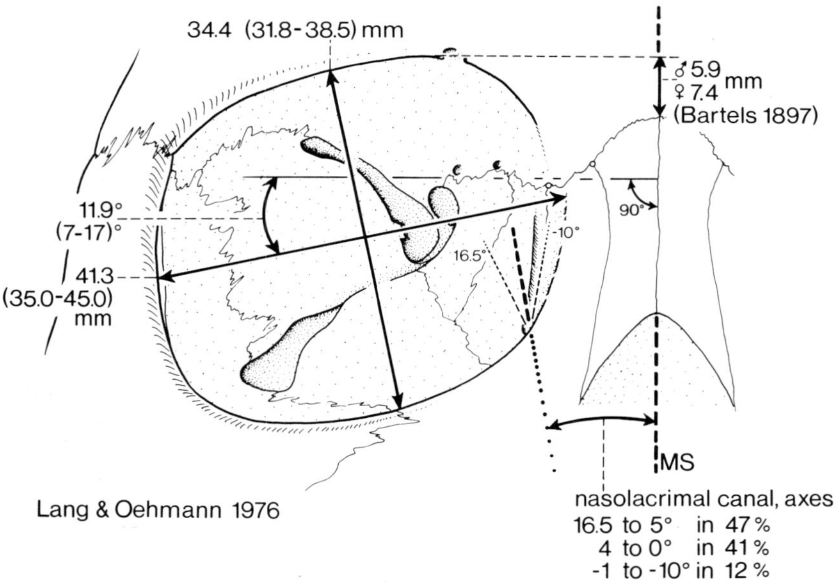

Fig. 1: Aditus orbitae, measurements. Seen is also, that the greatest width of the aditus is developed from medially above to laterally below. The angle with a transverse plain of the skull was measured with 11.9 (7 - 17)°. Seen is also the axis of the nasolacrimal channel to the medial-sagittal plain and the distances between the nasion and the upper margin of the aditus orbitae (BARTELS, 1887)

It was observed that the vertex of the cornea of the left was ordinarily further away from the lateral orbital rim than on the right [34], Figure 3 shows our measurements. Furthermore, the diagram depicts the distance of the ciliary ganglion to the lateral orbital rim as well as the course of the ophthalmic artery above or below the optic nerve.

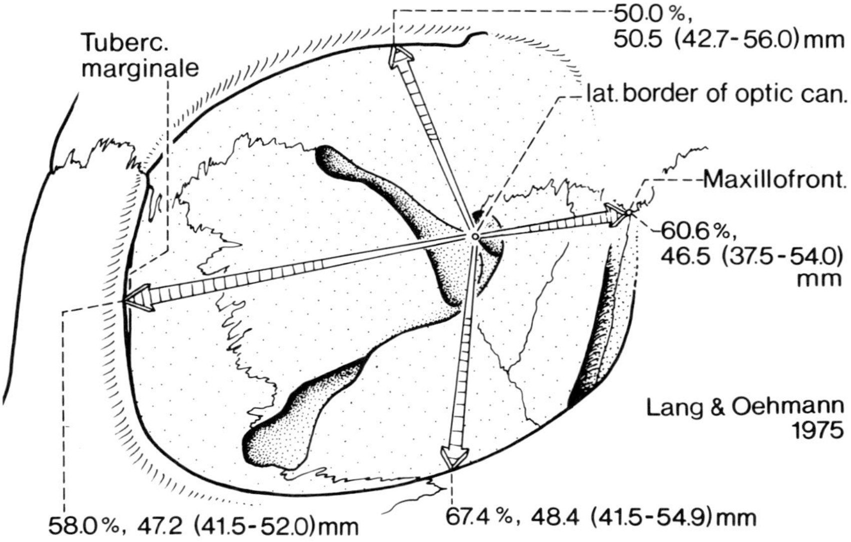

Fig. 2: Postnatal growth of the orbital walls and measurements of the length of the orbital walls

Orbital rim region, portals for nerves (and vessels)

In the region of the supraorbital margin we [32] actually found out only one portal zone in 44 %, two portals in 50 % and three portals in 6 %. These portals can be developed as incisures or as foramina (or as intermediate stages between incisures and foramina with spine formations). In the case of incisures these are defined below by the origin region of the orbital septum. If two portals are present the distance between both is measured to be 6.17 (0.5 - 13) mm. The lateral portal is described as foramen respectively incisura supraorbitalis for the lateral ramus of the supraorbital nerve (and its accompanying artery), the medial portal is the incisura/foramen frontalis for the medial branch of the nerve of the same name. Once again the paramedian distances of these portals were examined in our material. In our skulls the supraorbital foramen has a distance to the median sagittal plane of about 24 (14 - 35) mm. In the case of incisures they are closer to the median plane for the most part. The incisura/foramen frontalis f.e. lies about 19 (8 - 29) mm paramedian. It should be stressed that the courses of nerves and vessels may pierce a large distance in the squama ossis frontalis and they can cross f.e. 17 mm above the supraorbital margin to the forehead. If these nerves are damaged (subfrontal access to the orbit) an anaesthesia of the forehead region can follow. As a rule the zygomaticotemporal ramus of the maxillary nerve comes to the surface and runs to the front around the area of the frontozygomatic suture. Frequently there are anastomoses with the ramus lateralis n. supraorbitalis as well as with main branches of the lacrimal nerve. In the lateral lower area of the orbital rim the zygomaticofacial ramus comes - occasionally doubled - to the surface of the bones. Anastomoses exist below the origin of the levator labii superioris muscle. This muscle covers up the infraorbital foramen and the twigs of the infraorbital nerve coming out of this foramen. An important anastomosis at this zone exists with a ramus buccalis superior of the facial nerve. In the medial upper edge of the orbit terminal twigs of the supratrochlear and infratrochlear nerves come to the surface.

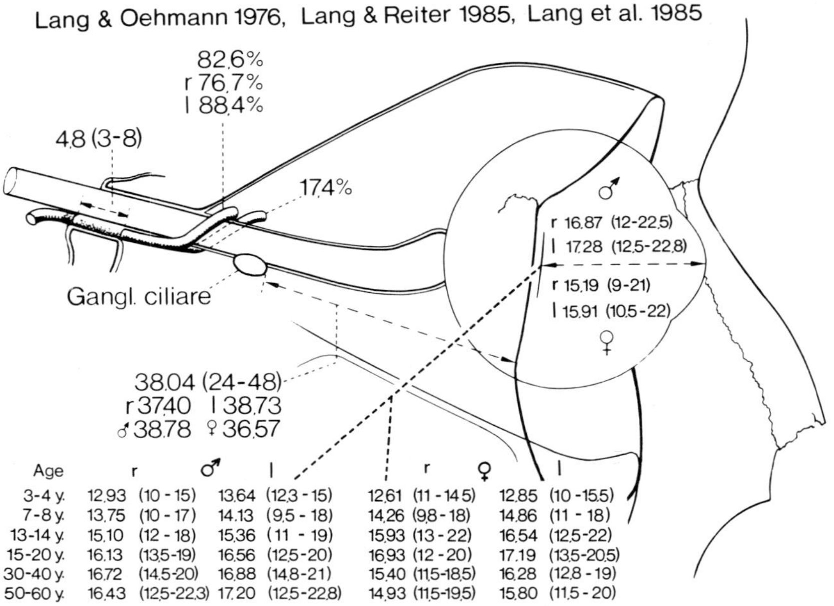

Age	♂ r		♂ l		♀ r		♀ l	
3-4 y.	12.93	(10 - 15)	13.64	(12.3 - 15)	12.61	(11 - 14.5)	12.85	(10 - 15.5)
7-8 y.	13.75	(10 - 17)	14.13	(9.5 - 18)	14.26	(9.8 - 18)	14.86	(11 - 18)
13-14 y.	15.10	(12 - 18)	15.36	(11 - 19)	15.93	(13 - 22)	16.54	(12.5 - 22)
15-20 y.	16.13	(13.5 - 19)	16.56	(12.5 - 20)	16.93	(12 - 20)	17.19	(13.5 - 20.5)
30-40 y.	16.72	(14.5 - 20)	16.88	(14.8 - 21)	15.40	(11.5 - 18.5)	16.28	(12.8 - 19)
50-60 y.	16.43	(12.5 - 22.3)	17.20	(12.5 - 22.8)	14.93	(11.5 - 19.5)	15.80	(11.5 - 20)

Fig. 3: Different measurements in the orbit. Seen is (from left to right) the length of the lower wall of the optic channel, the first intraorbital part of the ophthalmic artery above or below the optic nerve, the distance of the ganglion ciliare from the lateral part of the aditus orbitae and the prominence of the cornea (measured according to HÄRTEL) in the postnatal time and in adults.

Orbital content, structures at the front

Above, laterally and below the orbital septum stands up from the orbital rim area and reaches the upper and lower rims of the tarsi. In the orbital rim area the orbital septum turns into the pericranium as well as into the periorbit. It consists of collagenous and elastic fibres and is developed with several layers in most of the cases. In old age the septum can regress and particularly in the medial part cause so-called fatty hernias. The terminal twigs of the ophthalmic nerve, the ophthalmic artery as well as the beginning of the ophthalmic vein penetrate the orbital septum. The attaching zone of the orbital septum is shown at Figure 4. From this figure follows also that at the medial area the origin zone of the orbital septum goes dorsally and that the muscles arising from there as well as the lacrimal sac are embraced by it from the back. The diagram also shows the different origins of the pars superior and pars inferior of the orbicularis oculi muscle as well as neighbouring muscles and the insertions of the aponeurosis m. levatoris palpebrae superioris and of the ligamentum palpebrale laterale. For a long time a pars superficialis is distinguished from a pars profunda at the ligamentum palpebrale mediale. The origins of the orbicularis oculi muscle and neighbouring muscles were examined by RUPP (1980) in our material.

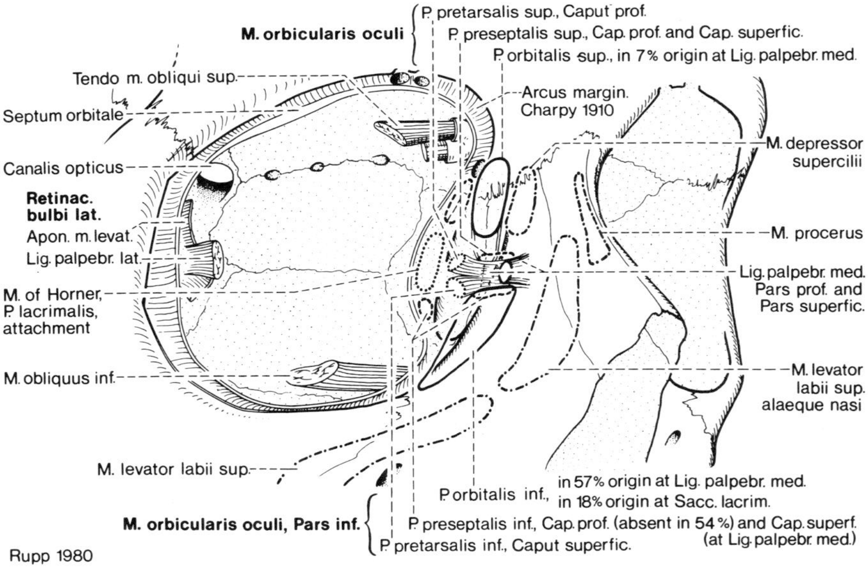

Fig. 4: Origin area of the orbicularis oculi muscle and neighbouring muscles and insertion area of some ligaments.

Figure 5 shows the first courses of parts of the orbicularis oculi muscle (a little bit extended from each other) (lateral view). It should be emphasized that a dilatation of the lacrimal sac by means of theses muscles is quite within the bounds of probability because of muscle parts originate from the lateral covering of the lacrimal sac (= diaphragma lacrimale). The superficial part of the ligamentum palpebrale mediale originates from the anterior lacrimal crista and a little bit in front of this at the processus frontalis maxillae and runs to the medial commissure of the eyelid as well as with two parts to the tarsi of the upper and lower eyelids. The ligament is measured to be 3.7 (2 - 6) mm in breath and 8.2 (6 - 13) mm in length.

The pars profunda likewise branches off the processus frontalis maxillae and the anterior lacrimal crista and runs then dorsally to the posterior lacrimal crista. This is also the segment which is described as diaphragma lacrimale.

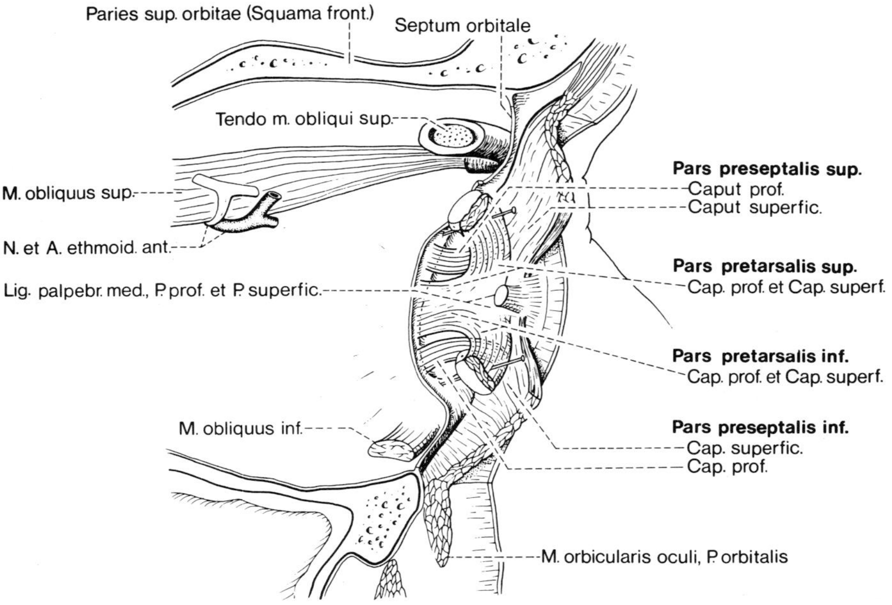

Fig. 5: Preparation of the origin areas of the orbicularis oculi muscle (lateral view)

B. Orbit, Walls

The paries superior orbitae is essentially built up by the frontal bone. Only in the posterior segment the ala minor ossis sphenoidalis, the original bone of the eye, is involved in its construction. This part is interspersed by the optic canal. The orbital roof is - especially in its medial segments - frequently doubled by the frontal sinus or by cellulae ethmoidales superiores. It can be rarefied sometimes and is often traversed by a meningoorbital foramen. Through this foramen (= canal) veins and arteries run through the bone to vasa meningea anteriora. Repeatedly we ascertained in our material that these vessels can also run through big frontal sinuses within folds of the mucous membrane or bony septa. Medially the os frontale borders the lamina orbitalis ossis ethmoidalis. In this area the ethmoidal foramina are situated. It should be stressed that it conformed to textbook anatomy (2 foramina and theirs canals) in only 50 % of the skulls in our material. In the remaining, either one foramen exists or there are up to 5 foramina. In not rare cases the foramina are situated in the region of the frontal bone, but they lie mostly in the border area of both bones.

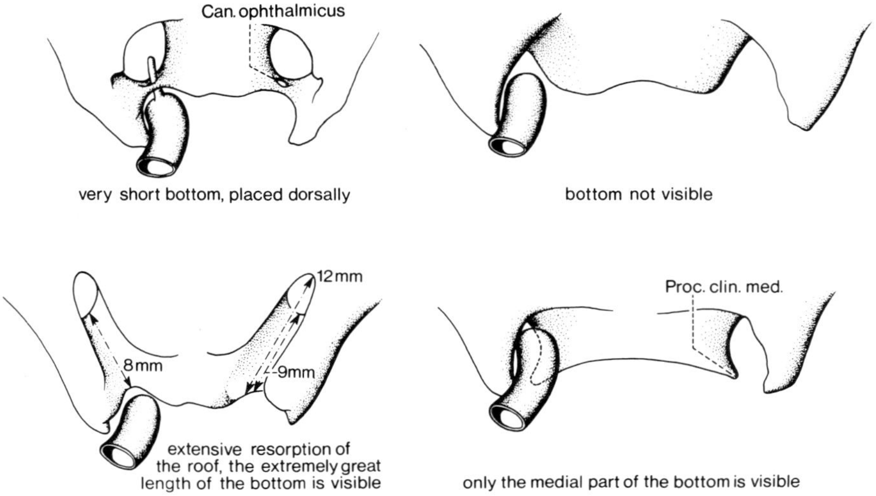

Fig. 6: Different shape of the optic channel and its relations to the internal carotid artery (viewed from above)

Paries lateralis

The paries lateralis is essentially built up by the ala major ossis sphenoidalis - in the region behind - and of the os zygomaticum - in the front region. In about 80 % of adults there is approximately in the middle of the lateral orbital rim, but behind the attachment of the orbital septum - a small protrusion which is described as tuberculum marginale ossis zygomatici. According to BUSCHKOWITSCH (1927) it is formed up to puberty in 72 % in male and 54 % in female skulls (Fig. 2). In the region of the tuberculum marginale ossis zygomatic is situated, about 11 mm below the frontozygomatic suture, are attached the retinaculum bulbi laterale, the lateral part of the aponeurosis of the levator palpebrae muscle, and the lateral palpebral ligament. The retinaculum bulbi laterale constitutes the strongest attachment zone of the ocular bulb. This fact is not surprising if one considers that the four straight eye muscles tend to pull the ocular bulb backwards and that the oblique muscles are exerting a tension to the front and medially. In the case of orbitotomia simplex as well as orbitotomia lateralis and other operations in this region the attachment zone of the eyeball and the eyelid should be taken into consideration.

C. Portals

The biggest portals of the orbit are the superior orbital fissure and the inferior orbital fissure. The former is marked by the ala minor ossis sphenoidalis at the top (occasionally in the lateral part also by the os frontale), and by the upper rim of the ala major ossis sphenoidalis at the bottom. It constitutes a connection between fossa cranii media and orbit and is - as a rule - wider in its medial part being formed by the body of the sphenoid bone than in its lateral. KORNBLUM and KENNEDY (1942) described the morphological types of the upper fissure of the orbit, we also measured and examined the superior and inferior orbital fissures. This fissure is marked by the ala major ossis sphenoidalis at the top, in the front border area also by the os zygomaticum, and by the maxilla at the bottom. In the most medial segment a small part of the lamina orbitalis ossis zygomatici can also reach this fissure. It should be emphasized that at the orbital side of the posterior part of the ala major ossis sphenoidalis there is often formed a small bony tongue originating a part of the m. rectus bulbi lateralis. In the medial upper border region of the superior orbital fissure a small bony spine may be found (Spina infraoptica).

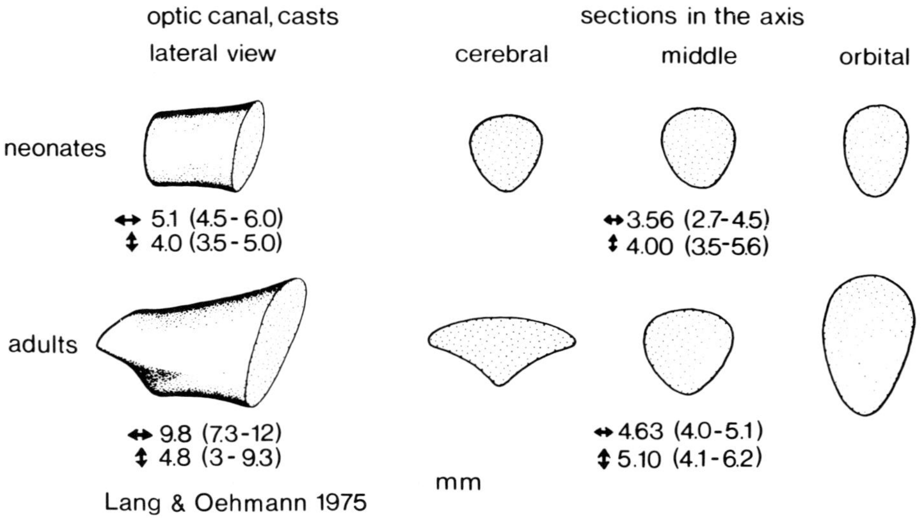

Fig. 7: Casts of the optic channel and measurements in neonates and in adults

From the middle part of the inferior orbital fissure a shallow bony sulcus commonly goes (seldom a canal already starts there) to the front and a little bit to the medial side and then forms itself into the inferior infraorbital canal from the top; it leads nerve and artery of the same name. Regularly the upper wall of the infraorbital canal has gaps or small canals for the passages of one or more small canals for the passages of one or more small twigs of the infraorbital artery to the orbital content.

Ethmoidal foramina and ethmoidal cells

The medial orbital wall is bluntly marked like the other orbital walls, too. From the top, the frontal bone roundly turns into the wall area being formed by the os ethmoidale. Below this area with its greatest region borders on the maxilla, posteriorly and above on the ala minor ossis sphenoidalis, posteriorly at the bottom on the lamina orbitalis ossis palatini and in front on the lacrimal bone. The lamina orbitalis ossis ethmoidalis is paper-thin: lamina papyracea - but supported by walls of the ethmoidal cells. These are variably numerous, and can be orientated vertically, anting or also horizontally.

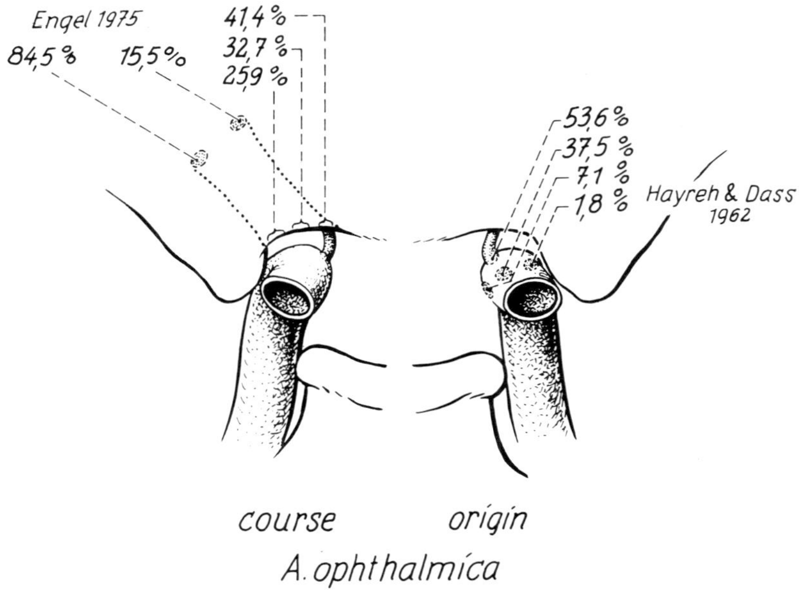

Fig. 8: Origin area of the ophthalmic artery according to HAYREH and DASS (1962) and enters and exit of the ophthalmic artery in the optic channel (ENGEL, 1975)

The ethmoidal foramina have a funnel-shaped appearance when examined from the orbital side, and lead canals of the same name. It should be stressed that the foramina can be situated in the region of the suture between the ethmoidal and the frontal bones or sometimes above. Clinically, especially important is the location of the posterior ethmoidal foramen which is found in the right orbit up to 2 mm at the orbital opening of the optic canal in our material, on the left side it was, in one instance, situated 1 mm in front of the orbital portal for the optic canal.

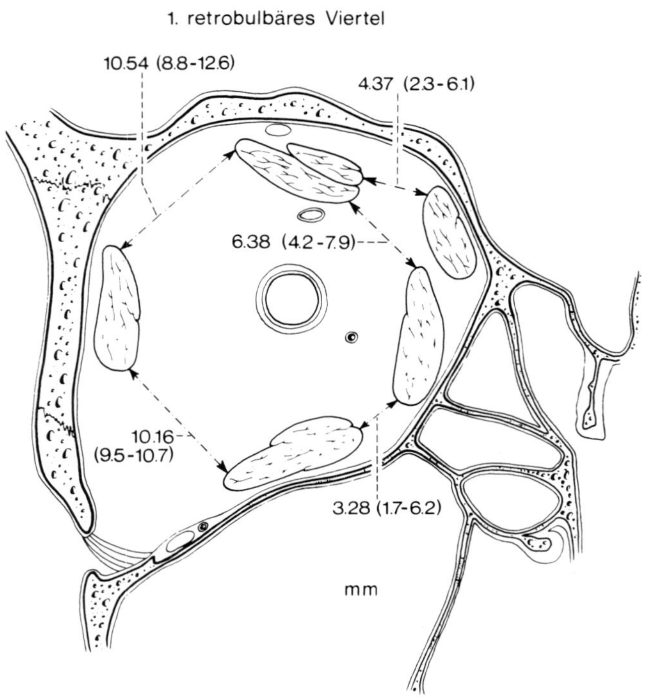

Fig. 9: Distances between the extraocular muscles in the first retrobular quarter immediately behind the bulb

Optic canal

Through the optic canal the optic nerve with its coverings and the ophthalmic artery run through the ala minor ossis sphenoidalis to the orbit. The upper wall of the canal is measured to be 9.8 (7.3 - 12) mm in length in our material (LANG and OEHMANN, 1976), the lower only 4.8 (3 - 9.3) mm. Only the lower wall of the canal is sharply bordered at the front and at the back. The length of the medial wall was determined to be 11.4 (8 - 16) mm that one of the lateral wall to be 10.8 (8.5 - 15) (LANG and REITER, 1985). Postnatally especially the upper wall of the canal grows up although reduction processes can be found at its posterior intracranial portal. On the other hand postnatally a part of the ala minor is included intraorbitally in the upper wall obviously. The rear segment of the upper wall is then covered with dura mater in which small bony tongues (as remnants of the former upper wall) are projecting. In the case of arteriosclerotic changes of the internal carotid artery, or dolichomegal internal carotid arteries, the optic nerve can be pressed from below on the sharp rim of this dural lamella and can be damaged. The reduction of the upper wall can progress to such an extent that the lower wall of the canal is visualized completely only in the superior view (see Fig. 9). It should be emphasized that so-called ophthalmic canals are present in 1 % of our material. In these cases the ophthalmic artery runs with a length of 1 - 2 mm below the optic canal in its own canal separately from the nerve (LANG, 1977). Figure 7 depicts the form of the optic canal in newborns and adults in the region of the intracranial opening, the middle segment, and the orbital portals as soon as the narrowest diameter in the region of the so-called waist of the canal.

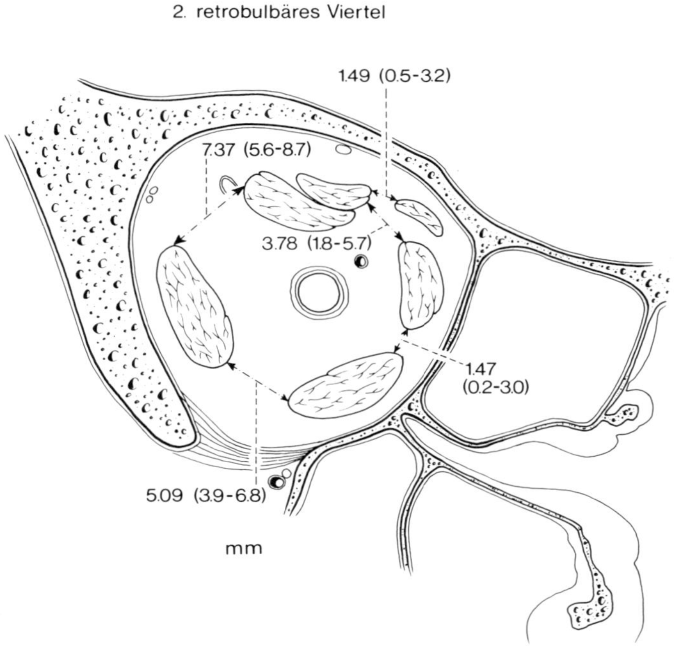

Fig. 10: Distances between the extraocular muscles in the second retrobulbar quarter behind the bulb

In our adult skulls the axis of the optic canal runs on an average at an angle of 39° (33 - 44.9) to the median plane laterally and with regard to the Frankfurt horizontal plane at an angle of 15.5° (3.2 - 28.5) down- and forwards. In our material one can see the wall of the optic canal from the sphenoidal sinus in approx. 80 %, that is to say that the sphenoidal sinus borders the canal for the optic nerve from which it is separated only by a thin bony lamella. The upper and lower walls of the canal can also be pneumatisized. In about 13 % a posterior ethmoidal cell reaches the medial wall of the canal for the optic nerve and the ophthalmic artery.

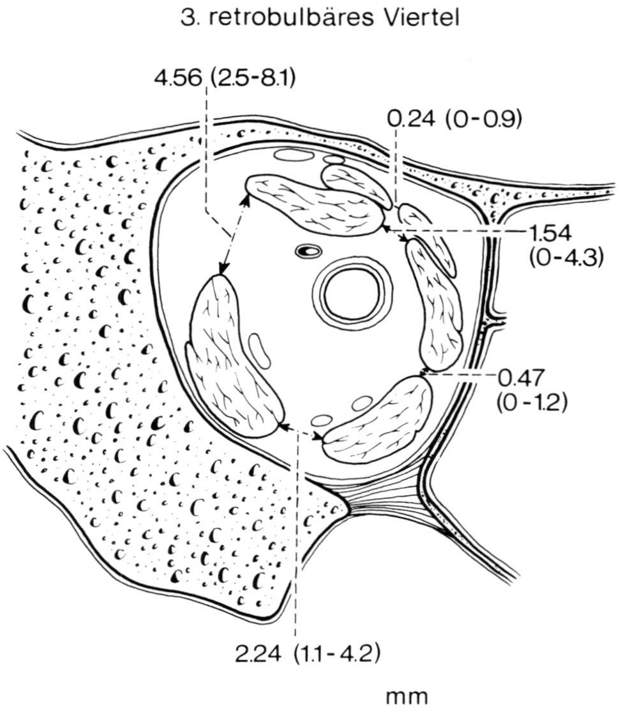

Fig. 11: Distances between the extraocular muscles in the third retrobulbar quarter of the orbit

D. Optic canal and orbit, contents

In the region of the intracranial portal of the optic canal the dura mater turns into a periosteal dural layer which covers the inner surface of the canal. At the intraorbital portal both the leaves are as it were diverging. The outer leaf extends as periorbit (= periosteum of the orbit), the inner one as dura mater n. optici. Inside the dura mater accompanies the arachnoidea (and a subarachnoidal space) as well as the pia mater accompanies the optic nerve to the sclera of the eyeball.

In the material of HAYREH and DASS (1962) the ophthalmic artery most frequently arises medially and below the knee region of the internal carotid artery, in the remainder something more above it (in very rare cases laterally). In our material [9]

the artery most frequently enters the optic canal medially and leaves the canal at the lateral region of the intraorbital portal (see Fig. 8).

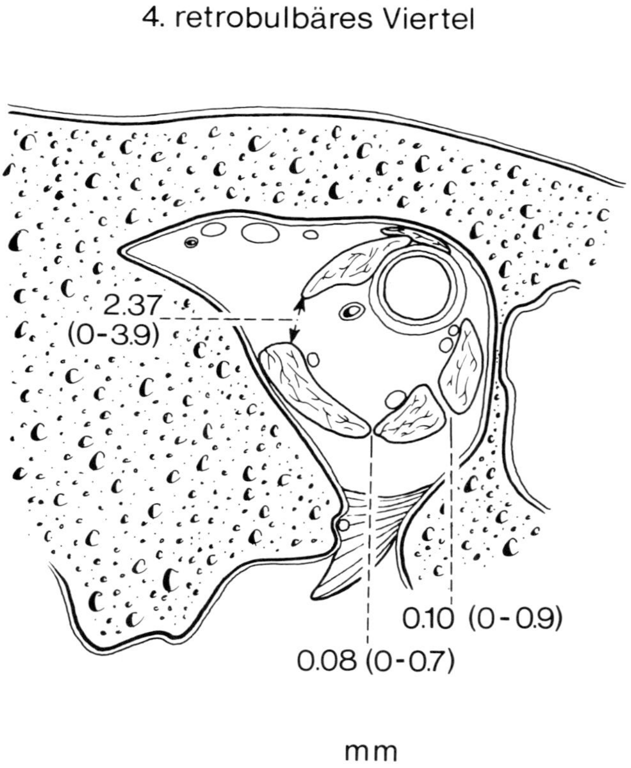

Fig. 12: Distances between the extraocular muscles in the fourth retrobulbar quarter of the orbit

According to HAYREH and DASS (1962) the diameter of the artery is found to be 0.7 - 1.4 mm. In our material, the outer diameter is 1.47 (0.9 - 2.1) mm [28] and we also found dolichomegal arteries with diameters up to 3 mm. The periorbit also closes the orbital fissures from the orbit. Therefore in the region of the superior orbital fissure is a connection with the dura mater of the middle cranial fossa as well as to the pterygopalatine fossa. The inferior orbital fissure is closed by the orbitalis muscle being mostly underestimated in its massiveness. At the orbital side this muscle is also covered by the periorbit. In the area of the infraorbital sulcus the periorbit runs into the periosteal layer of the infraorbital sulcus and canal. The same relationships are found at the ethmoidal, orbitofacial, and orbitotemporal canals as well as at the region of the menigoorbital foramina. It should be stressed that the vessels of the periorbit have connections with the orbital content as well as the orbital bone and the neighbouring paranasal sinuses (spreading of inflammations etc.).

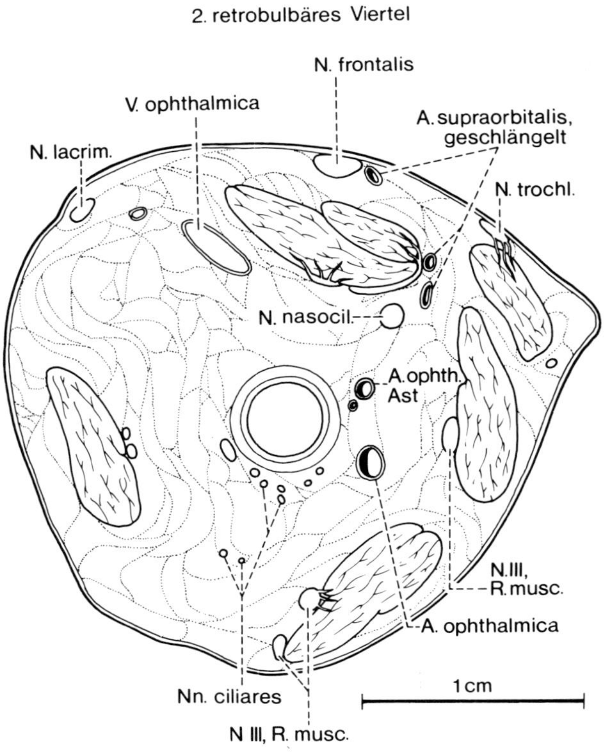

Fig. 13: Connective tissue membranes in the orbit (second quarter of the area behind the bulb)

Straight external eye muscles, origin area - nerves and vessels

The straight external eye muscles, including the levator palpebrae superioris muscle arise from the annulus tendineus communis in the top region of the orbit. The origin area is formed by a tendious funnel with a medial upper portal for the optic nerve and the ophthalmic artery. Through its lateral and lower portal the oculomotor (mostly divided into a superior and a inferior ramus), abducent and nasociliary nerves are running.

The upper and medial portal was called pars optica, the lower and lateral pars oculomotoria. The tendinous original ring also embraces the medial part of the superior orbital fissure in addition to the apertura orbitalis canalis optici. Lateral to the tendinous ring the lacrimal nerve, being often accompanied by a twig of the medial meningeal artery;, goes through the superior orbital fissure, below from it the ophthalmic vein, and further medially frontal and the trochlear nerves. Numerous variations of the course of the ophthalmic vein are well-known [22].

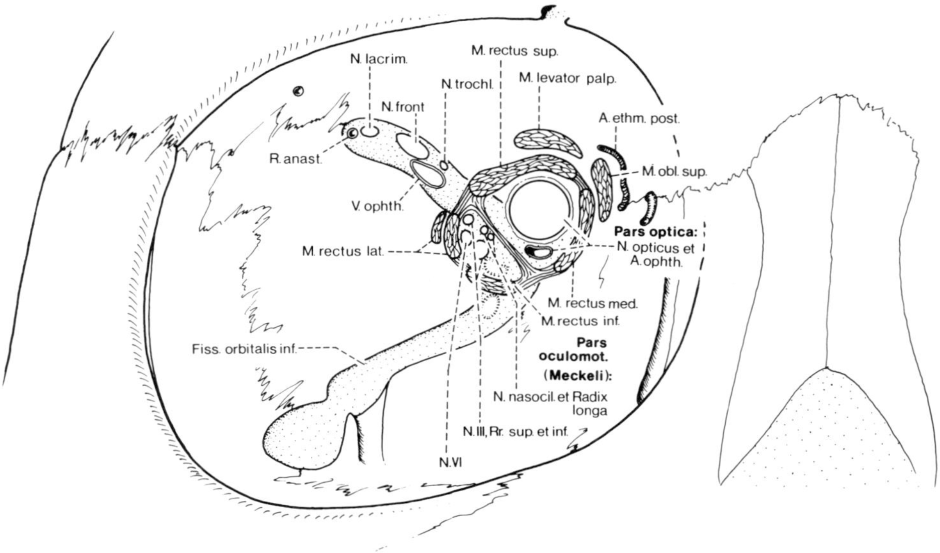

Fig. 14: Annulus tendineus and course of nerves and vessels in the apex orbitae

E. Frontal (subfrontal) access to the orbit

After cutting through the skin of the head in the region of the forehead-hairline-border its frontal part can be reflected downwards. It should be emphasized that the venter frontalis of the m. epicranius has no bony attachment. Therefore, the skin of the head (and the upper part of the orbicularis oculi muscle) then hangs at the origin region of this muscle as well as at the m. depressor supercilii and the m. procerus. For further details see Figure 4. After a craniotomia the dura mater is raised from the roof of the orbit and the roof area is opened. It should be stressed that the frontal sinus, just as the superior ethmoidal cells, pneumatise the roof of the orbit in different ways [26]. In our skulls the length of the region above the orbit (without opening the optic canals and without orbital rim) is measured to be 39.53 (32 - 45) mm [33]. Up to the middle of the upper orbital rim this length is 48.8 mm on an average in European males, and 52.5 mm in Japanese males. The measurements of ADACHI (1904) were 47.5 mm in European females, and 51.1 mm in Japanese females.

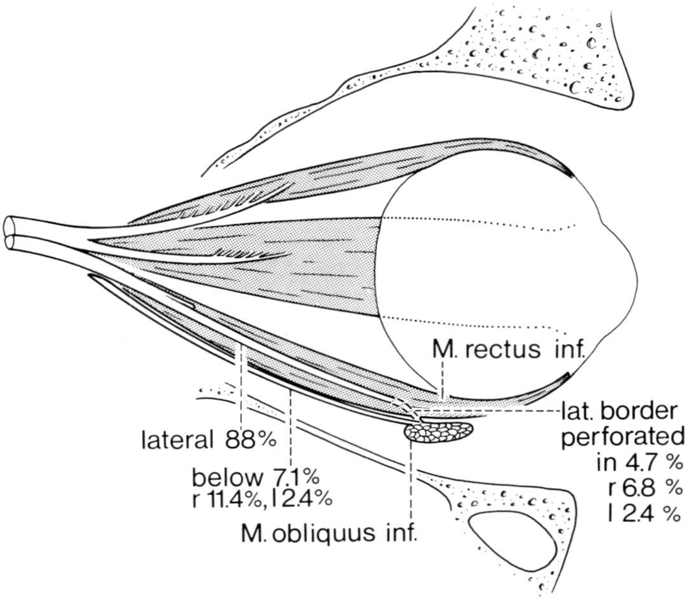

Fig. 15: Branch of the oculomotor nerve to the inferior obliquus muscle

At most, 730 (423 - 960) square mm of the inferior part of the anterior cranial fossa borders the orbit directly or separated through paranasal sinuses [33]. If one puts a tangent onto the frontomalare of the orbit and the lateral rim of the superior orbital fissure, it forms angles of 35 (25.5 - 52.0)° with the median sagittal plane. Laterally from it there is a cavity for the lacrimal gland and the remaining content of the orbit with an extension of 4.51 (0 - 7.5) mm: fossa glandulae lacrimalis. Frequently after removing the orbital roof in its close proximity twigs of the ophthalmic nerve and the trochlear nerve are already to be seen through the periorbit. In other cases flat layers of fat are situated between periorbit and nerves which were interpreted as displacement apparatus [20]. In our skulls [32] the frontal nerve has a breadth of 2.57 (1.0 - 5.0) mm in the dorsal section. It should be emphasized that the frontal nerve separates itself off the ophthalmic nerve already in the cavernous sinus, and also the lacrimal nerve. In the sidewall of the cavernous sinus, the trochlear nerve already crosses the oculomotor nerve from laterally to above and reaches medially and behind the superior oblique muscle at its upper side. The entry zone of its nerve fibres into the muscle has an average length of approx. 7 mm and a distance from the medial orbital rim region of 29 (21 - 40) mm. In our material we found 11.8 (4 - 21) mm nerve fibres which supply the muscles [31]. Also, after shifting the frontal nerve and removing further fatty tissue the levator palpebrae superioris muscle is to be seen. According to JONES et al. (1975) the muscle varies in about 20 %. The roughly triangular muscle has approx. a length of 41 (34 - 48) mm and a thickness of 1.12 (0.5 - 3.0) mm in its middle region. At the transition zone into its aponeurosis the breadth of the muscle was measured to be 15 (7 - 23) mm [27]. In the dorsal origin region immediately above the annulus tendineus its breadth was 3.6 (2 - 23) mm. In 14 % of our material this voluntary elevator of the eyelid has shown many variations.

During the access to intraconic regions the nerve running to the levator palpebrae superioris muscle should be preserved. In 83 % the nerve embraces the medial border of the superior rectus muscle and reaches the levator palpebrae superioris muscle from below. In the remainder, the nerve runs through the superior rectus muscle at different zones for penetrating the muscle. It should be stressed that the approach between the rectus bulbi lateralis and the levator palpebrae superioris muscles as well as the superior rectus muscle is dorsally broader than that one between m. obliquus bulbi superior and m. rectus superior respectively m. levator palpebrae superioris. The fasciae of the eye muscles are closely woven in the front region of the bulb (cingulum bulbi), they are relatively thin behind in the apex region of the orbit. At figures 9 - 12 the distances of the outer eye muscles from each other and the compartments of the intraorbital fatty tissue are shown. In these diagrams is also to be seen that the description of the orbit as a four-sided pyramid is not accurate for the following reason:

1. The ethmoidal bone is in upper segments narrower than in lower ones. Also the frontal medial border of the apertura orbitalis canalis optici is similar. In our material the paramedian distance of this border was measured to be 16.1 (11 - 20) mm at the right and 14.94 (11 - 19) mm at the left orbit. According to ADACHI (1904) the upper breadth of the whole ethmoidal bone is 26.2 mm in European specimens. This value corresponds well with our measurements. According to this researcher the lower breadth of the ethmoidal bone, however, is in European specimens 37.2 mm on average. It means that the lamina orbitalis ossis ethmoidalis runs down and laterally, and in the dorsal region of the orbit there exists a three-sided - and not a four-sided - pyramid with its top going down and laterally.

The orbital volume was found to be 27.14 (22.8 - 31.0) mm^3 in our adult skulls. This space is taken up by the eyeball and its adnexa. In the fatty tissue, one can distinguish an intraconic from an extraconic part. The intraconic part may be interpreted as a device to minimize friction during the movements of the optic nerve, and the muscles as well as a ball-and-socket joint for the eyeball. HUGO and STONE (1974) weighed the intraorbital fatty tissue of 54 orbits and found a weight of between 5 and some more than 10 g. Right-left differences up to 2 g occur, the difference between the sexes is not significant. According to ROHEN (1953) the septa of the connective tissue between the fatty lobuli are orientated more in an equatorial-transversal direction in frontal parts of the orbit, and more in a sagittal direction in posterior parts of the orbit. In addition to the cingulum bulbi, KOORNEEF (1977) very regularly ascertained circular arrangements of connective tissue septa between periorbit and vagina bulbi in the posterior third of the bulb in the case of frontal sections. At this level, such structures could not be so rigourously confirmed in our material (see Figs. 9 - 13). Besides, KOORNEEF pointed out that no border of connective tissue exists between intraconic and extraconic fatty tissue behind the bulb. Our material revealed the same results. According to JOHNSON and HADLEY (1964) (as well as PICKRELL, 1968 and others) 5 intraorbital fat compartments are distinguishable. Two parts shall be accessible through the upper eyelid, three through the lower eyelid. According to examinations by HUGO and STONE (1974) and KOORNEEF (1977) such a differentiation of special parts of fat is impossible in this way. In our material as well there was no such subdivision present.

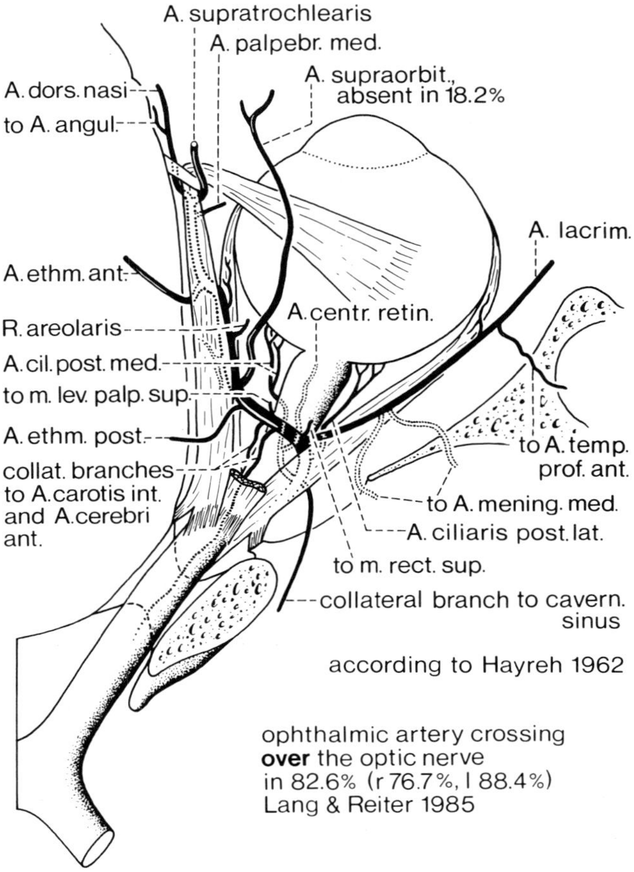

Fig. 16: Most common course and twigs of the ophthalmic artery

The optic canal can also be opened subdurally by using the frontal access.

Intradural access to the roof of the orbit

In the case of using the intradural access the frontal lobe of the brain over the hypophyseal area is raised and the dura mater of the orbital roof is opened from above. The most important arteries of the frontal love are: medially the medial frontobasal branch emerging from the anterior cerebral artery, and laterally the lateral frontobasal ramus from the middle cerebral artery. Usually in the medial part the a. centralis longa

(Heubneri) takes part in supplying the gyrus rectus and its vicinity. The outflow of the veins to the front occurs into the superior sagittal sinus, and to the back into the formation region of the basal vein. It should be stressed that in some cases small arteries of the first subarachnoidal course of the internal carotid artery are found which supply the posterior parts of the dura mater above the lesser wing of the sphenoid bone and the roof of the optic canal. Incidentally, the dura mater is medially supplied by small branches of the ethmoidal arteries and laterally by the frontal ramus of the medial meningeal artery. In the bordering area of the lesser wing of the sphenoid bone mostly the meningoorbital rami go through the bone to the orbit. In rare cases we found an anterior artery to falx cerebri coming out of the anterior cerebral artery immediately distal to the anterior communicating artery, and running to the falx cerebri in the medial region of the anterior cranial fossa.

Superolateral access to the orbit

McCARTY and BROWN (1964), PERSUIET et al. (1963) and recently AL-MEFTY and FOX (1985), too, removed not only the orbital roof but parts of the orbital sidewall. This separation also takes place in the region of the origin of the temporalis muscle being removed and replaced downwards and backwards. Via this approach tumors located in the orbital apex can be exposed. SCHÜRMANN pointed out that by this approach also intraorbital tumors extending through the optic canal in a intracranial direction can be removed. During this access the ocular bulb can easily be displaced. We stressed (LANG and REITER, 1985) that the optic nerve has an overall length of about 4 mm. Being unstretched the nerve together with its coverings has f.e. a length of 22.94 (17.5 - 31.0) mm, being stretched its length is measured to be 26.78 (21.0 - 34.5) mm. This intraorbital length of the optic nerve shows clear differences between the sexes. A displacement of the eyeball is also possible, of course, using the optic nerve at its intraorbital course like a stalk. Obviously we indicated the ampulla vaginae n. optici behind the eyeball for the first time (LANG, 1981). This enlargement of the outer coverings of the optic nerve was observed in 82.5 %. On an average it is 1.12 mm [31]. It is conceivable that the liquor accumulates here in the case of intracranial rise in pressure. The intracranial portals of the medial border of the optic canal are situated to be 7.0 (4.5 - 12.5) mm paramedian. It should be emphasized that the cross-section of the optic nerve is usually round within the orbit and the near the orbit but it is oval at the intracranial aperture of the optic canal and in its intracranial sector. In our material (255 preparations) the height of the intracranial nerve was measured to be 3.16 (1.5 - 5.0) mm and the breadth 5.03 (2.5 - 7.0) mm [35]. We determined the breadth of the optic chiasm to be 11.57 (8.5 - 15.0) mm.

Lateral approach to the orbit (operation after KRÖNLEIN and BERKE)

In front the lateral orbital wall is formed by the zygomatic bone and a lateral part of the frontal bone, and further dorsally by the ala major ossis zygomatici. The superior orbital fissure is situated in the region of the upper border of the ala major, and the longer inferior orbital fissure in the lower region. The ala major also forms a part of the lateral wall of the skull in the region of the temporal fossa. This zone is called fossa because it seems to be somewhat caved in comparison with other parts of the skull, and the zygomatic arch overlaps this region and the temporalis muscle.

The sensory supply of the skin in this region occurs by twigs of the maxillary nerve (zygomaticotemporal and zygomaticofacial rami) in the anterior sector, and by the means of the auriculotemporal nerve in back sectors. Numerous variations of the distribution zone of these nerves (which can replace one another) are found. Chiefly the temporal superficial artery takes on the arterial supply of the skin and the scalp at this region. Its course and its branches are extraordinarily variable.

Normally a frontal ramus, however, with a width of (1.38 $\pm$ 040) mm [43] is differentiated from a parietal ramus. The for a long time well-known, zygomatico-orbital artery merits mention, leaving the frontal ramus 1 - 10 mm above the zygomatic arch and running in the direction of the lateral orbital rim. This twig occurs in approx. 80 %.

The temporal rami of the facial nerve should be preserved as far as possible by using the lateral approach to the orbit [8]. In our material, 2 - 3 temporal rami were found most frequently. The uppermost twig provides the venter frontalis of the m. epicranius; if it is paralysed frowning is no longer possible. The next lower twigs penetrate the orbicularis oculi muscle from below, and in fact its orbital part and its superior palpebral part. It may be assumed that especially the superior palpebral part is important for the closure of the eyelid. Lower sectors of the orbitcularis oculi muscle are supplied by zygomatic rami of the facial nerve. These twigs run via the region of the zygomatic bone and reach at first the mm. zygomaticus major, zygomaticus minor and other muscles of the zone from below. These twigs are also responsible for the proper eyelid closure and its blinking and are responsible for the flow of tears from the conjunctival sac. Lesions of these branches of the facial nerve result not only in paralysis of the orbicularis oculi muscle but sometimes also in ectropium paralyticum because of the pars lacrimalis of the eyelid no longer touches the lacrimal fluid.

By the operation after KRÖNLEIN (1889) modified after BERKE (1954) the lateral orbital wall is removed after cutting the skin and taking cosmetic aspects into consideration as far as possible (and preserving the branches of the facial nerve). At the lateral orbital rim the orbicularis oculi muscle together with its periosteum is pushed away to the front. Thereafter, the lateral orbital rim is sawn in and luxated to the front and outwards. It should be stressed here that the important lateral fastening apparatus of the eyeball (retinaculum bulbi laterale) and of the eyelid (lateral palpebral ligament) have to be torn if this action takes place. It would be more advisable to preserve the lateral orbital rim in the frontmost section or to replant the fastening apparatus of the eyeball later on. The most frontal section of the temporalis muscle is dissected from its origins and pushed backwards. The more dorsally the opening of the orbit (and of the middle cranial fossa) is carried out the deeper becomes the rim between zygomatic arch and lateral orbit respectively wall of the skull. In newborns from our material the depth between arch is f.e. 14.2 mm on average, in four to five-year-old children 17.1 mm, and in adult specimens 21.1 mm [25]. As a rule in our skulls fatty tissue is situated in the frontmost part of the temporal fossa near the bones to the temporalis muscle. Also the middle temporal vein and the aa. and nn. temporales profundae anteriores can be damaged during this action. At the lower rim of this approach there is the inferior orbital fissure. Occasionally in the region of the frontal and broader end of the fissure protrusions of the intraorbital fatty tissue were found which ADACHI (1904) described as fatty hernias. Traction of this tissue can result in the loss of the eyeball. Through the lateral roof part of the orbit up to 0.8 mm thick intra- and extraorbital anastomoses can run between the ophthalmic artery and the deep temporal arteries.

After removing the lateral orbital wall the periorbit is available. Frequently in the upper part the lacrimal nerve and artery shine through the periorbit as well as a posterior part of the lacrimal gland, in the lateral posterior part the m. rectus bulbi lateralis. In the front part the lateral rectus muscle is increasingly covered by connective tissue of the cingulum bulbi and therefore (in anatomical preparations) not visible. Woven into the periorbit or below it the ramus communicans cum n. zygomatico runs supplying the lacrimal gland with its secretory fibres from the pterygopalatine ganglion. Frequently, in our skulls also exist arterial anastomoses between twigs of the infraorbital artery below and the lacrimal artery above. After cutting through the periorbit a thin fatty tissue commonly lies on the lateral rectus muscle. The breadth of this muscle at its middle region and measured somewhat more than 10 (5 - 15) mm in our material [27]. It is supplied by the abducent nerve having an entry zone with a length of 6.43 (3 - 10) mm. The frontmost nerve fibre to the lateral rectus muscle enters muscle 30 (18 - 44) mm behind the lateral orbital rim. It should be stressed that SCHÜRMANN (1974) pointed out that the orbitotomia lateralis constitutes a favourable approach particularly in the case of laterally lying tumors which do not reach the orbital apex. Ophthalmosurgical authors, however, [7, 36] consider it to approach up to the top of the orbit by using this access.

In this connection the slant of the lateral orbital wall should be stressed once more. In our material this wall forms with the median sagittal plane maximum angles of 46.02° on the right side and on the left angles of 45.08°. The limits of these angles are 35° and 56°. In other words the orbital apex region is situated deep and far medially in the operation area, and the ala major ossis sphenoidalis has to be removed during this access. But this also forms a part of the floor of the middle cranial fossa. HÜWEL and VORWERK (1986) analysed the Mainz material and found out that most of the processes concern the upper orbit and the orbital funnel (more frequently temporally, seldom nasally). BERKE pointed out that depending on the position of the tumor the lateral rectus muscle can be moved upwards or downwards and the tumor should be removed microsurgically by protecting the orbital contents. An overview of the most important guiding courses in the retrobulbar region is anatomically possible after removing the lateral rectus muscle (Fig. 15). According to HÜWEL and

VORWERK postsurgical functional disorders are shown frequently by abduction weakness (damage of the rectus bulbi lateralis, its lateral attachment or its nerve supply from the abducent nerve), diplopia (different cause), enophthalmus (not enough fatty retrobulbar tissue), and occlusion of central arteries. Figure 15 shows twigs of the upper and lower branches of the oculomotor nerve to the external eye muscles. It should be emphasized that especially the nerve running to the inferior oblique muscle should be preserved by using the access to the lower retrobulbar space. In our material this nerve runs in nearly 90 % lateral to the inferior rectus muscle, more seldom below this muscle or through its lateral rim. The origin of this muscle is situated only 1.54 (0 - 3.8) mm laterally to the lowest end of the lacrimal sac and 0.73 (0 - 2.5) mm behind the inferior orbital rim [28]. This muscle and the superior oblique muscle have to be spared during anterior inferior or anterior superior approaches to the orbit. Figure 16 depicts the arteries of the orbit with their regular twigs and anastomoses.

References

[1] Adachi B: Topographische Lage des Augapfels der Japaner. Z. Morph. Anthrop. 7, 481 - 501 (1904)

[2] Adachi B: Die Orbita und die Hauptmaße des Schädels der Japaner und die Methode der Orbitalmessung. Z. Morph. Anthrop. 7, 379 - 490 (1904)

[3] Al-Mefty O, Fox J L: Superolateral orbital exposure and reconstruction. Surg. Neurol. 23, 609 - 613 (1985)

[4] Bartels P: Über Geschlechtsunterschiede am Schädel. Med. Diss., Berlin 1897

[5] Berke R N: A modified Krönlein operation. Arch. Ophthalmol. 51, 609 - 632 (1954)

[6] Buschkowitsch W J: Über das Tuberculum orbitale des Jochbeins des Menschen. Anat. Anz. 63, 353 - 357 (1927)

[7] Buschmann W, Linnert D: Wandel der Indikation und der Technik in der Chirurgie retrobulbärer Orbitatumoren. Klin. Mbl. Augenheilkd. 172, 1 - 12 (1987)

[8] Dollinger J: Die Druckentlastung der Augenhöhle durch Entfernung der äußeren Orbitalwand bei hochgradigem Exophthalmus (M. Basedowii) und konsekutiver Hornhauterkrankung. Dt. Med. Wschr. 37, 1888 - 1890 (1911)

[9] Engel A: Ursprungs- und Verlaufsvariationen der ersten Ophthalmica-Strecke. Med. Diss., Würzburg 1975

[10] Hayreh S S, Dass R: The ophthalmic artery. I. Origin and intra-cranial and intra-canalicular course. Brit. J. Ophtal. 46, 65 - 98 (1962)

[11] Hayreh S S, Dass R: The ophthalmic artery. II. Intra-orbital course. Brit. J. Ophthal. 46, 165 - 185 (1962)

[12] Hüwel N, Vorwerk D: Intraorbitale Raumforderungen und ihre operative Behandlung. In: Neurochirurgia Moguntiaca 1985. D. Voth (ed.). Walter de Gruyter, Berlin, New York 1986

[13] Hugo N E, Stone E: Anatomy for a blepharoplasty. Plast. Reconstr. Surg. 53, 587 (1974)

[14] Hyrtl J: Onomatologia Anatomica. W. Braumüller, Wien 180

[15] Johnson J B, Hadley R C: The aging face. In: Reconstructive Plastic Surgery. Edited by J.M. Converse. W.B. Saunders, Philadelphia 1964

[16] Jones L T, Quickert M H, Wobig J L: The cure of ptosis by aponeurotic repair. Arch. Ophthalmol. 93, 629 - 634 (1975)

[17] Koornneef L: New insights in the human orbital connective tissue. Arch. Ophthalmol. 95, 1269 - 1273 (1977)

[18] Kornblum K, Kennedy G R: The sphenoidal fissure. An anatomical, Roentgenological and clinical study. Am. J. Roentgenol. Radium Ther. 47, 845 - 858 (1942)

[19] Krönlein R U: Zur Pathologie und operativen Behandlung der Dermoidcysten der Orbita. Klin. Chir. 4, 149 - 163 (1889)

[20] Lang J: Über die Vascularisation der Periorbita. Gegenbaurs morph. Jahrb. 121, 174 - 191 (1975)

[21] Lang J: Angioarchitektonik der terminalen Strombahn. In: Meesen, H.: Handbuch der allgemeinen Pathologie 111/17 Mikrozirkulation. Springer, Berlin, Heidelberg, New York 1977

[22] Lang J: Praktische Anatomie: Ein Lehr- und Hilfsbuch der anatomischen Grundlagen ärztlischen Handelns. Begr. von T. von Lanz, W. Wachsmuth. Fortgef. und hrsg. von J. Lang, W. Wachsmuth. Teil 1. Bd. 1 Kopf. Teil B Gehirn- und Augenschädel von J. Lang. In Zsarb. mit K.-A. Bushe, W. Buschmann und D. Linnert. Springer, Berlin, Heidelberg, New York 1979

[23] Lang J: Klinische Anatomie des Kopfes: Neurokranium, Orbita, kraniozervikaler Übergang. Springer, Berlin, Heidelberg, New York 1981

[24] Lang J: Neue Ergebnisse zur Anatomie der Orbita. Fortschr. Ophthalmol. 79, 3 - 10 (1982)

[25] Lang J, Götzfried H P: Über praktisch-ärztlich wichtige Maße an der Fossa cranialis media. Anat. Anz. 151, 433 - 453 (1982)

[26] Lang J, Haas R: Neue Befunde zur Bodenregion der Fossa cranialis anterior. Verh. Anat. Ges. 73, 77 - 86 (1979)

[27] Lang J, Horn Th, von den Eichen U: Über die äußeren Augenmuskeln und ihre Ansatzzonen. Gegenbaurs morph. Jahrb. 126, 817 - 840 (1980)

[28] Lang J, Kageyama I: Some measurements of the ophthalmic artery and its branches. Surgical and Radiologic Anatomy (in press)

[29] Lang J, Kageyama I: Über die Ursprungsregion des M. obliquus bulbi inferior. Klin. Monatsbl. Augenheilkd. (in press)

[30] Lang J, Oehmann G: Formentwicklung des Canalis opticus, seine Maße und Einstellung zu den Schädelebenen. Verh. Anat. Ges. 70, 567 - 574 (1976)

[31] Lang J, Reiter W: Über praktisch-ärztlich wichtige Maße des N. opticus, des Chiasma opticum und des Tractus opticus. Gegenbaurs morph. Jahrb. 131, 777 - 759 (1985)

[32] Lang J, Reiter W: Über die dem Orbitadach und -rand angelagerten Strecken des N. ophthalmicus und seiner Äste. Neurochirurgia 30, 129 - 134 (1987)

[33] Lang J, Roth Ch: Über die Fläche des Bodens der vorderen Schädelgrube und des Augenhöhlendaches. Anat. Anz. 156, 1 - 19 (1984)

[34] Lang J, Schäfer W D, Grafen W, Wallner B: Über Seitenunterschiede der Lage des Hornhautscheitelpunktes zum lateralen Orbitarand (Messungen mit dem Exophthalmometer nach Hertel). Klin. Mbl. Augenheilkd. 187, 521 - 524 (1985)

[35] Lang J, Stefanec P, Breitenbach B: Über Form und Maße des Ventriculus tertius, von Sehbahnteilen und des N. oculomotorius. Neurochirurgia 26, 1 - 5 (1983)

[36] Maaron J C, Kennerdell J S: Lateral microsurgical approach to intraorbital tumors. J. Neurosurg. 44, 556 - 561 (1976)

[37] MacCarty C S, Brown D N: Orbital tumors in children. Clin. Neurosurg. 11, 76 - 88 (1964)

[38] Pertuiset B, Morax P V, Aron D, Cabezas C: La voie frontotemporale extradurale sa place dans l'abord des tumeurs de l'orbite (d'après 18 observations). Ann. Ocul. 196, 917 - 933 (1963)

[39] Pickrell K L: Reconstructive plastic surgery of the face. Clinical Symposia. Edited by J.H. Walton, Vol. 20, Ciba Ltd. Canada 1968

[40] Rohen J: Morphologische Studien zur Funktion des Lidapparates beim Menschen. Gegenbaurs morph. Jahrb. 93, 43 - 97 (1953)

[41] Rupp R: Über die medialen Ansatzstellen des Musculus orbicularis oculi. Med. Diss., Würzburg 1980

[42] Schürmann, K.: Neurochirurgische Aufgaben in der Orbita. Arch. Otorhinolaryngol. 207, 253 - 282 (1974)

[43] Stock A L, Collins J P, Davidson T M: Anatomy of the superficial temporal artery. Head & Neck Surg. 2, 466 - 469 (1980)

Microsurgical anatomy of the ophthalmic artery

R. Renella, S. Hussein, M. Waidner

Introduction

Since the first comprehensive description in 1847 [1] numerous anatomical studies have extensively reported the origin as well the intracranial and the intracanalicular course of the ophthalmic artery [2, 3, 4, 5, 6, 9, 10, 11, 12, 13]. It is generally accepted that the ophthalmic artery is the first intracranial branch emerging from the wall of the internal carotid artery at its exit from the cavernous sinus, first coursing medially forward, inferior to the optic nerve, and then crossing it within the optic canal. However, contradictory descriptions regarding the visualisation of the origin and the first intracranial segment of this vessel during surgery and the relationship of its intracranial course to the basal dura are still found in the literature. Discrepancy between anatomical and surgical findings may occasionally result from the peculiarity of the anatomy and techniques but it is more likely to be explained by the different approaches to the basal region. As a matter of fact many surgeons have encountered major problems in presenting the first portion of the ophthalmic artery during microvascular procedures or tumor removal in the parasellar area. With introduction of microsurgery and the development of new surgical approaches a more accurate knowledge of the ophthalmic artery and especially of its osseous, dural and nervous relationships has important practical implications. In this report we present the results of our microanatomical studies of the ophthalmic artery related to selective microsurgical procedures.

Material and Methods

The origin and the intracranial and the intracanalicular course of the ophthalmic artery were studied in 50 human orbits obtained from 25 cadaver specimens. The ophthalmic artery was selectively cannulated via the internal carotid artery and perfused with hypoxid (Biodur^R, Heidelberg, FRG) after being perfused with warm Ringer's solution. The skull basis were fixed using a Mayfield-Kees three-points head holder and positioned according to a pterional approach. The preparations were carried out using microtechniques. In every specimen the basic anatomical relationships were measured and the surgically important landmarks were documented by photographs.

Results and Discussions

The point of origin of the ophthalmic artery was usually situated in the subdural space at the emergence of the internal carotid artery from the cavernous sinus (47 of 50 specimens). The vessel arose more frequently from the anterior medial or from the superior medial wall of the carotid, but other points of origin e.g. from its anterior or even superior aspects were also observed in the present series (Tbl. I). According to HARRIS and RHOTON (1976) [8] the origin of the ophthalmic artery can be located in relationship to the tip and the medial side of the anterior clinoid process. In our material the vessel was found to originate between 4 mm anterior and 8 mm posterior to the clinoid tip and 0.5 - 5 mm medially to its medial aspect. Therefore the origin of the ophthalmic artery was clearly seen directly or after mobilisation of the optic nerve in only 8 specimens. On the contrary in most cases removal of the anterior clinoid process using an high-speed electrodrill was required in order to present ophthalmica branching (Fig. 1, 2).

Tab. I: Site of origin of the ophthalmic artery in 50 specimens. ICA: A. carotis interna, AMM: A. meningea media

ICA Intradural				ICA Extradural	AMM
Anterior	Antero-Medial	Superior	Supero-Medial		
4	23	3	17	2	1

In 2 specimens the vessel arose from the upper intracavernous bend of the internal carotid, close to its point of penetration of the basal dura. In both instances the ophthalmic artery entered the optic canal through a separate opening in its floor without coursing into the subdural compartment.

Although anatomosis with the middle meningeal artery was regularly demonstrated in our material, the orbital meningeal branch being enlarged in 9 specimens, we were able to find only a single case of abnormal origin of the ophthalmic artery from the middle meningeal branch. In this case connection with the internal carotid artery was absent and the ophthalmic artery entered the orbita through the superior orbital fissure.

According to HAYREH [9, 10] the intracranial and intracanalicular course of the ophthalmic artery may be divided into a short limb, a long limb and a distal part up to the orbital apex. In the present series the average short segment measured 1.5 mm in length (0.8 - 3 mm) and coursed forwards and slightly downwards in the subdural space under the medial aspect of the optic nerve. Intracanalicular location of this portion was never observed in this series (Tab. II, Fig. 3). The average long segment measured 2.5 mm in length (1.2 - 4.9 mm) and ran forwards and laterally, following the direction of the optic nerve. The main portion was located subdurally or intradurally, depending on the length of the vascular portion. Segments of 20 mm in length coursed almost entirely in the subdural space (18 specimens). On the contrary the main portion disappeared in the dural sheath of the optic nerve when the whole segment measured less then 20 mm in length (28 specimens, Tab. II).

Concerning the point of penetration of the dural sheath of the optic nerve our observations confirm the results of WOLF [14] and HAYREH [9, 10]. As a rule the ophthalmic artery entered the inferior lateral aspect of the dural sheath at the cranial end of the optic canal. In 3 specimens, however, the point of penetration was situated in the subdural space, 0.5 - 1 mm proximally to the optic canal.

Tab. II: Length and direction of the intracranial segments of the ophthalmic artery in 47 specimens with subdural point of origin

	Length MM	Direction	
Short segment	1.5 (0.8 - 3)	Forwards Upwards	8
		Forwards Downwards	18
		Forwards Laterally	2
		Forwards Medially	7
		Forwards Upwards Medially	11
		Forwards Upwards Laterally	1
G. Ophthalmica			
Long segment	2.5 (1.2 - 4.9)	Forwards Laterally	39
		Laterally	8

When the origin of the ophthalmic artery was situated extradurally, the vessel entered the proximal part of the optic canal through a separate opening in its floor and coursed between the two dural layers laterally to the optic nerve (2 specimens). The deep dural layer, separating the vessel from the optic nerve, was less defined and more irregular in its texture then the superficial layer. Therefore the artery could be easily dissected and also displaced according to surgical requirements (Fig. 4).

With regard to the relationship between the ophthalmic artery and the optic nerve in the optic canal our observations diverge from the classical descriptions of WOLF [14] and HAYREH [9, 10]. Although the most frequent penetration point of the dural sheath was located on its inferior lateral aspect, the ophthalmic artery was observed to cross under the optic nerve in 40 specimens, running then medially in 28, on the midline in 11 and laterally in only 9 specimens.

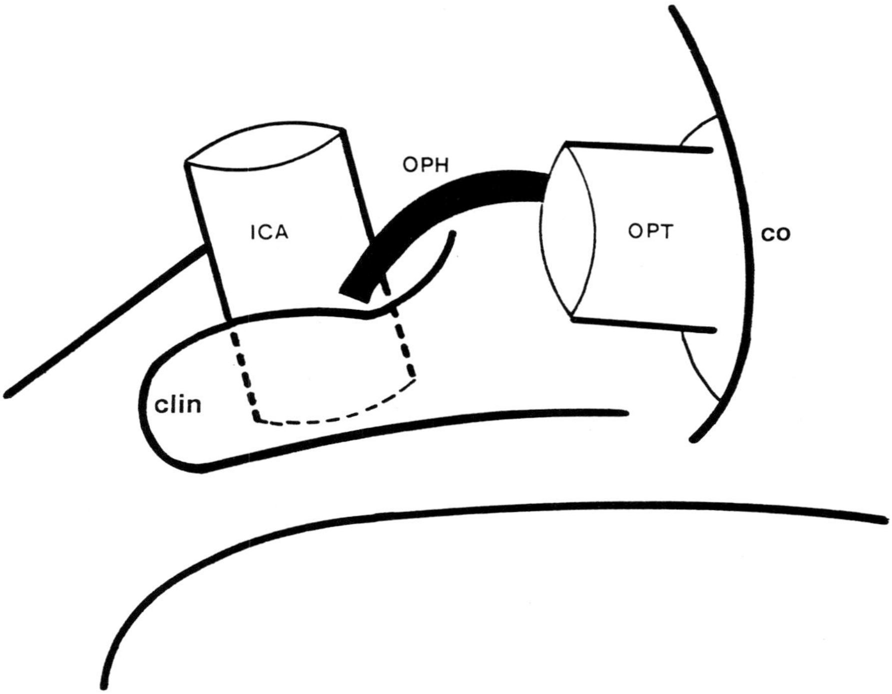

Fig. 1: The point of origin as well as the initial (short) segment of ophthalmic artery may be directly visualised only when the anterior clinoid process is hypoplasic (rare variant)

The overlying objectives in surgery of the sellar and parasellar areas relate to obtaining maximal exposure and intraoperative flexibility for lesion access and manipulation without injury of normal neuro-vascular structures. The pathological spectrum involving the ophthalmic artery include carotid-cavernous fistulas, aneurysms arising from the medial or the supero-medial aspect of the internal carotid artery as well as mass lesions extending from the anterior clinoid process to the optic canal.

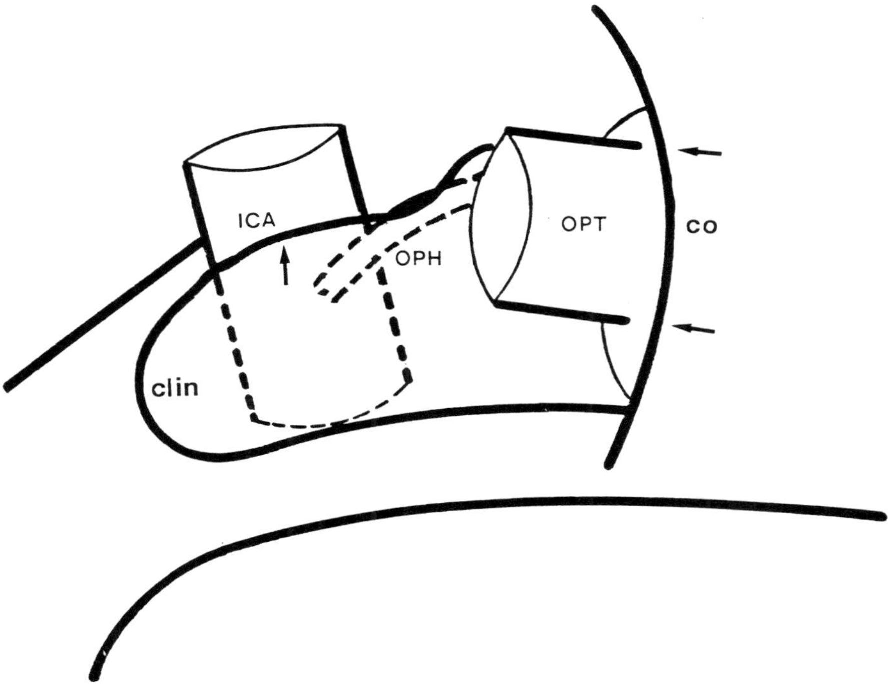

Fig. 2: The point of origin of the ophthalmic artery and its proximal part are hidden by a well developed anterior clinoid process (most frequent variant)

According to HAMBY and GARDNER [7] a carotid-cavernous fistula may be treated by extracranial ligature of the internal carotid artery combined with its occlusion proximally to the origin of the ophthalmic artery (trapping procedure). In carotid-cavernous fistulas, however, vascular anatomy is distorted by the engorgement of the anterior compartment of the cavernous sinus, which displaces the internal carotid artery in superior and posterior direction and stretches the epidural segment of the ophthalmic artery. In our opinion a trapping procedure without sacrifice of the ophthalmic artery seems to be almost impossible as the ophthalmic artery courses closely to the dura and the visualisation of its origin requires bone removal even in absence of pathological conditions.

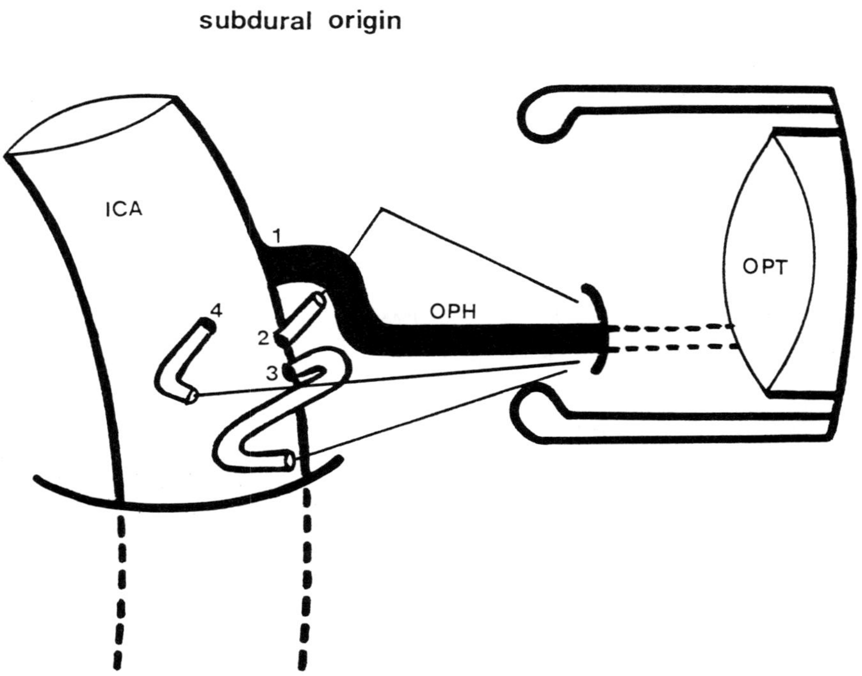

Fig. 3: Intracranial and intracanalicular course of the ophthalmic artery (subdural origin): 1,2: most frequent variants, 3,4: rare variants

Aneurysms arising from the medial or superior-medial aspect of the internal carotid artery (so called carotido-ophthalmic aneurysms) act as a mass displacing the short limb of the ophthalmic artery toward the cavernous sinus. Since the vessel is fixed at the level of the optic canal, attempts to visualise the neck of the malformation without bone removal may eventually reduce or interrupt the blood flow toward the orbita. On the other hand, visualisation of the ophthalmica branching is required to confirm a suspected extension of the aneurysm into the cavernous sinus as well as to check the carotid wall for a possible temporary clipping. Therefore drilling of the anterior clinoid process and enlargement of the optic canal should be performed as a first step in aneurysms hidding the origin of the ophthalmic and the proximal portion of the internal carotid artery.

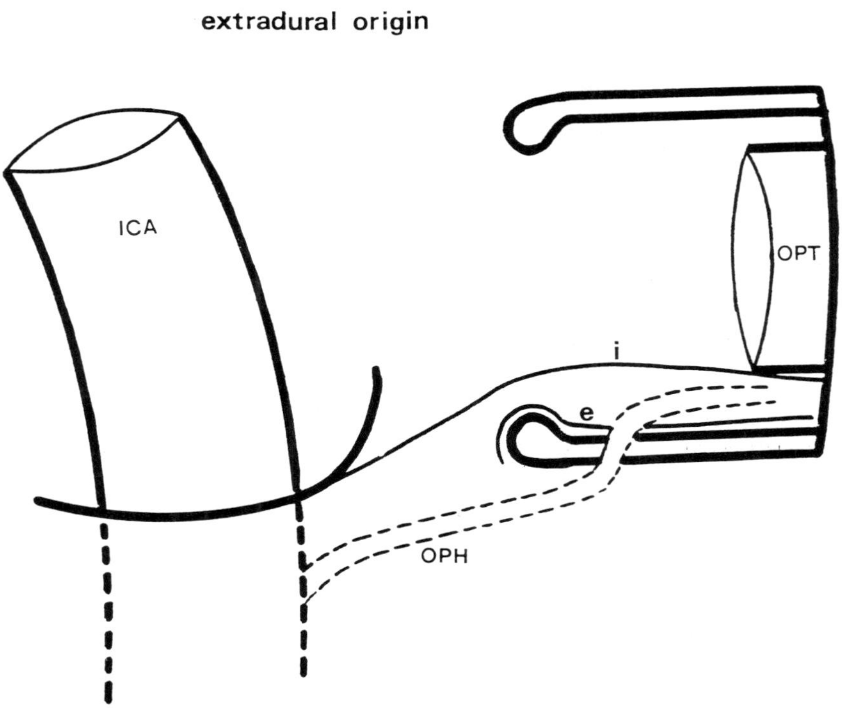

Fig. 4: The ophthalmic artery may occasionally originate in the extradural space. In this instance it courses extradurally and enters the optic canal through a separate opening in its floor. The internal dural layer separates the vessel from the optic nerve. i: internal dural layer, e: external dural layer

Tumors invading the optic canal usually squeeze the ophthalmic artery in the space between the optic nerve and the carotid artery, especially when the optic nerve is fixed by a superimposed fold of dura mater. In this instance it may by helpful to unroof the optic canal, to dissect the dural attachments and to mobilise the optic nerve before starting the preparation to the wall of the internal carotid artery.

When the ophthalmic artery remains invisible after drilling the clinoid process and lifting of the optic nerve an extradural origin should be considered. In this case it may be helpful to drill the optic canal from medially to laterally, mobilising the optic nerve from the lateral wall, in order to avoid injury of the ophthalmic artery at its penetration point.

References

[1] Arnold F: Handbuch der Anatomie des Mensch, Band 2, Teil 1. Herder Verlag, Freiburg i.B., 1847

[2] Böck J, Schwarz-Karsten H: Bericht über die 58. Zusammenkunft der Deutschen Ophthalmologischen Gesellschaft, Band 58, 1953

[3] Böck J, Schwarz-Karsten H: Further investigating on the anatomy of the origin ophthalmic artery Graefes Arch. Ophtal 199 (1975) 302 - 310

[4] Decker K, Schlegel HJ: Normalbilder und Normvarianten der A. ophthalmica im Röntgenbild. Albrecht von Graefes Arch. Ophtal., 159 (1955) 160 - 164

[5] Di Chiro G: Ophthalmic arteriography. Radiology, 77 (1961) 948 - 957

[6] Dilenge D, Fischgold H, David M: L'angiographie par soustraction de l'artère ophthalmique et de ses branches. Masson, Paris, 1965

[7] Hamby WB, Gardner WJ: Treatment of pulsating exophthalmos with report of two cases. Arch. Surg., 27 (1933) 676-685

[8] Harris FS, Rhoton AL: Anatomy of the cavernous sinus. J. Neurosurg., 45 (1976) 169-180

[9] Hayreh SS: The ophthalmic artery. Section I. Normal gross anatomy. In: Newton, T.H., Potts, D.G.: Radiology of the Skull and Brain, Vol. II, Book 2, Mosby, St. Louis, 1974

[10] Hayreh SS, Dass R: The opthalmic artery. I. Origin and intracranial and intracanalicular course. Brit. J. Ophthal. 46 (1962) 65 - 98

[11] Renn WH, Rhoton AL: Microsurgical anatomy of the sellar region. J. Neurosurg. 43 (1975) 288 - 298

[12] Salamon G, Guerinel G, Louis R, Guidicelli G, Finidori F: Etude radioanatomique de l'artère ophthalmique. Ann. Radiol. 8 (1965) 557 - 569

[13] Vignaud J, Aubin ML, Clay C: La vascularisation de l'orbite. I. Arteriographie normale l'artere ophthalmique. Amer. Radiol. 18 (1975) 171 - 180

[14] Wolf E: The Anatomy of the Eye and the Orbit, 4. Ed., Lewis, London, 1954

The topography of the orbit as demonstrated by High-Resolution Computed Tomography and multiplanar reconstructions

J.P. Haas, G. Kahle, W. Draf

Abstract

A precise knowledge of the variable normal orbital borders and even more the pathologically altered borders is essential before any therapeutic approach can be attempted.

High-Resolution Computed Tomography is now able to outline the delicate bony structures and the preshaped communicating pathways. With reformatting techniques - generating reconstructed multiplanar slices or pseudo 3D-images - CT can produce any desirable view of the orbital topography.

Introduction

The introduction of computed tomography (CT) into clinical practice CCT proved very useful for the exploration of the orbit and numerous excellent papers (see for examples [1] - [14]) have enriched our knowledge of an appropriate and with regard to the examination's aim a modified modality of scanning. The characteristic normal and pathologic morphologic pattern of the soft tissue contents of the orbit are now well known.

Numerous preformed communications and the paranasal sinuses, which are surrounding the orbit, are often pathways for pathologic transmission.

Diseases, reaching the orbit by those channels are frequently subject to multidisciplinar therapeutic efforts.

The radiologist has to delineate the extent of the pathologic invasion and the delimitation of the normal conditions and its alteration. HR-CT rendering a maximum spatial resolution of 0.4 mm offers an effective tool for defining the integrity of osseous limitations of the orbit.

In the following the osseous orbit will be discusses in relation to its surroundings.

Three dimensional (3D) reconstructions of the whole facial skull or of parts of it deliver a radio-anatomical survey over the bony walls of the orbit and their relationship to each other.

Considering the actual degree of technical development the delicate osseous structures of the lateral orbital walls in their fronto-occipital extension can only be distinguished in axial CT-scans, whereas the cranio-caudal extension is best demonstrated in coronal scans or reconstructions (Fig. 1).

The greater wing of the sphenoid bone and the zygomatic bone are separated from each other by the spheno-zygomatic suture, while the frontal bone and the zygomatic bone are separated from each other by the fronto-zygomatic suture.

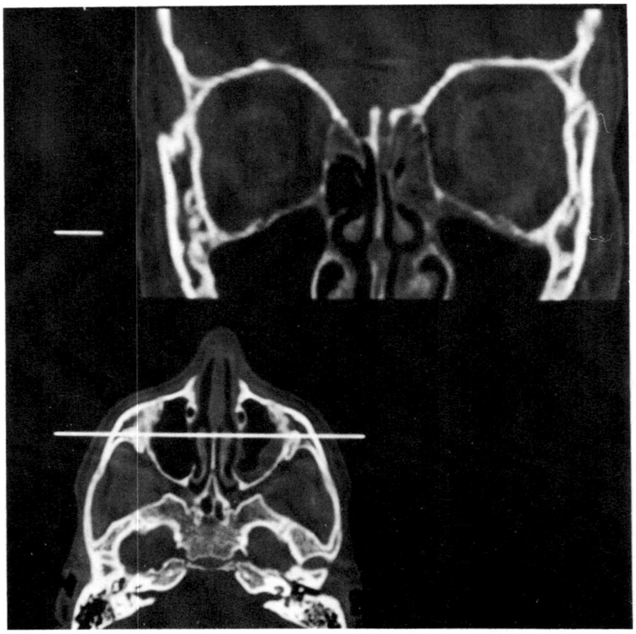

Fig. 1: Coronal reconstruction, lateral orbital wall

The relationship of the fronto-lateral orbital wall to the extracranial temporal fossa and of the occipito-lateral orbital wall to the intracranial middle cranial fossa are best demonstrated by coronal reconstructions.

Vessels are crossing the lateral orbital wall via the meningo-orbital foramina, running between the orbit and the middle cranial fossa.

A large pneumatization of the sphenoid bone, reaching into the greater wings of the sphenoid, can result in a close vicinity of the sphenoid sinus and the lateral orbital wall (Fig. 2).

The orbital roof is almost exclusively formed by the orbital parts of the frontal bone. A small part of the dorsal aspect is part of the lesser wing of the sphenoid bone.

The connecting suture, the sphenofrontal suture, is best to be studied in sagittal reconstructions (Fig. 3).

Pneumatization can also reach the lesser wings of the sphenoid bone, and clearly demonstrated by the pneumatized anterior clinoidal processes.

Posterior ethmoidal cells can contribute to form the dorsal aspect of the medial cranial parts of the orbital roof, refered to as Onodi's cells.

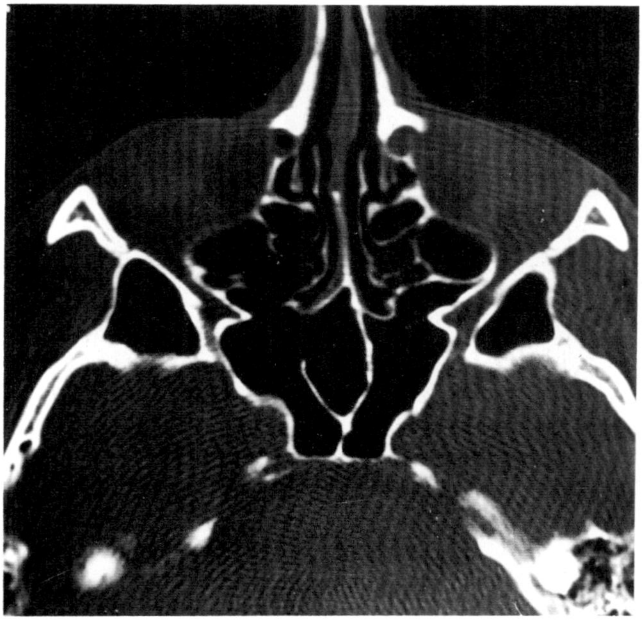

Fig. 2: Axial CT scan, pneumatization of the greater wings of sphenoid

In cases of an aplastic frontal sinus the orbital roof consists of solid bone. On the other hand, in cases of wide spreaded pneumatization the frontal sinus can fill the whole orbital roof, and reaching the lateral orbital wall. Unlike all other orbital walls the orbital floor has a constant relationship to the maxillary sinus, which is extremely rarely aplastic. This relationship can be studied in 3D-reconstructions from different points of view.

The major part of the orbital floor is a part of the wall of the maxilla (facies orbitalis maxillae) as can be demonstrated in coronal reconstructions.

The lateral part of the orbital floor formed by the zygomatic bone, the inferior orbital fissure. The most posterior portion of the orbital floor is formed by the orbital process of the palatine bone well recognisable in sagittal (Fig. 4) and coronal (Fig. 5) reconstructions. The infraorbital foramen and the infraorbital canal are delineated in axial scans.

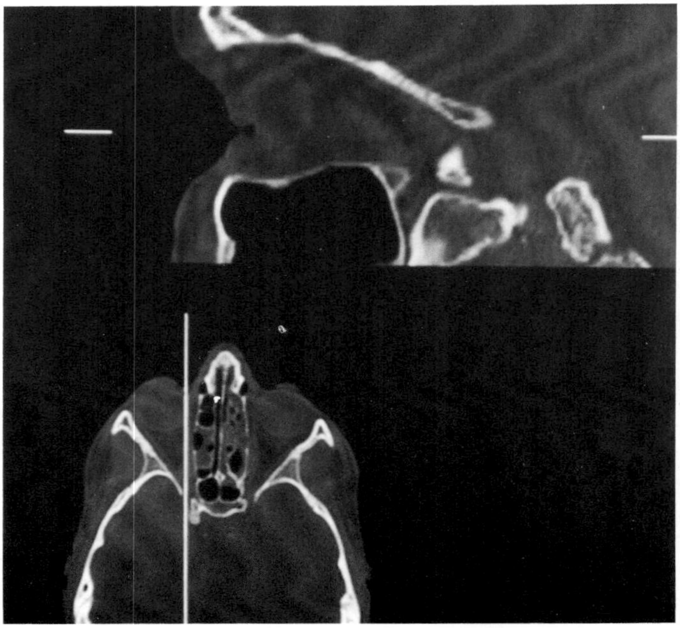

Fig. 3: Sagittal reconstruction, sphenofrontal suture

The groove of the lacrimal sac is visible in 3-D reconstructions in sectional images and is best demonstrated in axial scans. The entire course of the draining lacrimal system with the nasolacrimal duct opening beneath the inferior turbinate is depicted in sagittal reconstructions.

Haller's cells are - if present - an important topographically related formation as they are in contact with the orbital floor as well as with the medial orbital wall. They can be seen in axial scans and in coronal reconstructions.

A very large portion of the medial orbital wall derives from the orbital lamina of the ethmoid bone, easily seen in 3D-reconstructions situated in close vicinity of the ethmoidal labyrinth and shown in 3D-reconstructions of the skull, in a coronal plane (Fig. 6).

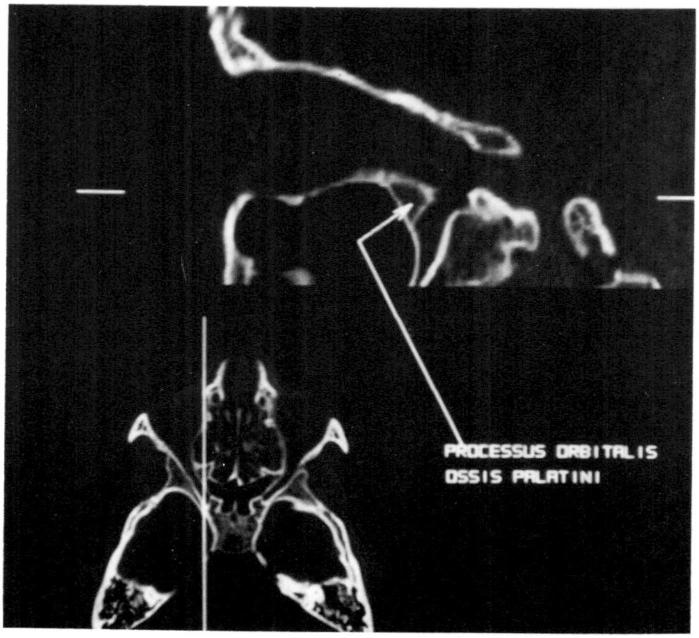

Fig. 4: Sagittal reconstruction, orbital process of palatine bone

Axial or coronal CT scans and reconstructions thus provide a complete survey of the spatial relationship between ethmoidal labyrinth and medial orbital wall.

The ethmoidal foramina, located near the fronto-ethmoidal suture allow the passage of ethmoidal nervs and vessels.

These foramina can be delineated in axial CT scans as anterior, posterior and - occasionally present - a third ethmoidal foramen.

The posterior portion of the medial orbital wall is closely connected to the sphenoid sinus, as the body of the sphenoid bone forms the posterior most aspect of the medial orbital wall. This view is depicted in axial CT scans as well as in coronal reconstructions. With the latter modality the superior orbital fissure is shown in its greatest extension.

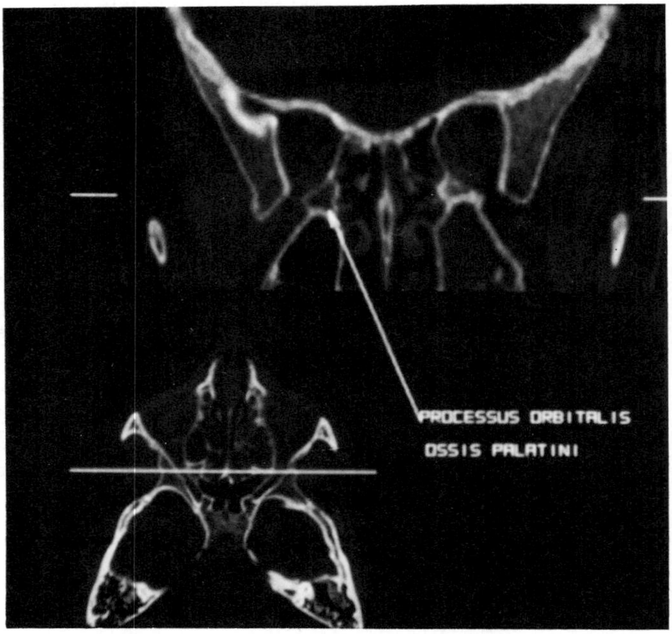

Fig. 5: Coronal reconstruction, orbital process of palatine bone

Frontally there is direct connection of the medial orbital wall with the nasal cavity. The same is valid for the region of the frontal process of the maxillary bone and for the lacrimal bone, a frontal relationship clearly seen in an axial CT-scans.

The orbital apex deserves our special interest, as a number of structures are running from the vicinity to the orbits.

From the middle cranial fossa there is a connection via the superior orbital fissure, outlined by coronal or sagittal reconstructions. The typical configuration of this fissure with its maximum seize in cranio-caudal extension medially and its upward directed course to the lateral aspect is to its best advantage shown in a 3D-reconstructions (Fig. 7).

Roof and floor of the optic canal are best assessed in oblique reconstructions, due to its oblique course through the lesser wing of sphenoid bone.

The lateral border is the anterior clinoidal process while the medial border, formed by the body of the sphenoid bone is depicted in axial sections.

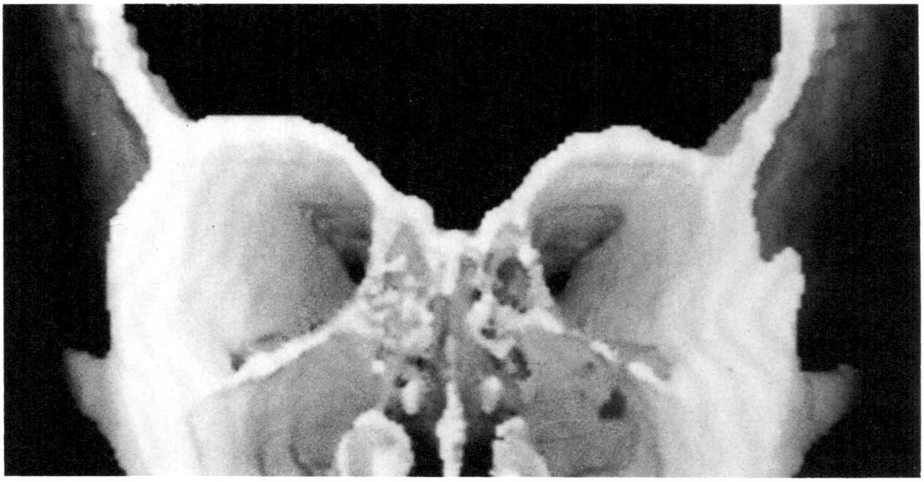

Fig. 6: 3D reconstruction, orbital lamina: cut off in coronal plane

The inferior orbital fissure gains special importance by leading medially into the pterygo-palatine fossa, shown in axial scans.

The pterygo-palatine fossa has various apertures, communicating with the facial skull as well as with the cranium. It connects the orbit with the nasal cavity and the medial cranial fossa. The sphenopalatine foramen reaches in a fronto-medial direction the nasal cavity, whereas the foramen rotundum runs backwards to the middle cranial fossa.

Surgeons who are dealing with the orbital region need a detailed radiologic delineation of the variable normal morphologic pattern and of the pathologic morphologic pattern of the osseous orbit before planning and executing a successful surgical approach.

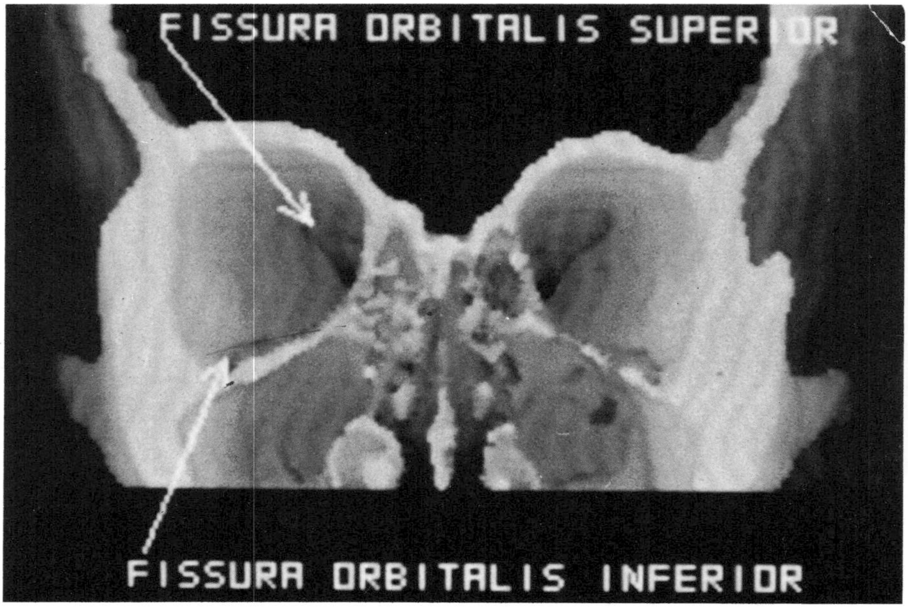

Fig. 7: 3D reconstruction, superior orbital fissure

This can be achieved with a High-Resolution-CT, supported by multiplanar reconstructions and eventually 3D-reconstructions. This procedure has been successful in great numbers of patients, in close cooperation the radiologist of ENT-, neuro, ophthalmic and maxillofacial surgeons.

References

[1] Enzmann D, Donaldson SS, Marshall WH, Kriss JP: Computed Tomography in orbital pseudotumor. Radiology 120 (1976) 597 - 601

[2] Enzmann D, Donaldson SS, Kriss JP: Appearance of Graves' Disease on orbital computed tomography. J. Comp. Assist. Tomogr. 3 (1979) 815 - 819

[3] Forbes GS, Earnest F, Waller RR: Computer tomography of orbital tumors. Radiology 142 (1982) 387 - 394

[4] Godde-Jolly D, Cabanis EA, Lopez A, Danicel V, Iba-Zizen MT, Sallolini U, Texeira KI: Anatomie et physiologie tomodensitometrique du cone musculaire. Bull. Soc. Ophthalmol. 80 (1980) 215 - 218

[5] Grove AS: Computed tomography in the managment of orbital trauma Ophthalmology 89 (1982) 433 - 440

[6] Healy JF: Computed tomographic evaluation of metastses of the orbit Ann. Ophthalmol. 15 (1983) 1026 - 1029

[7] Johns TT, Citrin CH, Black J, Sherman JL: CT evaluation of perineural orbital lesions. AJNR 5 (1984) 587 - 590

[8] Lallemand DP, Brasch RC, Char DH, Norman D: Orbital tumors in children: characterization by computed tomography. Radiology 151 (1984) 85 - 88

[9] Lemoine JJ, Trokel SL: Tomodensitometrie et pathologie orbitaire inflammatoire non Basedowienne. Bull. Soc. Ophthalmol. 1983, 113 - 132

[10] Manelfe C, Psquini U, Bank WO: Metrizamide demonstration of the subarachnoid space surrounding the optic nerves. J. Comp. Assist. Tomogr. 2 (1987) 545 - 547

[11] Peyster RG, Hoover ED, Hershey BL, Haskin ME: High resolution CT of lesions of the optic nerve. AJNR 4 (1983) 169 - 174

[12] Salvolini U, Cabanis EA, Rodellec A, Menichelli F, Pasquini U, Iba-Zizen MT: Computer tomography of the optic nerve. Part I: Normal results. J. comp. Assist. Tomogr. 2 (1978) 141 - 149

[13] Unsoeld R, De Groot J, Newton TH: Images of the optic nerve: Anatomic-CT correlation. AJNR 1 (1980) 317 - 323

[14] Wende S, Aulich A, Nover A, Lanksch W, Kazner E, Steinhoff H, Meese W, Lange S, Grumme T: Computed tomography of orbital lesions. Neuroradiology 13 (1977) 123 - 134

MRI of the orbit and optic chiasm

A. Markl, K. G. Riedel, T. Vogl

Abstract

The purpose of this study was to evaluate the improvement of MR Imaging of orbital diseases using fast sequences, surface coils, and contrast agents.

170 patients with a wide range of orbital pathology (primary and secondary orbital tumors, inflammatory and vascular diseases, Graves' diseases) were examined by MR Imaging, in most cases performed with surface coils.

48 patients were studied before and after intravenous administration of Gadolinium-DTPA with T1- and T2-weighted spin-echo sequences and a multi echo sequence in transverse, frontal, and paraxial section orientation.

Additionally short sequences (FISP, FLASH) were performed in 10 cases.

The use of frontal and paraxial (oblique-sagittal) views allowed for better visualization of the optic nerve and the region of the optic canal, as well as tumor infiltration into the surrounding anatomical structures.

The use of the paramagnetic contrast agent allowed for better delineation and differentiation of pathology. Particularly hemangiomas and vascular diseases showed a marked increase of the signal intensity.

Short sequences are sometimes useful to shorten the examination times.

Introduction

Before the development of diagnostic imaging techniques like ultrasound (US) and high-resolution computed tomography (CT) it was difficult to investigate the orbit, the optic nerve and chiasm and related space-occupying lesions.

The available techniques for investigating the orbit were either relatively poor in information (plain X-rays, phlebography of the orbit) or risky (angiography of the orbit).

After the advent of ultrasound noninvasive examination of the eye and the anterior half of the orbit became possible; but the apex and the bony borders remained inaccessible by ultrasound investigation.

High-resolution computed tomography allows a delineation of the entire orbit, its bony borders, and of the optic chiasm. There are difficulties, however, in the region of the optic canal because of partial volume effects.

In addition the exposure of the lens to ionizing radiation must be taken into consideration, especially in cases of multiple CT-reexaminations.

Magnetic resonance (MR) imaging has further improved the investigation of the orbit and the optic chiasm.

Particularly the use of surface coils, multiaxial views, and the application of a paramagnetic contrast agent in several cases provides a good delineation of the orbital anatomic structures and diagnostic accuracy of orbital diseases.

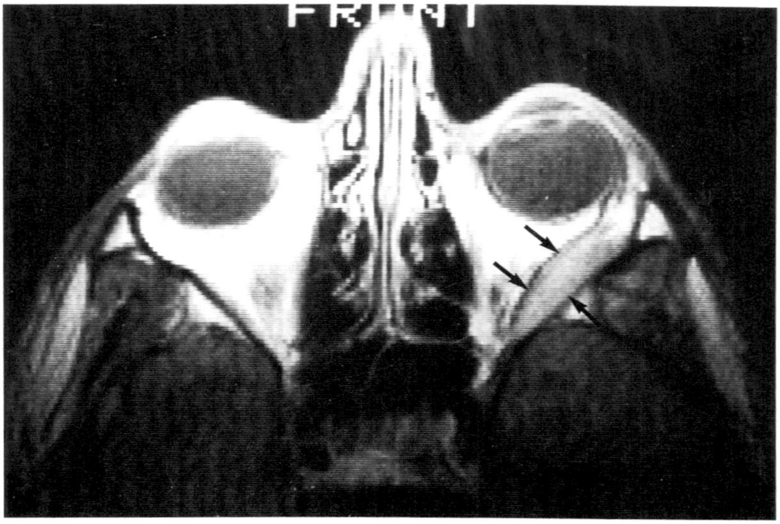

Fig. 1a: Transverse slice orientation, with Gadolinium-DTPA

Patients and Methods

170 patients with suspected orbital or chiasmatic space-occupying lesions were examined by MR.

In some patients reexaminations resulted in a total number of 209 investigations with 213 findings.

97 of the patients were female, 73 male (sex distribution 1,3 : 1,0). The youngest patient was 1, the oldest 87 years of age (mean value: 43 years of age).

48 of the patients were scanned before and after administration of a paramagnetic contrast agent. 26 of these patients were female, 22 male (sex distribution 1,2 : 1,0). The youngest of these patient was 21, the oldest 84 years of age (mean value: 48 years of age).

MR images were obtained by means of a 1.5 Tesla superconductive magnet (MAGNETOM/Siemens AG, Erlangen), which was operated at 0.35 Tesla (96 examinations) and 1.0 Tesla (113 examinations).

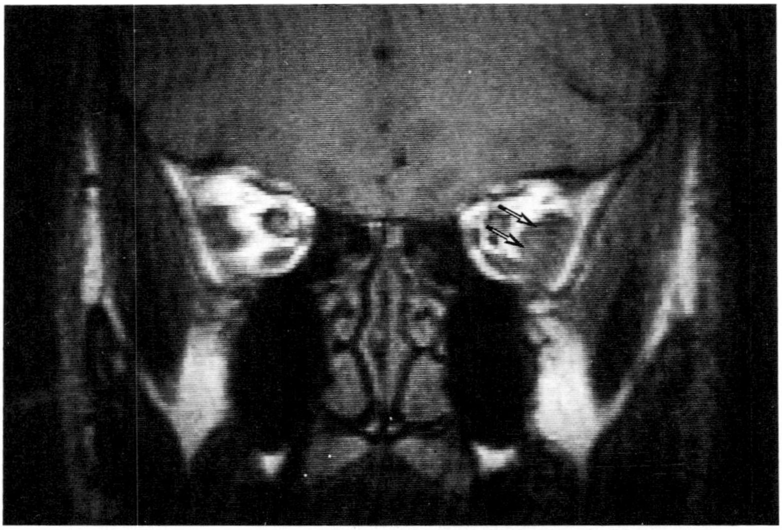

Fig. 1b: Frontal slice orientation, with Gadolinium-DTPA

The patients were examined using either the head coil or various surface coils of our own design.

The acquisition matrix size was 256 x 256 pixels. The slice thickness was 5 mm and the zoom-factor (hardware zoom) was set to 1.4. Data acquisition utilized 2 averages of signal. The spatial resolution of the head coil was 1 x 1 x 5 mm, the one of the surface coils 0.5 x 0.5 x 5 mm.

In all patients a spin echo technique was used with T1- and T2-weighted pulse sequences (Table I). The multi echo sequence was only applied in plain MR. Additionally short sequences like FISP and FLASH with various flip angles were used in 10 patients.

The contrast medium was Gadolinium-DTPA-Dimeglumine (aqueous solution of the di-N-methylglucamine-salt of the DTPA-complex with Gadolinium), manufactured by Schering AG/Berlin. The dosage was 0.1 mmol GD-DTPA/kg Bodyweight = 0.2 ml Gd-DTPA/kg BW),injected in a cubital vein.

Results

The orbital and chiasmatic space-occupying lesions of all patients were separated into 5 groups (Table II).

25 patients showed no pathological findings.

All space-occupying lesions of the orbit and optic chiasm could be identified by plain MR with T1-weighted, T2-weighted and multi echo sequences.

The diseases of the patients examined before and after application of Gadolinium-DTPA included 222 primary and secondary intraorbital tumors, 17 cases with external tumor infiltration of the orbit, 6 inflammatory and vascular diseases, 1 tumor of the optic chiasm and 1 case with Graves' disease (Table III).

1 patient showed no pathological findings.

In 15 cases the application of the paramagnetic contrast agent Gadolinium-DTPA provided important additional information in comparison to the plain MR examination.

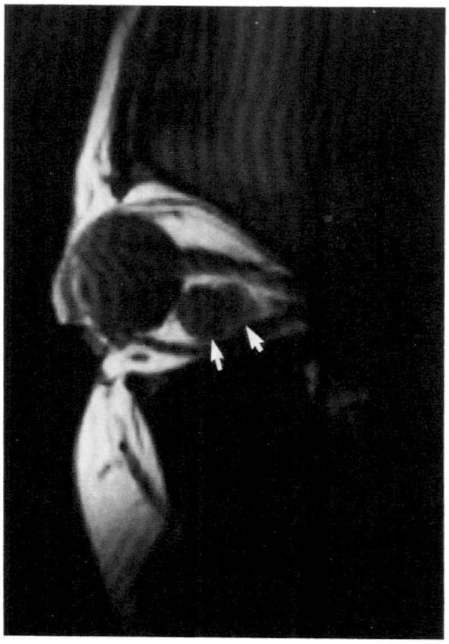

Fig. 2: Intraorbital metastasis of a rhabdomyosarcoma, arrows = tumor, T1-weighted images (TR/TE : 600/30); paraxial slice orientation, with Gadolinium-DTPA

As shown on table III in the group 1 (primary and secondary intraorbital masses) the hemangiomas showed the highest increase of the tumor signal on the T1-weighted images with Gadolinium-DTPA (Fig. 1).

Also a monorphed adenoma of the lacrimal gland showed a significant enhancement. Both of these tumors had a marked increase in signal intensity in the T2-weighted images before application of the contrast medium. The signal intensity, however, did not reach the level of the T1-weighted contrast scan.

Intraorbital metastases (Fig. 2), mainly of breast and lung cancer, only showed a moderate increase in the signal intensity after Gadolinium-DTPA as well as tumors of the optic nerve like optic nerve gliomas (Fig. 3) and optic nerve sheath menigiomas.

The enhancement of choroidal melanomas was very small.

The advantage of paramagnetic contrast agents was shown by the tumors of the second group in table III.

By only moderate increase of the signal intensity of the carcinomas and meningiomas infiltrating the orbit, the differentiation between the tumors and the surrounding anatomical structures was better in the contrast scans in comparison to plain MR.

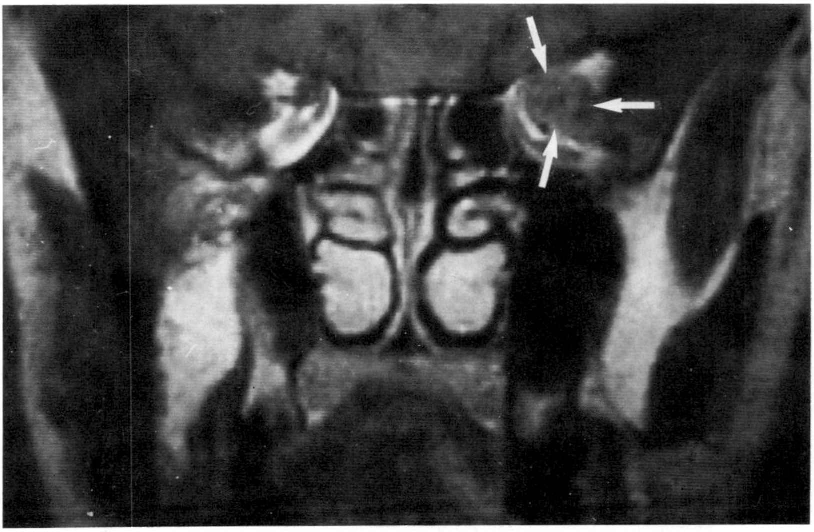

Fig. 3: Optic nerve glioma, left orbit, arrows = tumor, T1 weighted images (TR/TE : 600/30); frontal slice orientation, with Gadolinium-DTPA

In case of a menigotheliomatous meningioma with infiltration of the orbit and the optic chiasm, the T1- and T2-weighted plain images and the multi echo images failed to demonstrate the intracranial portion of the tumor exactly. This was only possible with the T1-weighted Gadolinium scan. As expected, interaorbital vascular diseases (e.g. orbital varices) showed a marked increase of the signal intensity after the application of Gadolinium-DTPA.

The contrast enhancement of the inflammatory diseases (group 3) was variable depending on the acuteness of the inflammation. Acute inflammation yielded a stronger signal intensity compared to a chronic inflammation due to an increased blood circulation.

Orbital pseudotumors appeared in T1-weighted images as a diffuse soft tissue infiltration of the orbital fatty tissue (Fig. 4).

In Graves' disease (group 5) the availability of MRI of multiaxial views without moving the patient, especially the coronal slice orientation, provided an advantage in measuring the muscle thickness in comparison to CT.

In one case of Graves' disease the application of Gadolinium-DTPA produced no change of the signal intensity of the enlarged rectus muscles.

Discussion

The first report using MRI of the eye and orbit are only a few years old [6 - 10, 16, 17].

Early MR images had only a small spatial resolution and were comparable to CT scans of the first generation.

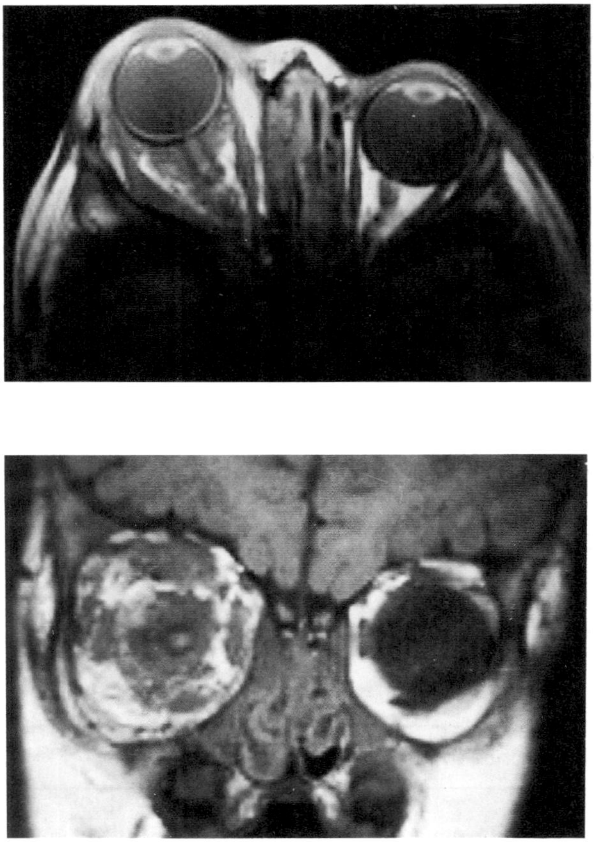

a)

b)

Fig. 4: Orbital pseudotumor, right orbit, diffuse soft tissue infiltration of the orbital fatty tissue, T1-weighted images (TR/TE : 600/30), plain; transverse (a) and frontal (b) slice orientation

The use of surface coils, specially designed for the orbit, lead to a higher signal to noise-ratio and an excellent spatial resolution. These MR images are as good as high resolution CT scans [1 - 5, 11 - 13, 15, 18 - 21].

Particularly within the orbital cone, the optic canal and the base of the skull MRI allows for good soft tissue visualization as there are no interferences at the soft tissue-bone interface.

The accuracy in the preoperative diagnosis of space-occupying lesions in the region of the optic canal and chiasma could thus considerably be increased. However, the identification of small calcifications, (e.g. in optic nerve sheath meningiomas), is still rather difficult.

Table I: Pre- and post-contrast pulse sequences

pre-contrast	0.35 Tesla TR/TE (msec)	1.0 TeslaTR/TE(msec)
SE T1-weighted	600/35	600/30
SE T2-weighted	1600/70	2000/90
SE multi echo	1600/30-240	1600/30-240
post-contrast		
SE T1-weighted	600/35	600/30
SE-T2-weighted	1600/70	2000/90
fast sequences		
FISP and FLASH with various flip angles		

Additionally an essential advantage of MRI is the availability of multiaxial views without moving the patient. Especially the paraxial (oblique-sagittal) view along the optic nerve allows for an optimal assessment of the optic nerve in its whole extent and of lesions in this structure from the eyeball to the chiasm, respectively.

Hoping to achieve a better tissue differentiation a paramagnetic contrast medium was developed for MRI.

Using this contrast agent, Gadolinium-DTPA however the advantage of MRI as a noninvasive method was to some extent given up. Contrast enhanced MR sometimes showed a better delineation between tumor and surrounding structures in T1-images. Contrast enhancement in tumors seemed to be similar to iodine enhancement in X-ray computed tomography. The amount of enhancement by itself provided additional information over plain MR in identifying the type of tumor, particularly in the case of vascular masses [11 - 15].

The application of paramagnetic contrast agents and the use of short sequences like FISP and FLASH shortened the acquisition time in patients, who did not tolerate the long examination times required for plain MR with T1- and T2-weighted sequences and a multi echo sequence. In most cases the signal to noise-ratio was lower in comparison to conventional SE sequences.

Orbital lesions larger than 1 cm could well be depicted in the images obtained with fast sequences. With smaller lesions we had some difficulties. These lesions (< 1 cm) could only be depicted in images acquired with SE sequences. In some cases significant image degradation was encountered due to artifacts caused by changes of the susceptibility close to the sinuses.

Table II: List of the space-occupying lesions of all patients examined

space-occupying lesion	n
1) primary and secondary intraorbital tumors	n = 54
optic nerve gliomas n = 12 metastases n = 11 optic nerve sheath meningiomas n = 9 choroidal melanomas n = 5 hemangiomas n = 5 tumors of the lacrimal gland n = 4 others n = 8	
2) external tumor infiltration of the orbit	n = 59
carcinomas (paranasal sinuses, pharynx, maxilla, parotid gland, petrous bone) meningiomas (meningotheliomatous, sphenoid bone) esthesioneuroblastoma fibroma others	n = 25 n = 19 n = 3 n = 3 n = 9
3) inflammatory, traumatic, vascular diseases	n = 25
inflammatory diseases (pseudotumor, myositis) traumatic diseases	n = 10 n = 9
(hematoma, foreign body) vascular diseases (varix, carotid-sinus cavernous-fistula)	 n = 6
4) tumors of the optic chiasm 5) Graves' diseases	n = 13 n = 37

Table III: List of diseases of the patients examined before and after application of the Gadolinium-DTPA and amount of the increase of signal intensity after injection of the paramagnetic contrast agent

space-occupying lesion	n	increase of signal intensity after Gadolinium-DTPA
1) primary and secondary intraorbital tumors	n = 22	
metastases	n = 6	+ +
choroidal melanomas	n = 5	+
tumors of the optic nerve	n = 4	+ + +
hemangiomas	n = 4	(+ + +)
immunoblastoma	n = 1	+ +
2) external tumor infiltration of the orbit	n = 17	
carcinomas (paranasal sinus, maxilla, parotid gland, pharynx, petrous bone)	n = 9	+ +
meningeomas (sphenoid bone, meningotheliomatous)	n = 5	+ +
esthesioneuroblastoma	n = 1	+ +
fibroma	n = 1	+ +
chondroma	n = 1	+
3) inflammatory and vascular diseases	n = 6	
orbital pseudotumor, myositis	n = 3	variable
varix	n = 2	+ + +
carotid-sinus cavernous-fiustula	n = 1	+
4) tumor of the optic chiasm		n = 1 +
5) Graves' disease	n = 1	0

References

[1] Atlas SW, Bilaniuk LT, Zimmermann RA, Hackney DB, Goldberg HI, Grossmann RI: Surface-coil MR imaging of the orbit at 1,5 Tesla: initial experience. Radiology 161 (P) (1986) 285

[2] Atlas SW, Grossmann RI, Savino PJ, et al.: Surface coil MR of orbital pseudotumor. Am J Neuroradiol 8 (1987) 141 - 146

[3] Axel L: Surface coil magnetic resonance imaging. J Comput Assist Tomogr 8/3 (1984) 381 - 384

[4] Beyer D, Steinbrich W, Friedmann et al.: Use of surface coils in magnetic resonance imaging of orbit and knee. Diagn Imag Clin Med 55 (1986) 84 - 91

[5] Bilaniuk LT, Schenck JF, Zimmermann RA: Ocular and orbital lesions: Surface coil MR imaging. Radiology 156 (1985) 669 - 674

[6] Daniels DL, Herfkins R, Gager R, Meyer WE, Koehler GA, Williams PR, Haughon VM: Magnetic Resonance Imaging of the Optic Nerves and Chiasm. Radiology 152 (1984) 79 - 83

[7] Edwards JH, Hyman RA, Vacirca SJ, Boxer MA, Packer S, Kaufman IH, Stein HL: 0,6 T Magnetic Resonance Imaging of the Orbit. Am J Roentgenol 144/5 (1985) 1015 - 1020

[8] Han JS, Benson JE, Bonstelle CHT,, Alfidi RJ, Kaufman B, Levine M: Magnetic Resonance Imaging of the Orbit: a Preliminary Experience. Radiology 150 (1984) 755 - 759

[9] Hawkes RC, Holland GN, Moore WS, Rizk S, Worthington BS, Kean DM: NMR imaging in the evaluation of orbital tumors. AM J Neuroradiol 4 (1983) 254 - 256

[10] Li KC, Poon PY, Hinton P, Willinsky R, Pavlin CJ, Hurwitz JJ, Buncic JR, Henkelman RM: MR imaging of orbital tumors with CT and ultrasound correlations. J Comput Assist Tomogr 8 (1984) 1039 - 1047

[11] Markl AF, Riedel KG, Naegele M, Vogl TH, Lissner J: MRI of the orbit and optic chiasm using surface coils and contrast agents. In: Lemke HU, Rhodes ML, Jaffee CC, Felix R (eds): Computer Assisted Radiology CAR `87. Springer-Verlag, Berlin -Heidelberg-NY 1987

[12] Markl AF, Riedel KG, Oeckler R, Naegele M, Hahn D, Lissner J: MR Imaging of orbital diseases using surface coils and contrast agents. Radiology 161 (P) (1986) 286

[13] Markl AF, Riedel KG, Oeckler R, Vogl TH, Hahn D, Lissner J: MRI of the diseases eye, orbit, and optic chiasm using surface coils and contrast agents. Magnetic Resonance Imaging, Suppl. I 6 (1987) 122 -123

[14] Markl AF, Riedel KG, Oeckler R, Vogl TH, Scheidhauer K: Kernspintomographie der Orbita: Erste Erfahrungen mit der Anwendung des paramagnetischen Kontrastmittels Gd-DTPA. Digit Bilddiagn 4/6 (1986) 151 -155

[15] Markl AF, Riedel KG, Vogl TH: Kernspintomographie orbitaler Erkrankungen unter Verwendung von Oberflächenspulen und Kontrastmitteln. In:

Lissner J, Doppman JL (eds): Internationales Kernspintomographie-Symposium, "MR '87", Garmisch-Partenkirchen, Referateband. Schnetztor-Verlag, Konstanz 1988

[16] Morrice GD, Smith FW: Early experience with nuclear magnetic resonance (NMR) imaging in the investigation of ocular proptosis. Trans Ophthal Soc UK 103 (1983) 143

[17] Mosely I, Brant-Zawadzki M, Mills C: Nuclear magnetic resonance imaging of the orbit. Br J Ophthalmol 67 (1983) 333 - 342

[18] Schenck JF: The surface Coil Approach. Magnetic Resonance Imaging of the orbit. General Electric Milwaukee (1984) 2 - 22

[19] Schenck JF, Hart HR, Foster TH, Edelstein WA, Bottomley Pa, Redington RW, Hardy CJ, Zimmermann RA: Improved MR Imaging of the Orbit at 1,5 T with Surface Coils. Am J Roentgenol 144/5 (1985) 1033 - 1036

[20] Sullivan JA, Harms SE: Surface-coil MR imaging of orbital neoplasms. Am J Neuroradiol 7 (1986) 29 - 34

[21] Sullivan JA, Harms SE: Characterization of orbital lesions by surface coil MR imaging. Radiographics 7 (1987) 9 - 28

MR imaging of space-occupying lesions in the orbit

M. Langer, CH. Zwicker, D. Grannemann, R. Felix

Abstract

MR imaging was used in 41 patients with space-occupying lesions in the orbital cavity. A correlation with CT was possible in 18 cases, in 10 patients high resolution ultrasound examinations were compared with the MRI results.

It could be seen that choroidal melanomas had an increased signal intensity in T1-weighted and a reduced signal intensity in T2-weighted images compared to normal tissue and could be differentiated from bleedings due to these characteristics. MRI gave a better diagnostic information than CT for orbital pseudotumors lesions. Examination of the extraocular tumors allowed no histological subclassification which could be based on MRI characteristics. Osseous destructions were better seen in CT scans than in MR images.

Introduction

For the evaluation of tumours lesions in the orbital cavity, ultrasound as well as computed tomography are established diagnostic procedures. A new imaging modality, magnetic resonance imaging, has proved to be valuable for the evaluation of intracranial diseases. Due to an increased spatial resolution in MR imaging by the application of specially designed superficial coils, the examination of space-occupying lesions in the orbital cavity using MRI seems advantageous.

The aim of the present study is to demonstrate the diagnostic information gained by MRI, computed tomography and high resolution B-mode ultrasound scanning.

Patients and methods

From January, 1985, to March, 1987, 40 patients (26 female, 14 male, mean age 58 $\pm$ 14 years) had an MRI examination of the orbital cavity. 35 pathological lesions were diagnosed (Tab. 1). The diagnosis for tumorous lesions was confirmed by operation and histology, for inflammatory diseases by the clinical follow-up and the regression of the lesion under therapy.

All MRI examinations were performed on a superconducting 0.5 T magnet (Magnetom, Siemens). For 34 patients, a specially designed orbital superficial coil with 12 cm diameter was used. The head coil (30 cm diameter) was used for comparative evaluations of both orbital cavities in 6 patients.

All examinations consisted of T1-weighted spin-echo (SE) sequences (TR 400 ms, Te 30 ms) and of progressively T2-weighted multi-echo sequences (TR 1600 ms, Te 30 to 240 ms). The slice thickness was 5 mm with 2 to 4 averages for T1-weighted images and was 10 mm for the multi-echo sequences. The mean examination time was 45 to 60 minutes per patient.

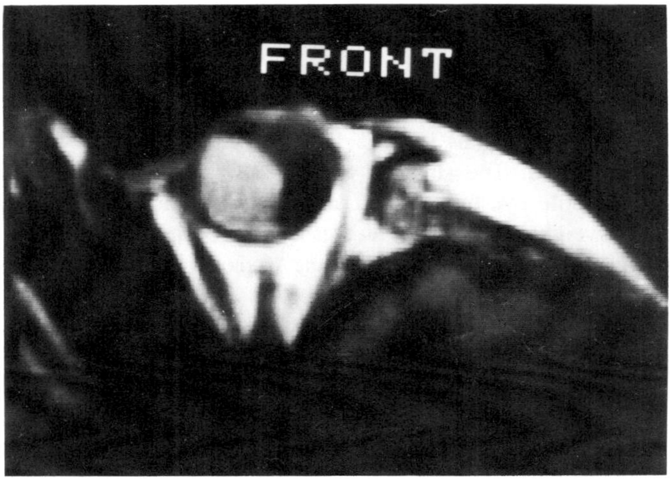

a)

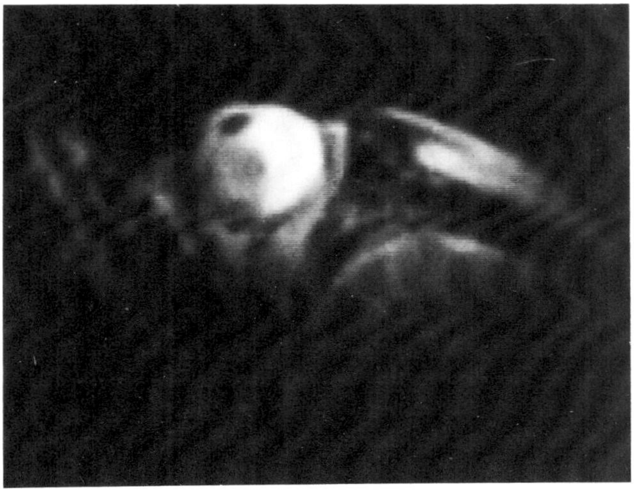

b)

Fig. 1a,b: Malignant melanoma of the right eye; a) T1-weighted sequence (400/30), high signal intensity of the medial tumor; b) T2-weighted sequence (1600/150), decreased signal intensity compared to the T1-weighted image.

In 17 cases, a comparison to high resolution computed tomography with and without application of intravenous contrast medium was performed. 10 patients had a high resolution B-mode ultrasound examination, additionally.

Results

Malignant Melanoma

In 9 patients, malignant melanoma (Figure 1) of the chorioid or, in one case, of the ciliar body were examined. The smallest tumor was 4 mm in diameter, the largest lesion occupied the whole eye bulb. In all melanotic melanoma using a high signal intensity in the T1-weighted images a decrease of the signal intensity in the T2-weighted image was seen when compared to the vitreous fluid. These characteristics were not present in one case of amelanotic melanoma.

Hemangioma

All 4 hemangiomas were of reduced signal intensity in the T1-weighted and of increased signal intensity in the T2-weighted sequences compared to the normal tissues. For a cavernous hemangioma, multiple tubulus-like structures with no signal in the T1- and T2-images could be seen. MR was not of sufficient diagnostic value for the detection of osseous destructions, but these could be diagnosed without a problem by computed tomography.

Meningioma

Three menigiomas of the optical nerve were examined. All tumors could not sufficiently be differentiated from the nerve itself on MR images. Neither was the differentiation from the orbital muscles at the orbital apex sufficient. A CT with contrast-enhancement gave a better differentiation of the tumor from the adjacent structures than MRI.

Orbital Pseudotumor

Three patients with inflammatory orbital pseudotumors were examined. The diffuse inflammatory infiltration of the retroocular space gave an inhomogeneous, slightly increased signal intensity in the T2-weighted images in comparison to the adjacent healthy tissue. No signal intensity changing could be seen in T1-weighted images compared to the normal surrounding tissues.

Under therapy, a normalization of the variation of the signal intensity in the T2-weighted image was demonstrated.

Hemorrhage

In 2 patients, intraocular or subretinal hemorrhages older than 5 days were examined. In both cases, a high signal intensity could be seen in T1- and T2-weighted images compared to the normal tissue (image 2).

Adenoma of the Lacrimal Gland

A pleomorphous adenoma of the lacrimal gland showed in the T1-weighted image a reduced signal intensity compared to the white matter of the brain and had an inhomogeneous signal increase in the T2-weighted multi-echo sequence (image 3). Due to this signal inhomogenity, MR could better delineate the size of the tumor than CT. Especially the sagittal projection gave further diagnostic informations.

Discussion

The MR examination of malignant orbital melanomas showed a characteristic increase in signal intensity in T1- and decrease in signal intensity in T2-weighted images compared to normal tissues. GOMORI (6) explained this by paramagnetic effects of free radicals of the melanin molecule. This was contradicted by EDWARDS (5), who only saw this so called characteristic signal intensity change in one of four melanomas, and was unable to differentiate the other three melanomas from chronic hemorrhages. For our own patients we saw these characteristic signal intensity changes in T1- and T2-images in 8 of 9 melanomas. All 8 were melanotic and the one with no change of the T1- and T2-signal intensity compared to a hemorrhage was amelanotic. This would support the theory of GOMORI (6) that free radicals in the melanin molecule have a certain paramagnetic effect. In our patients as well as for other groups (2, 3, 7, 8, 9, 11, 15, 17), MRI was superior to CT in diagnosing chorioidal melanomas due to the changes of signal intensity in MRI.

Intraocular and retrobulbar hemangiomas, the most frequent orbital tumors (8), cannot be differentiated from adenocystic carcinomas, lymphomas or basal cell carcinomas in MRI because all these space-occupying lesions have long T1- and T2-times (10, 13, 15, 17, 19). For our own patients, all hemangiomas showed this signal behaviour. In all three cases, CT and MRI were equivalent, but only CT was able to demonstrate the osseous destruction of a large cavernous hemangioma.

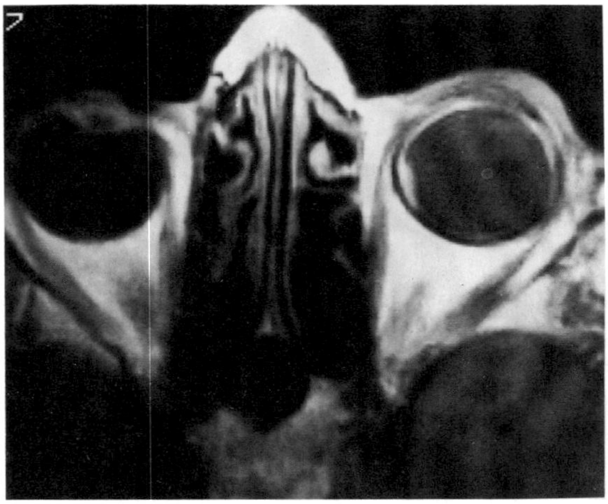

a)

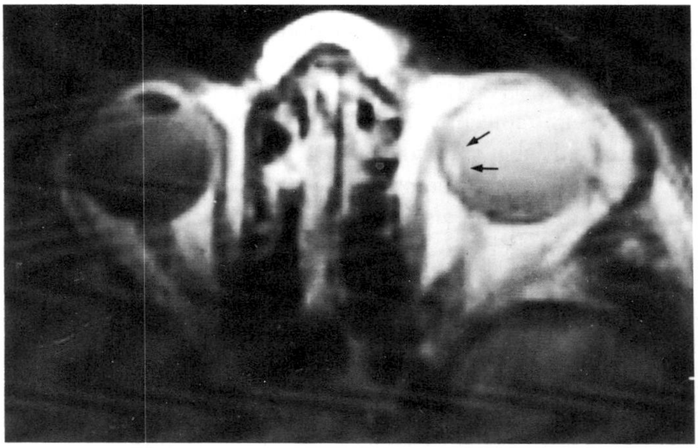

b)

Fig. 2a,b: Subretinal hemorrhage of the right eye; a) T1-weighted sequence (400/30), high signal intensity of the hemorrhage; b) T2-weighted sequence (1600/90), persistent high signal intensity of the hemorrhage compared to the T1-image.

The diagnostic procedure for diagnosing an optic meningeoma is, still a contrast-enhanced CT scanning. In concordance with LEE (10) and BILANIUK (2), we do not see that MRI without the use of Gd-DTPA gives any further information in optic meningeomas compared to CT. If Gd-DTPA is used, a characteristic enhancement as demonstrated by TREISCH (18) for intracranial meningeomas can be expected and the diagnostic accuracy could be enhanced. Small tumors close to the optic nerve could be obscured by chemical shift artefacts (3, 4, 14, 16) due to different resonance frequencies of water and liquid-bounded protons.

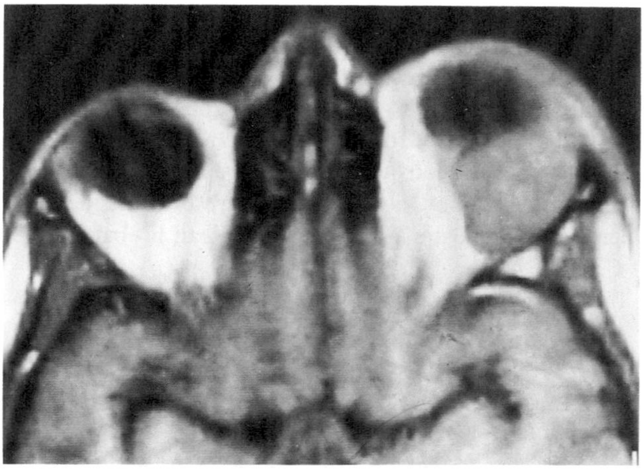

a)

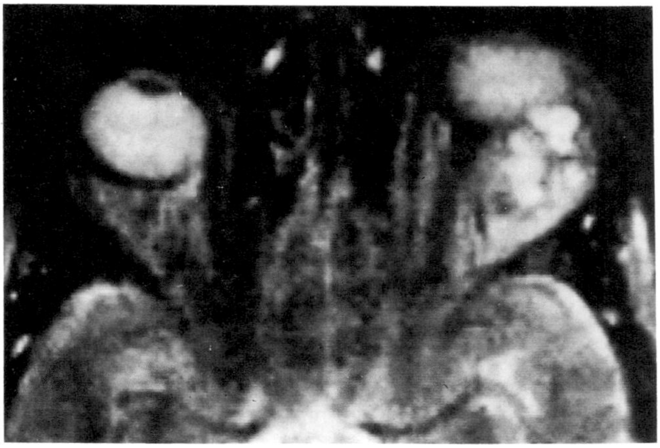

b)

Fig. 3a,b: Adenoma of the lacrimal gland; a) T1-weighted sequence (400/30), only insignificant difference of signal intensity of the tumor compared to the brain; b) T2-weighted sequence (1600/180), inhomogeneous signal of the tumor

Orbital pseudotumors produce an inflammatory edema of the retrobulbar space which is the reason for a reduced signal intensity in the T1-weighted image (1, 15). In our patients, we saw a small inhomogenous increase in signal intensity in the T2-weighted image in comparison to the retroorbital fat. This small increase in signal intensity in the T2-weighted image could probably be explained by the inflammation while malignant tumors usually have a rather strong increase in the T2-time.

Conclusion

J. MRI is superior to CT in the diagnostic of malignant melanotic melanomas and for the differentiation of this tumor from subretinal hemorrhage.

K. Pathologic space-occupying lesions in the apical portions of the orbital cavity can exactly be demonstrated by MRI due to the multiplanar imaging modalities.

L. All tumors with simultaneous osseous destructions are better diagnosed by CT than MRI. Up to now, meningeomas of the optic nerve are best diagnosed by CT with contrast enhancement, the diagnostic accuracy of MRI can probably be enhanced by the application of Gd-DTPA.

Tab. 1: Diagnoses of 35 pathologic MRI examinations of the orbital cavity

Diagnosed malignant melanoma	9
Hemangoma	4
Meningoma	4
Pseudotumors	3
Adenoma	1
Neurofibroma	1
Endocrine orbitopathy	3
Myositis	1
Chronic hemorrhage	2
Retinal detachment	2
Caverneous fistula	2
Neuritis of optic nerve	2
Cataract	1

References

[1] Atlas SW, Grossmann RJ, Savino PJ, Sergott RC, Schatz NJ, Bosley TM, Hackney DB, Goldber HJ, Bilaniuk LT, Zimmermann RA: Surface - coil MR of orbital pseudotumor. AJNR 8 (1987) 141 - 146

[2] Bilaniuk LT, Schenk JF, Zimmermann RA, Hart HR, Foster TH, Edelstein WA, Goldberg HJ, Grossmann RJ: Ocular and orbital lesions: surface coil MRI imaging. Radiology 156 (1985) 669 - 674

[3] Daniels DL, Herfkins R, Gager WE, Meyer GA, Ruben Koehler P, Williams AL, Haughton VM: Magnetic resonance imaging of the optic nerves and chiasm. Radiology 152 (1984) 79 - 83

[4] Daniels DL, Kneeland JB, Shimakawa A, Pojunas KW, Schenk JF, Hart H, Foster T, William AL, haughton VM: MR imaging of the optic nerve and sheath: correcting the chemical shift misregistration effect. AJNR (1986) 249 - 253

[5] Edward JH, Hymann RA, Vacira SJ, Boxer MA, Packer S, Kaufman JH, Stein HL: 0,6 T magnetic resonance imaging of the orbit. Amer. J. Roentgenol. 144 (1985) 1015 - 1020

[6] Gomori JM, Grossmann RJ, Shields JA, Augsburg JJ, Joseph PM, De Simone D: Choroidal Melanomas: correlation of NMR spectroscopy and MR imaging. Radiology 158 (1986) 443 - 445

[7] Han JS, Benson JE, Bonstelle CT, Alfidi RJ, Kaufmann B, Levine M: Magnetic resonance imaging of the orbit: a preliminary experience. Radiology 150 (1984) 254 - 256

[8] Hawkes RC, Holland GN, Moore WS, Riszk S, Worthington BS, Kean DM: NMR imaging in the evaluation of orbital tumors. AJNR 4 (1983) 254 - 256

[9] Krahe Th, Gieseke J, Herter M, Trier H-G, Wolf HH, Lackner K: Magnetische Resonanztomographie (MRT) der Orbita. Fortschr. Röntgenstr. 146, 3 (1987) 267 - 273

[10] Li KC, Poon PY, Hinton P, Willinsky R, Pavlin CJ, Hurwith JJ, Buncic JR, Henkelmann RM: MR imaging of orbital tumors with CT and ultrasound correlations. J. Comput. Assist. Tomogr. 8, 6 (1984) 1039 - 1046

[11] Markl A, Seiermann B, Riedel KG, Mayr B, Hahn D, Lissner J: Orbitale Raumforderungen - Vergleich von Kernspin- und Computertomographie. In: Vogler E, Schneider GH (ed.). Digitale bildgebende Verfahren. Integrierte digitale Radiologie. S. 251 - 255. Schering, Berlin 1986

[12] Reuther G, Requardt H: Kernspintomographie der Orbita mit Oberflächenspulen. Fortschr. Röntgenstr. 145, 4 (1986) 386 - 392

[13] Schenck JF, Hart HR, Foster TH, Edelstein WA, Bottomley PA, Redington RW, Hardy CJ, Zimmermann RA, Bilaniuk LT: Improved MR imaging of the orbit at 1, 5 T with surface coils. Amer. J. Roentgenol. 144 (1985) 1033 - 1036

[14] Seiler T, Müller-Stolzenburg N, Wollensak J: Phase transitions in ocular tissue = NMR and temperature measurements. Graefe's Arch Clin Exp Ophthalmol 221 (1983) 122 - 125

[15] Sobel DF, Mills C, Char D, Norman D, Brant-Zawadzki M, Kaufman L, Crooks L: NMR of the normal and pathologic eye and orbit. AJNR 5 (1985) 345 - 350

[16] Stolle E, Kühnert A, Luska G: Artefaktanalyse in der bildgebenden Kernresonanzdiagnostik. In: Vogler E; Schneider GH (ed.). Digitale bildgebende Verfahren. Integrierte digitale Radiologie. S. 109 - 114. Schering, Berlin 1986

[17] Sullivan JA, Harms SE: Surface-coil MR imaging of orbital neonplasms. AJNR 7 (1986) 29 - 34

[18] Treisch J, Schörner W, Laniado M, Felix R: Characteristika intrakranieller Meningeome in der magnetischen Resonanztomographie. Fortschr. Röntgenstr. 146, 2 (1987) 207 - 214

[19] Zimmermann RA, Bilaniuk LT, Yanoff M, Schenk JF, Hart HR, Foster TH, Edelstein WA, Bottomley PA, Redington RW, Hardy CJ: Orbital magnetic resonance imaging. Am. J. Ophthalmol 100 (1985) 312 - 317

MRI in lesions of the visual pathway and surrounding structures

F. Koschorek, H. Gremmel, G. Brinkmann

Abstract

113 patients with lesions in the region of the visual pathways or of the visual pathways have been studied at 0.35 T, at 0.5 T, and at 1.5 T from 1984 through summer 1987. The patient population consisted of 60 tumors in the region of the sella, 25 cases of multiple sclerosis with impairment of the visual pathway, 10 cases of vascular processes in the brainstem or in the occipital lobe, 11 lesions in the orbit, 3 midline tumors, 1 case of toxic atrophy of the optic nerve, and 1 contusion in the region of the lamina quadrigemina. 2 cases were suspected to suffer from arachnopathia optico-chiasmatica. Gadolinium-DTPA (GD-DTPA) and Fast Field Echo imaging were helpful in further characterizing the lesions. DIXON's proton spectroscopic imaging technique seems to be helpful to demonstrate orbit lesions.

Introduction

Visual disturbances need a very meticulous diagnostic approach, since many different diseases may cause visual impairment, and thus, a precise diagnosis is essential for treatment planning. The main diagnostic modalities are: clinical examination, plain X-ray films, ultrasound and CT. The advent of magnet resonance imaging (MRI) challenges well established imaging modalities, such as ultrasound and CT, as MRI has the ability of multiplanar imaging with virtually anatomic quality. However, especially in the orbit, a major disadvantage of MRI has to be considered: motion artefacts, which lead to image degradation. On the other hand, as in ultra-sound, no ionizing radiation is applied. The introduction of gradient echo sequences as FLASH [3], FFE and GRASS seems to overcome this short-coming of MRI in the diagnostic work-up of visual impairment. The following gives our experience gained in 13 cases of lesions of the visual pathways or the region of the visual pathways.

Tab. I: Methods

Superconducting magnet operating at 0.35 T, 0.5 T, 1.4 T
SE-sequences: 400/35; 500/30; 1600/35/140; 3000/30/100
Fast Field Echo (FFE) imaging: 850/17.2, flip-angle 23°/60°
Dynamic Gd-DTPA enhanced MRI using FFE sequences with 36/17.2, flip-angle 45°
Proton spectroscopic imaging

Material and Method

From 1984 through summer 1987 111 patients with visual disturbances were studied first by MRI at 0.35 T and 0.5 T in the Radiological Institute Oldenburg/Old.Later, since January 1987 at 1.5 T in the Dept. of Radiology, University of Kiel. Tab. I and II show the patient population and the applied techniques. In addition to common spin echo sequences dynamic Gd-DTPA enhanced MRI, FFE imaging and proton spectroscopic imaging [1] was used in several cases to achieve more information about different lesions.

Tab. II: Preliminary results of dynamic MRI

Tumors in the sella region		60
Pituitary tumors(giant)	30	
Meningeoma	14	
Craniopharyngeoma	13	
Epidermoid/Dermoid	3	
Multiple sclerosis		25
Lesion in the orbit		11
Hemangioma	5	
Adeno-Carcinoma	2	
M. Wegener	1	
M. Boeck	1	
Splinter of glass	1	
Metastasis	1	
Infarction (brainstem/occipital lobe)		10
Midlinetumors		3
Contusion in lamina quadrigemina		1
Atrophy of optic nerve (toxic)		1
Suspecion of arachnopathia optico chiasmatica		2
Total		113

Gd-DTPA enhanced MRI

As reported previously in detail [5, 6], immediately after boluslike injection of 0.1 mMol/KG bodyweight Gd-DTPA serial MRI started. First, at 0.5 T a SE sequence with TR = 100 ms, matrix 128^2 was used. Then, at 1.5 T a FFE sequence with TR = 36 ms TE = 17.2, matrix $128^2$was applied. In every case the time period of measurement was from 0 s to 160 s. During this time at least 9 or up to 54 images were acquired. 5 para-meters were determined: ascent to peak, time to peak, height of peak, per-percentage of height of peak in the end of measurement, and area under curve (fig. 1).

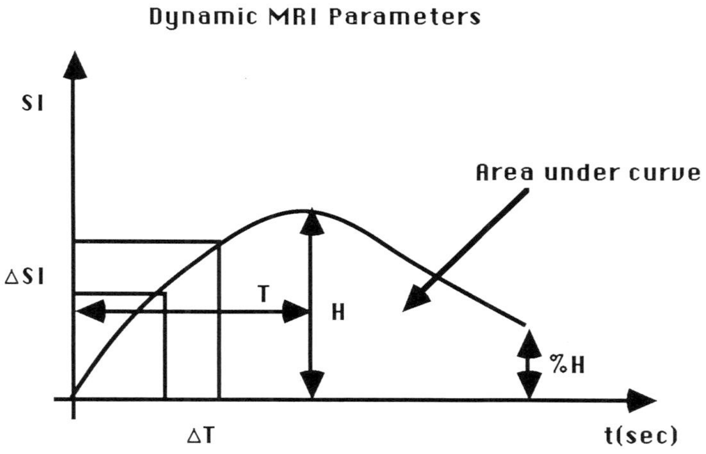

Fig. 1: Dynamic Gd-DTPA enhanced MRI parameters

FFE imaging

In order to reduce motion artefacts a gradient echo sequence, FFE [8], was applied at 1.5 T. The imaging parameters were: TR = 850 ms TE = 17.2 ms, multi-slice, slice thickness 4 mm, no gap.Matrix 256^2. A flip angle of 23° was used. This technique resulted into a remarkable signal to noise improvement. FFE uses an excitation pulse with relatively small flip-angle, produces echoes by means of gradient inversion, instead of a 180° refocussing pulse, and generates the profiles extremely fast, without interaction with the computer.

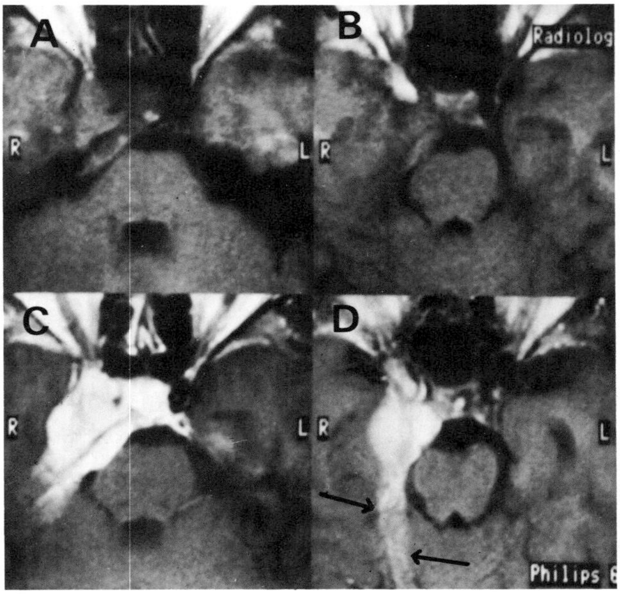

Fig. 2: Sphenoidmeningeoma pre and post Gd-DTPA-Fig.2A and fig. 2B: Pre Gd-DTPA. The tumor is almost isosignalintenive to the surrounding brain tissue. Fig.2C and fig.2D: Post Gd-DTPA. The extension of the tumor is clearly deliniated. The relationship to the tentorium is well depicted (arrow)

Proton spectroscopic imaging

At the end of a 90°pulse the magnitization of the protons in water and the magnitization of protons in fat CH2 groups point in the same direction. Since the water protons precess between 3 to 4 parts per million faster than the protons of fat, this situation does not last. Initially the magnetization is a maximum when water and fat magnetization point in the same direction but soon goes through a minimum when water and fat magnetization point in opposite directions. An imaging sequence finished at the minimum results in a new type of image: the brightness of a pixel depends of the difference between the water and fat magnetizations. An image taken at the maximum shows the sum of water and fat . The sum of both images is an image of water only, the difference of fat [1]. Components less abundant than water and fat contribute some intensity to both the new types of images as to the conventional or inphase image.

Results

Our results are in line with the findings of other authors [2, 4, 7] concerning spin echo sequences. Anatomic details both in the orbit as in the visual pathways and surrounding structures usually were well demonstrated. Thus, the relationship of pathologic findings to visual structures was clearly delineated.

The application of Gd-DTPA enhanced information as the extension of a lesion and the relationships to nearby visual structures were clearly delineated (Fig. 2). The further characterizing of lesions was also improved, as vascular lesions may be differentiated from tumors by application of dynamic Gd-DTPA enhanced MRI (Tab. III). Using the WILCOXON, WHITNEY and MANN test the values of time to peak and of percentage of height in the end of measurement were significant different at the 95 percent level from those observed in tumors.

FFE imaging demonstrated in a case of a glass splinter the lesion and the intraorbital structures accurately. However, the application of this technique seems to have a further advantage, namely functional studies by NMR movies. The application of proton spectroscopic imaging was helpful in one case of an edema within the optic nerve (Fig. 3) because of postsurgical scar formation.

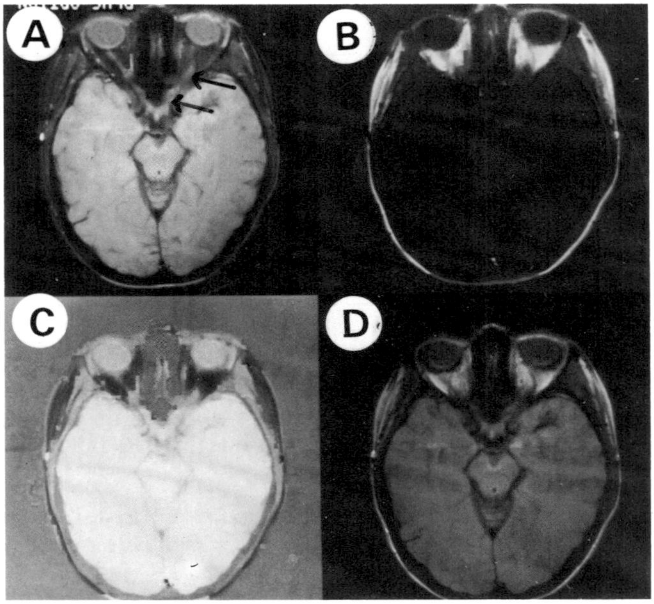

Fig. 3: Proton spectroscopic imaging. A: Water image. B: Fat image. C: Opposed image. D: In-phase image. Fig.3A demonstrated edema of the optic nerve (arrow)

Discussion and Conclusions

MRI lesions of the orbit and the visual pathways seems to achieve more accurate information on the pathology [9]. Virtually anatomic image quality of structures in the orbit can be gained when the field of view is adapted. In line with recent findings of other authors [2, 7] in some of our cases the precise diagnosis was achieved by MRI. Since MRI avoids ionizating irradiation there will be no known harmful effects on the refracting structures of the eye, which are very sensitive to X-rays [4]. In cases of meningeomas and of bony tumors however MRI had some shortcomings. Thus, MRI with its multiplanar capabilities seems to be a good support for CT, when such lesions are suspected. However, the application of Gd-DTPA will hopefully overcome these disadvantages. Despite ultrasound and CT, MRI will have a leading part in the diagnostic procedure of visual disturbances, since the relationship of vascular structures to tumors can be demonstrated, especially in the region of the chiasma opticum, and since proton spectroscopic imaging may lead to a further characterization of lesions. In cases of inflammatory or degenerative diseases of the CNS with involvement of the visual pathways MRI is most sensitive to demonstrate morphological changes. In future the use of MR movies may facilitate functional studies of structures in the orbit and the blood-flow in vascular malformations and in vascular tumors.

Tab. III: Patient Population

Lesion	Ascent	Time to peak	Height of peak	% Height of peak	Area of peak	#cases
AVM	4.982	40.300	269.42	48.253	31.78	10
Tumor	3.141	98.938	297.80	66.783	37.141	16

References

[1] Dixon WT: Simple proton spectroscopic imaging. Radiology 153 (1984) 189 - 104

[2] Guthoff R, Terwey B, Sautter R, Domarus D von: Erste Erfahrungen mit der Kernspintomographie der Orbita. Fortschr Ophthalmol 82 (1985) 481 - 483

[3] Haase A, Frahm J, Matthaei D, Hänicke W, and Merboldt K-D: Flash imaging. Rapid NMR imaging using low flip-angle pulses. J. Mag. Res. 67 (1986) 258 - 266

[4] Hünermann B: Neue Aspekte bildgebender Verfahren: Kernspintomographie. Diagnose & Labor 35 (1985) 91 - 101

[5] Koschorek F, Jensen H-P, Terwey B: Dynamic MR imaging: A further possibility for characterizing CNS lesions. AJNR 8 (1987) 259 - 262

[6] Koschorek F, Gremmel H, and Brinkmann G: The value of MRI in vascular malformations: Studies with and without gadolinium-DTPA. In: A Calabro and M Leonardi (eds): Computer aided Neuroradiology, pp 271 - 274, CIC Edizioni Internazionali, Rome, 1987

[7] Schenck F, Duncker G and Koschorek F: Magnetische Resonanztomographie bei Prozessen im Bereich des Chiasma opticum und der Orbita. Spectrum Augenheilk 1: 187 - 190, 1987

[8] Van der Meulen P, McKinnon GC, In der Kleef JJE, and Cuppen JJM: Fast field Echo Imaging: MR imaging with very short acquisition time. Radiology 157 (P) (1985) 335

[9] Van Nieuwenhuizen O, Abbing PR, Ziedses des Plantes BG, et al: Role of MRI scanning in the diagnosis of cerebral visual disturbance. Pediatr. Neurol. 2 (1986) 363 - 366

Single photon emission tomography of the cranium

B. Nägele-Wöhrle, O. Nickel, H. Höhrmann, S. Fischer, K. Hahn

Introduction

Nuclear medical studies - bone scintigraphy in particular- are able to detect disturbed metabolic function as well as the actual location of the causal lesion. The technique represents the ideal synthesis of function and localization without the necessity for further invasive procedures.

Like any other method there are limitations for planar bone scintigraphy. In case of small lesions located in large organs loss of detailed information occurs due to signal averaging of a large volume. SPECT is a multiplanar imaging technique making it possible to scan an organ in a defined slice thickness. The system consists of a rotating gamma-camera as well as a computing system for putting the gained digitized information into images comparable with CT or MRI technology.

The examination of a patient necessitates the intake of radioactive labelled substances, such as Technetium 99 m which can be bound to an organ specific carrier (in case of bone scans: phosphate complex).

The advantage of SPECT lies in the elimination of the background noise, resulting in a high contrast between the lesion and the surrounding anatomical structures depicted with an improved spatial resolution. This approach is advantageous for scanning the visceral cranium and the base of the skull.

The SPECT technique has been applied with great success in bone scintigraphy. The aim of our study was the evaluation of the diagnostic potential of SPECT and to correlate the results to conventional planar scintigraphy of the cranium.

Method

From January 86 till 87 we examined 77 patients with planar bone scintigraphy and SPECT technique.

The planar examination was performed using a large field camera, high resolution collimator, SPECT was carried out with a double head camera and a high resolution collimator.

After administration of 10 to 15 mCi (370 -555 MBq) 99 TC DPD the bone scan of the cranium was performed in two - or three - phase technique. The SPECT examination followed immediately. We used a 64 x 64 Matrix and 64 angle increments. The pixel size was 4.2 mm with a zoom factor of 1.5 to get improved spatial resolution. The examination time was 21 minutes.

Patients

33 Metastases
10 Malignant bone tumors
15 Benigne bone tumors
7 Inflammatory bone lesions
22 Diverse lesions (Sinusitis, Tinnitus, M. Paget, Hyperostosis, Eosinophilic granuloma)

Results

Table I

	77 patients			
	planar scintigraphy		ECT	
	positive	negative	positive	negative
right	44	17	54	18
false	7	12	3	2
sensitivity	78 %		96 %	
specificity	70 %		86 %	

77 patients were examined by both modalities, 54 SPECT-scans proved to be positive, 18 cases negative, 2 false negative and 3 false positive.

The planar scintigraphy was 44 times positive, 17 times negative, 7 times false positive and 12 times false negative. The sensitivity of the planar scintigraphy reached values of 78 % and 70 % only.

The results were correlated to histology or CT.

SPECT proved to be superior to planar imaging especially when the lesion is located centrally or in the visceral cranium.

SPECT was able to detect lesions even in an early stage when conventional radiological procedures were initially negative and showed positive results only during later control examinations.

First case: Left sided malignant otitis. In the first examinations increased bone metabolism was found in the region of the left petrous bone and in the sphenoid cavity (Fig. 1).

The control scintigram half a year later showed only an affliction of the left petrous bone (Fig. 2). In spite of the therapy no improvement of the clinical symptoms was gained. Half a year later additional CT controls failed to prove any further significant change or progression. The concomitant SPECT scan however showed progression of disease in the region of the medial aspect of the right petrous bone (Fig. 3). The histological diagnosis proved osteomyelitis of the right and left petrous bone as well as in the sphenoid cavity.

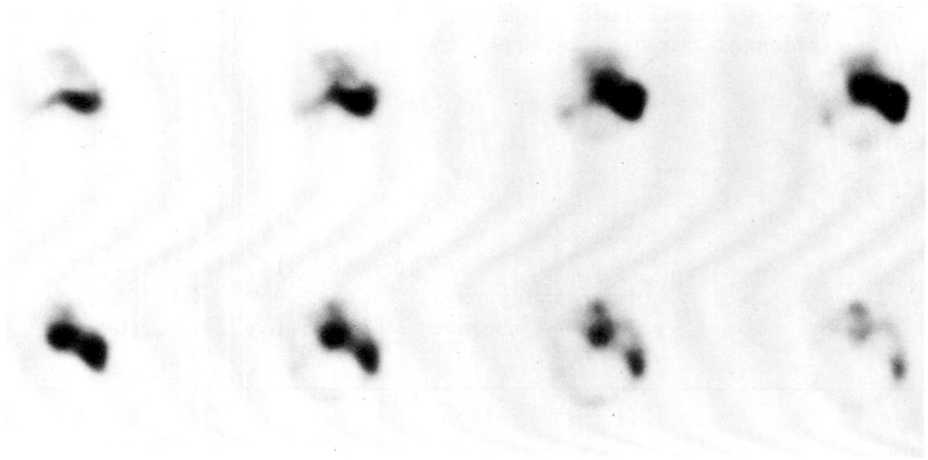

Fig. 1

Discussion

SPECT is superior to planar scintigraphy especially in centrally located lesions [3]. The reason for that is a high contrast to noise ratio and a superior spatial resolution of the normal and pathological anatomical structures [6, 1].

The planar scintigraphy locates focal spots with a high sensitivity just when they are located close to the detector surface.

The spatial resolution of SPECT is definitely inferior to CT. The purpose of SPECT is not gaining perfect morphological information but the detection of pathological bone metabolism patterns and there exact location [2]. The use of double head camera systems improved the signal to noise ratio and reduced the examination time by the half [4].

We can confirm the statement of KÖNIG and BIELER (4) that SPECT detects lesions which are not regarded as pathological structures by planar scintigraphy. After STRASHON et al. [5] SPECT is able to detect lesions earlier than CT.

The SPECT technique is an important and useful modality for follow up studies. Even when planar scintigraphy detects the lesion it is often not possible to judge the progression and the exact location of disease. SPECT is able to give these answers even in cases where CT and conventional X-rays fail to give a diagnostic help.

Indication for SPECT

1. Diagnostic following up of inflammatory bone lesions of the skull (focal osteomyelitis) especially in the region of the base of the skull and the visceral cranium.
2. Suspected primary bone tumors of the skull where early detection is vital for adequate therapeutic approach.
3. Suspected bone metastases of the skull.
4. Follow-up studies under therapy.

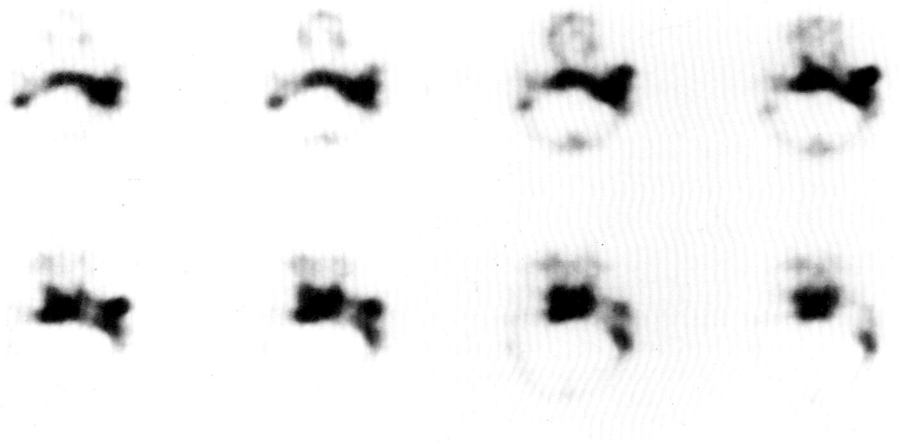

Fig. 2

Conclusion

SPECT often provides additional clinically important information of inflammatory bone lesions, primary bone tumors and bone metastases regarding extension, infiltration and progression of disease. SPECT is an additional imaging tool when planar scintigraphy or CT fails to detect the suspected lesion. Follow up studies by SPECT play an important role in inflammatory lesions, primary bone tumours and bone metastases.

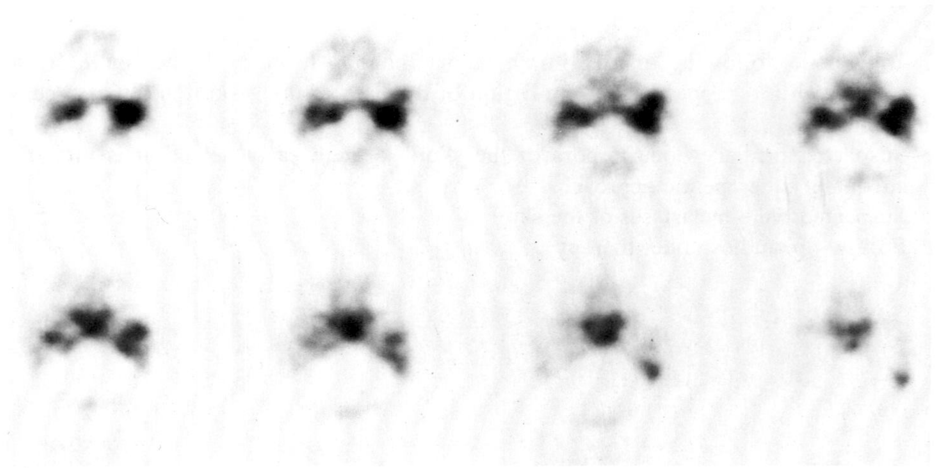

Fig. 3

References

[1] Bieler EU, Vox K, Rummeny E, Pfannenstiel P: Die Einzel-Photonen Emissions-Computer- Tomography (SPECT) bei Patienten mit benignen und malignen Erkrankungen der Wirbelsäule. Fortschr. Röntgenstr. 145, 2 (1986) 182 - 188

[2] Büll U, Kirsch CM, Roedler HD: Die Single-Photon-Emissions-Computertomographyie in der Knochenszintigraphie (SPECT). Fortschr. Röntgenstr. 138, 4 (1983) 391 -402

[3] König H, Feine U, Müller-Schauenburg W: Klinische Bedeutung der Schädel-Emissions-Computertomographie in der Knochenszintigraphie. Fortschr. Röntgenstr. 143, 4 (1985)

[4] Jaszczak RJ, Whitehead FR, Lim CB, Coleman RE: Lesion Detection Emissions Computertomography (SPECT) compared conventional imaging. J. Nucl. Med 23 (1982) 97 - 102

[5] Strashon A, Masood N, Nejatheim S, Stranley J, Goldsmith B: Malignant External Otitis: Early Scintigraphic Detection. Radiology 1984, 150 : 541 - 54

[6] Wust R, Golde G, Schneider R, Fiegler W, Hedde PJ: Optimierung der Nachweisbedingungen von fokalen Aktivitätsschwankungen in der SPECT mit rotierender Gammakammer. Fortschr. Röntgenstr. 144, 6 (1986) 659 - 707

Videoangiography - a new technique for the quantification of the Retinal circulation

G. Richard

Summary

The new method of videoangiography makes is possible to quantify retinal and choroidal circulation in the one area of the body where vessels are constantly observable under physiological conditions. The enabling factor is the use of fluorescein;-filling of the blood vessels during slow-motion playback of the angiogram. The progress of choroidal filling can be exactly followed, so that different precisely defined sectors and retinal and choroidal circulation times are determinable. By this means the arterial, capillary and venous circulatory phases of the retina can be isolated for studying and is based on a division of the overall circulation interval of a bolus through the retinal vessel into arterial, early venous and late venous circulation times, by this, a quantitative determination of the blood flow in retinal arteries in human beings is possible. Television fluorescein angiograms are used and no further procedures since all the necessary information is taken from the image itself. The patients' eye movements do not cause errors because their influence is excluded by the computer programming.

Introduction

The study of physiological and pathological haemodynamics in the retinal and choroidal blood vessels requires that the intervals between photography are shorter than in conventional serial fluorescein angiography. Videoangiography offers this possibility, and our goal in the last years has been to improve the image quality of this method to the point where high-quality pictures are possible with slight brightness stress for the patient.

Although this method was first developed for routine use in the clinic, it soon became evident that it opens up new possibilities for scientific research.

Videoangiographical technique

Computer-aided videoangiography is an improved method of fluoresceinangiography developed and introduced into clinical practice by us (1). The fluoresceinangiogram is recorded continuously, while the patient suffers little discomfort and the picture quality is good.

In the near future a continuous digital display will be added with increased precision in measuring the flow of fluorescein and even wider application for videoangiography in research and clinical practices will be offered.

In videoangiography a specially-developed adapter makes it possible to use a highly sensitive residual light amplification (low-light) camera, so that much less light is required for videoangiography than in conventional sequential angiography.

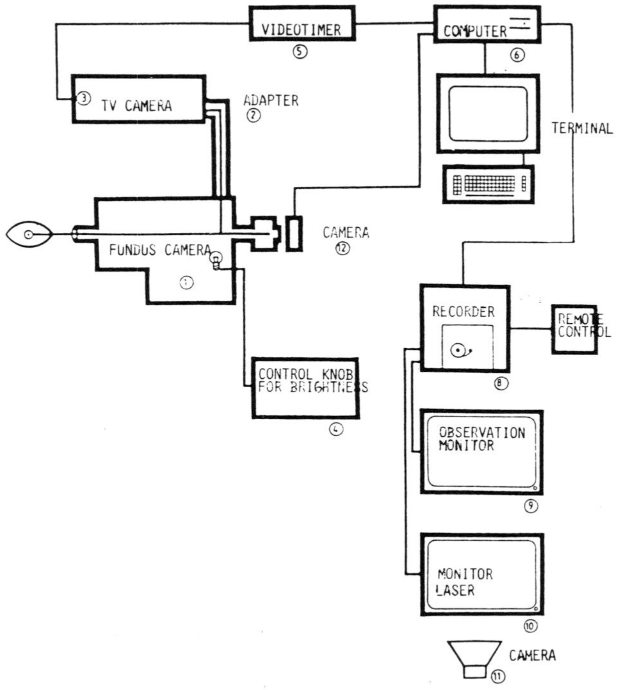

Fig. 1: Videoangiographical System

The examination unit consists of the following part: A video camera (3) is coupled to a diagnostic camera (1) with the special adapter. A brightness control (4) allows light intensity to be adjusted continuously during the videoangiography. The video camera signal is fed through a video timer (5) and a computer (6) to a monitor (7), where the picture appears with a patient code and a time signal. A video recorder (8) simultaneously stores the picture on tape for a later frame-by-frame or slow-motion evaluation. The angiography can be observed both in the central monitor and in a control monitor, where an instant camera (11) stands ready to photograph individual frames. A simple switchover allows a miniature camera (12) to make sequential pictures of the angiography simultaneously with the video recording (Fig. 1).

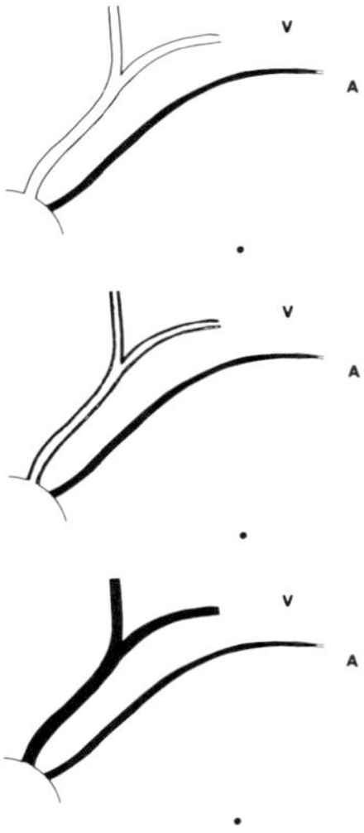

Fig. 2: Top: Arterial circulation time. Middle: Early venous circulation time. Bottom: Late venous circulation time

Advantages of videoangiography over sequential angiography

The angiographic pictures are stored on videotape and are immediately available for playback whenever desired. Since film development is not required, both patient and physician are spared waiting till a later date to discuss the pictures. Each phase of the angiogram can be studied at actual speed, in slow-motion, or frame-by-frame and can be recorded on polaroid film. The ease of recording a wide range of intraocular information opens new opportunities for medical training. A further monitor can be placed directly beside the laser, allowing the therapist to refer instantly to the actual intraocular situation while lasering. The quality of the picture can be adjusted at will at any time during the angiography.

The unpleasant flashes - characteristic of sequential angiography - are eleminated. Particularly at the beginning of a conventional angiogram these flashes often cause rapid blinking by the patient, so that the all-important first few seconds of the angiogram are photographed either poorly or not at all. With videoangiography this problem is solved.

Retinal circulation times

Slow-motion analysis of videoangiography introduces a new degree of precision into assessment of the retinal circulation times: it permits an accurate determination of the flow-rate of fluorescein through the retinal vessels.

The use of this method has led us to divide the overall retinal circulation time into 3 subcategories: (1) arterial circulation time; (2) early venous circulation time, and (3) late venous circulation time (Fig. 2).

Arterial circulation time

The arterial circulation time is defined as the interval between the arrival of fluorescein at a point in the temporal vessels 4 disk diameters away from the disk and its arrival at the disk itself. By this means the velocity of arterial flow can be determined in millimeters per second: this in turn serves as a criterion for the condition of the arterial circulation. We took the disk as a standard because its diameter (1,5 mm) is independent of refraction and other factors. It therefore serves as an objective unit measurement. The arterial circulation time for the arteria temporalis superior in our healthy controls average 0,62 s, for the arteria temporalis inferior 0,65 s. The arteria temporalis superior filled generally a little earlier than the arteria temporalis inferior. On this basis the average speed of flow in the arteria temporalis superior was 10,3 mm/s, in the arteria temporalis inferior 10,8 mm/s.

Early venous circulation time

The early venous circulation time is defined as the interval between the arrival of flourescein at the disk and the onset of the laminary venous border flow at the disk. The average early venous circulation time for both vena temporalis superior and inferior was 3,44 s in our healthy controls.

Late venous circulation time

The late venous circulation time is defined as the interval between the arrival of fluorescein at the disk and the complete filling of the vena temporalis superior and inferior at the disk. The average late venous circulation time for the healthy controls (n = 100 was 7.87 s).

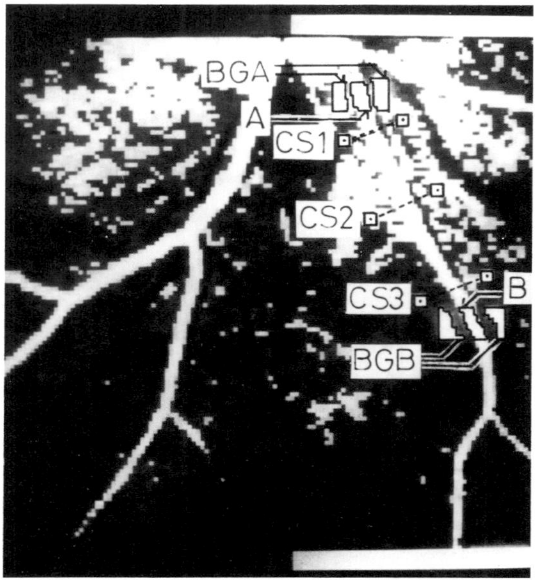

Fig. 3: Retinal arteries: The proximal (A) and distal (B) region and corresponding background (BGA, BGB) are marked. Three cross-sections (CS1, CS2, CS3) are defined.

Choroidal circulation time

Because of its ability to capture images rapidely, videoangiography permits an analysis of circulation times with a precision of 1/50 second (1, 2). This opens the way to an analysis of choroidal circulation. The aim of this paper is, to find a demarcation line between physiological and pathological filling of the choroid, in order to define the syndroms of primary choroidal occlusion and the its clinical findings.

Quantitative measurement of retinal blood flow, by application of digital image-processing methods to videoangiograms

In the following sections we will briefly describe the individual steps of data processing needed to produce the desired result.

Data preparation. Firstly, the data have to be processed by the digital image method. Each individual image is divided into 512 - 512 picture elements (pixels) with a depth of 8 bits. This means that an intensity value between 0 and 255 is given to each pixel. There is no information loss in the process of analogue to digital conversion because the dynamic range of the recording camera is only about 7 bits. Within the frame of the TV norm used the camera takes 25 of these full images per second. The computer program automatically allows a complete sequence of eye-movement corrections.

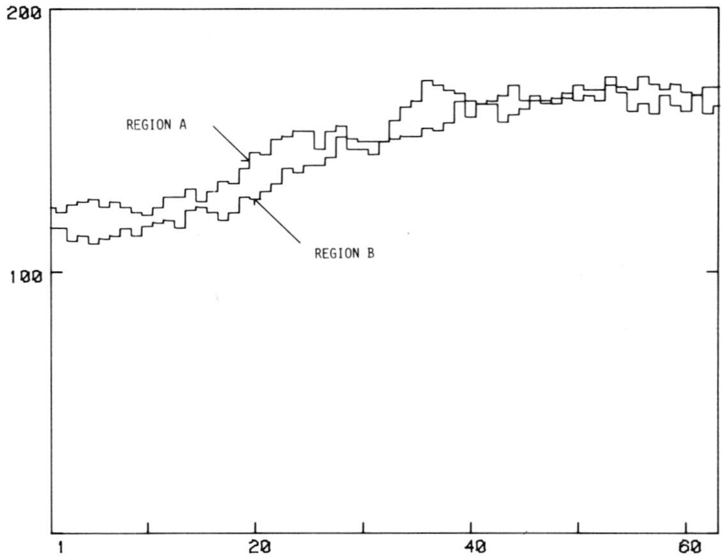

Fig. 4: Intensities (arbitrary units) as functions of time (frames, 1 frame = 0,04 s) for regions A and B in Fig. 1

Flow in an arterial vessel. The flow through a branchless artery can be simply calculated by $F = (D/2)^2 * \pi * L/T$ with D = diameter of the vessel, L = length of the part concerned. T = flow-time over the length L. It is assumed that the diameter of the vessel is almost constant over the length L. An example is shown in Fig.3. The flow is studied between the regions A and B. L can be simply read from the image. The determination of the diameter D, and especially of the flow-time T, needs more effort and will be shown in the following. The flow-time T can be calculated from the timedependent intensity curves of the regions A and B. Figure 2 shows these time curves normalized to one pixel area. These curves depend on many parameters (injection velocity, resampling of the injection bolus in the lung, amount of fluorescein, blood pressure amplitude, camera sensitivity, other nonlinear interferences of the data recording process, etc.). However, their shape has to be nearly identical for all parts of one artery except for the time shift between different parts. To calculate this time shift T properly, the curves have to be corrected for the local background defined by the regions BGA and BGB in Fig. 1 and normalized in such a way that both curves fill the same dynamic range. The latter can be simply achieved by subtracting the minimum of each individual curve and then dividing by the maximum. Now the two curves are iteratively shifted against each other in time direction. For each individual shift the sum of the absolute differences between the intensities, normalized to the overlapping range, is calculated. This sum has a minimum for the time shift.

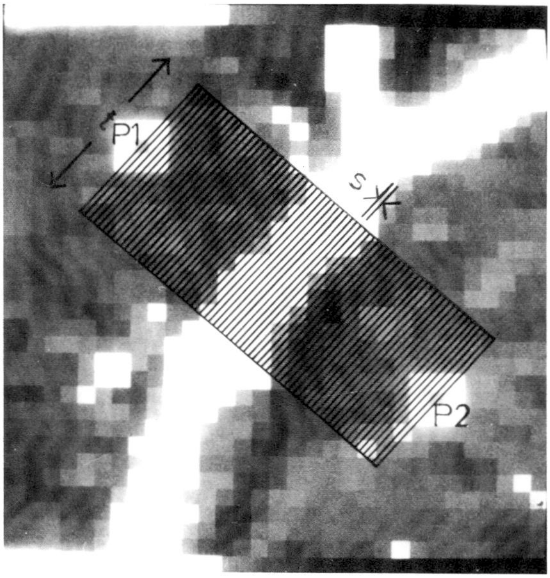

Fig. 5: Extraction process to calculate a cross-section of a vessel

From Fig. 5 it can be seen how the vessel diameter D is calculated. The two points P1 and P2 are interactively set using the cursor. Also, the thickness T and the slit width s have to be defined interactively. Typical values are t = 10 and s = 0,1 pixel units. The program now calculates for each individual slit, the pixel fractions falling into that slit. These fractions are multiplied by the corresponding intensity values and summarized over the slit. From the resulting vessel profile the vessel width can be easily determined. Normally, this cross-section is taken at different locations of the vessel (see Fig. 3) and the mean over the results is taken. The whole procedure requires some numerical effort. However, it allows a calculation of D with an accuracy of about 0,2 pixel units.

In the example shown, the flow-time from A to B is four frames, i.e. 0,16 s, the vessel diameter is D = 0,13 mm within a mean error of only 5 % for the different locations. The velocity is 13,5 mm/s and the total flow comes out to be 0,18 μl/s.

With the method presented here the retinal blood flow in human beings can be well determined. However, up to now there has been a uncertainty in the results, typically 25 %. This error is due the time resolution of the TV camera being 0,04 s corresponding to the TV norm. To reach a higher resolution, the recording velocity has to be increased by using other hardware equipment, which will be built up in the near future. However, the method itself, especially the logistic structure of the computer programs, is not affected by these hardware changes.

References

[1] Richard G: Die klinische Anwendung der Videoangiographie der Retina. Klin. Mbl. Augenheilkunde: 185 (1984) 119

[2] Richard G: Differentiation of Retinal Circulation times by videoangiograpy Ophthalmologica (Basel) 191 (1985) 161

[3] Richard G, Darrelmann O, Kreissig I, Schubring G, Weber J: Videoangiographische Unterteilung der Netzhaut-Kreislaufzeit. Ihre Bedeutung für die Diagnostik von Durchblutungsstörungen der Netzhaut. Fortschr. Ophtalmol. 81 (1984) 592

[4] Richard G, Kreissig I: Der Einfluß der Lasertherapie bei Retinopathia diabetica auf die Hämodynamik der Netzhautgefäße. Klin. Mbl. Augenheilk. 186 (1985) 107

[5] Preußner PR, Richard G, Darrelmann O, Weber J, Kreissig I: Quantitative measurement of retinal blood flow in human beings by application of digital image-processing methods to television fluorescein angiograms. Graefe's Arch Ophthalmol 221 (1983) 110 - 112

Measurement-based, reproducible ultrasonography of the orbit

W. Buschmann, W. Haigis

Introduction

Routine ultrasonography of the orbit is now mainly done using B-scan equipment with small, hand-held transducer probes and facilities for A-scan examination of areas selected from B-scans. Digitized signals and video-techniques are used nowadays in ophthalmology as well. But, contrary to other application areas of ultrasonography, no array scanner for ophthalmic use is commercially available at present. Electromechanical sector scan is preferred.

The entirely empirical approach, still widely used in ultrasonography of other body areas, is presently replaced by measurement-based examination conditions to yield reproducible, comparable results. This became possible by international agreement on measurement methods for the diagnostically important parameters of ultrasonic pulse-echo equipment. They are described in the Document 854 of the International Electrotechnical Commission.

Clinically applicable measurement procedures

The sensitivity adjustments at the apparatus are comparable only if the relation to a standard test reflector echo is given. The IEC Document recommends echoes from steel or glass test reflectors. Such reflectors are generally available, but the resulting echoes are so powerful that they cannot be brought down to a measurable level with the built-in dB attenuators of our apparatus. Therefore, we use a standard test reflector made from the material of soft corneal contact lenses (hydroxyethylmetacrylate, water content 38 percent). This material is commercially available in a very constant, pure quality. Contact lens manufacturers can easily provide us with plane test reflectors of constant quality. The amplitude of the echo from such a reflector is 17 dB below that of a steel reflector, and therefore it is in the control range of the built-in attenuators. On the other hand, the correlation to the IEC-recommendation is maintained. The necessity of such equipment checks is demonstrated by the results achieved in two equipment series from different manufacturers (see Tables I and II).

The working frequency can be determined simply by counting the HF oscillations of the reflector echo per microsecond. A braid damage of a transducer cable seemed to have no influence on its function, and in many hospitals it would be "repaired" by an adhesive tape bandage only. However, the measurement of working frequency proved that this damage already caused a frequency shift which could well influence diagnostic criteria in the echograms.

The lateral and depth resolution is determined using a filament echo and the - 6 dB-criterion. This suffices for practical purposes in A-scan. For B-scan, filament series or cages, like the test-cage of the American Institute of Ultrasound in Medicine, can be used, but the dimensions must be adjusted to conditions of ophthalmic ultrasonography. The minimum filament distance for presentation of clearly separated echoes at a given adjustment of equipment sensitivity is used.

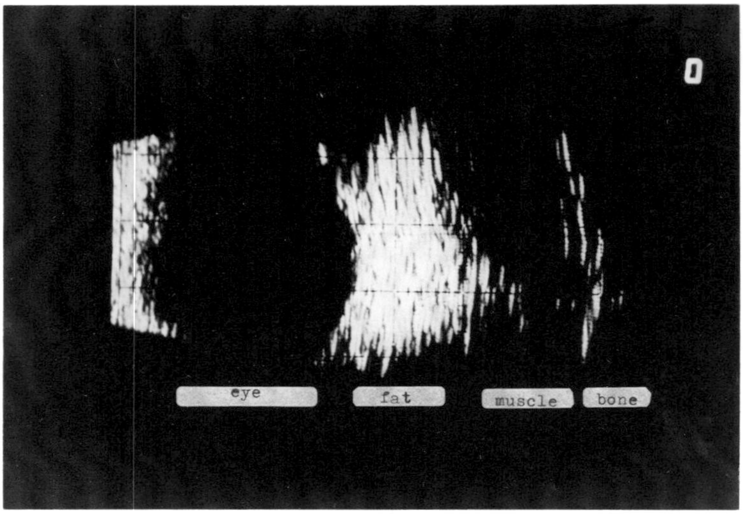

Fig. 1a: B-scan demonstrating eye, orbital fat (partially displaced) and swollen external eye muscle with enhancement of orbital bone-wall echo and without echographic signs of muscle fibrosis (nearly no internal structure echoes from the muscle area at a sensitivity of ΔV W38 = 52 dB).

Additional electronic measurements can, of course, be made using an oscilloscope, but experienced staff would be required. Much simpler this can be done using the ECHOSIMULATOR developed by REUTER and TRIER (3), which can be used by medical aids. It permits to check the accuracy of the B-scale and the dynamic range of the amplifier in A- and B-scanning; furthermore, the frequency spectrum can be measured. The dynamic range, however, could be determined as well using the echo of the W 38 test reflector - provided that the dB scale of the diagnostic equipment is accurate.

Indication for orbital ultrasonography

Orbital ultrasonography should be applied as first special technique following general eye and orbit examination. This way, the final diagnosis can be achieved in many patients. If further information is needed, additional X-ray computertomography and/or MRI with techniques especially adapted to orbital problems would be indicated. To apply these techniques prior to ultrasonography is not justified - not only because of the cost/benefit ratio.

Ultrasound exophthalmometry enables the examiner to differentiate with very high reliability between pseudo-protrusion (resulting from unilateral or bilateral enlargement of the eye in myopia, posterior sptahyloma, or buphthalmos) and real protrusion (exophthalmos). The Hertel readings are entered into a scheme of a transversal section of the skull, giving the cornea vortex position. From this point, the axial length of the eye (measured ultrasonically) up to the posterior pole is marked. The half of this distance is taken by us as position of the eye center. Thus, in addition to the position of the cornea vortex, one can also compare the positions of the eye center of both sides, and the positions of the posterior poles. Recommended technique for axial length measurement: Transducer probe of 3.5 to 5 mm diameter, working frequency 10 MHz, coupling via water-bath, equipment sensitivity adjusted to Δ V W38 = 39 dB, linear amplification.

Sonom. Ocuscan 400
10 MHz, w.f. 9.7 MHz

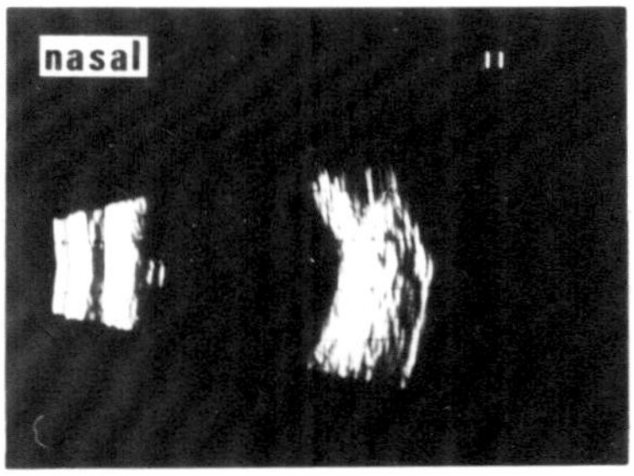

horizontal, 50° n. unten
ΔV (W38) = 43 dB

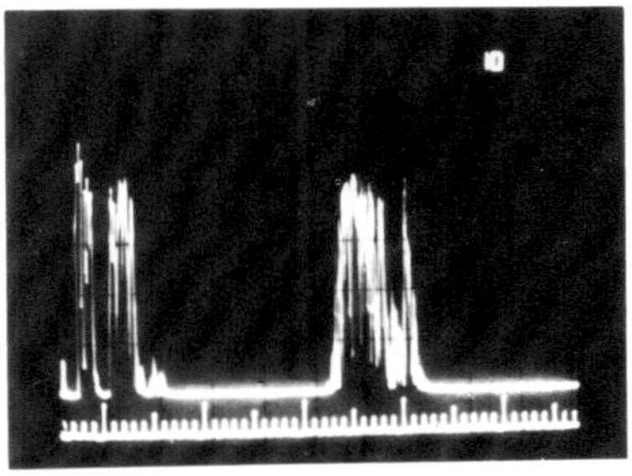

horizontal, 50° n. unten
ΔV (W38) = 44 dB

Fig. 1b: B-scan and A-scan in another patient, medium degree of muscle fibrosis (see muscle structure echo amplitudes, at sensitivity of ΔV W38 = 44 dB).

In case of unilateral protrusion (exophthalmos) not only the corneal vortex, but also the eye center and the posterior pole are displaced anteriorly. Often, the bulbus is impressed from behind by the space-occupying lesion resulting in shortening of the axial length (and hyperopization). Then, the posterior pole is shifted ahead even somewhat more than the corneal vortex.

Sonom. Ocuscan 400
10 MHz, w.f. 9.7 MHz

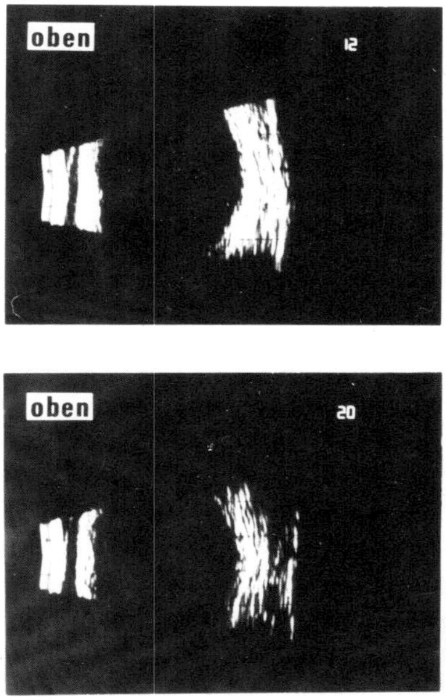

vertikal, 45° n. nasal
ΔV (W38) = 42 dB

vertikal, 45° n. nasal
ΔV (W38) = 35 dB

Figure 1c: Only slight enlargement of muscle diameter, but high degree of fibrosis. at the sensitivity level used in the upper echogram (and in Figure 1b), differentiation of fat and muscle area is nearly impossible, due to intensive muscle structure echoes. With further reduction of sensitivity (ΔV W38 = 35 dB, echogram below), fat and muscle area become clearly separated.

In pseudoprotrusion, however, resulting from enlargement of the eye, the corneal vortex is displaced anteriorly as well, but not the eye center. The posterior pole of the larger eye is usually even more posteriorly located in the orbit than the posterior pole of the other (normal) eye. This eliminates any suspicion of a space-occupying orbita lesion. Ultrasonography of the orbita tissues, CT scan and MRI would be unnecessary. Results are shown in Table III.

If, however, a real protrusion (exophthalmos) is found, B- and A-scan examination of the orbital tissues becomes indispensable. We examine in transbulbar and parabulbar directions using contact coupling, 10 MHz working frequency, and several 10 dB-steps of equipment sensitivity ranging from Δ V W38 = 70 dB to 40 dB.

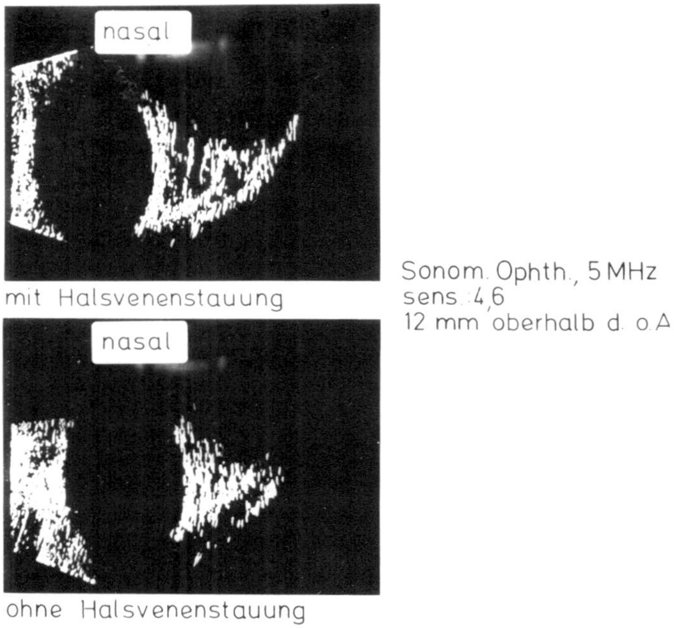

Figure 2: Orbital varicosis, intermittent exophthalmus

The most frequent cause of unilateral as well as bilateral exophthalmos is Graves' opthalmopathy. The orbital involvement is found before, simultaneously with, or after the beginning of the thyroid disease. If the latter was already proven, ultrasonic detection of multiple swollen muscles and of fat tissue involvement may suffice for the final diagnosis. Reduction of visual acuity, visual field defects, dilated retinal veins, or changes of the optic disc and/or the echographic findings of a dilated optic nerve sheath diameter would indicate compression neuropathy of the optic nerve, requiring additional X-ray computertomography (preferably direct coronary scans) of the posterior third of the orbit. This area cannot be evaluated sufficiently in the echograms.

The ultrasonic diagnosis of Graves' opthalmopathy is easy and safe, if an increased diameter of several external eye muscles, perhaps combined with some degree of fibrosis, are found. Even in patients with clinically unilateral Graves' ophthalmopathy usually some muscle dilatations are found in the fellow orbit as well. We evaluate them using B-scan cross sections from all parts of the muscle. The higher the degree of fibrosis, the more the equipment sensitivity has to be reduced in order to see the muscle separated from the orbital fat. If only one or two muscles in one orbit are involved, differentiation from myositis has to be considered, especially in an acute phase of the disease.

The ultrasonic diagnosis of Graves' ophthalmopathy is more difficult if (nearly) exclusively the fat tissue is involved and marked swelling of muscles is missing. The echographic findings of fat tissue edema with coarse, inhomogeneous structure and reduced sound attenuation would allow the correct diagnosis, if the thyroid disease were already detectable. Should, however, such an ophthalmopathy precede the thyroid disease, a safe diagnosis of the orbital disease would be more difficult, and all diagnostic means have to be used - especially X-ray computertomography and MRI - to differentiate inflammatory pseudo-tumors of the orbit and other possible causes.

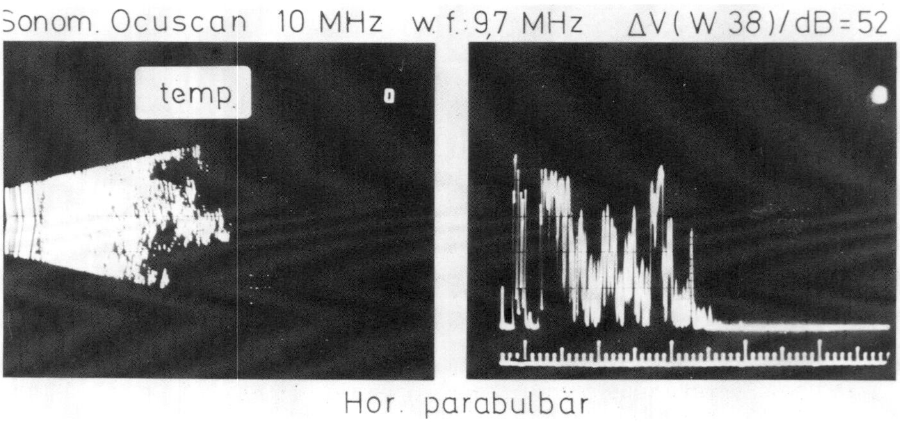

Figure 3: Parabulbar hemangioma in a child, age 3 years. Ocuscan 400, working frequency 9.7 MHz, ΔV W38 = 52 dB. Parabulbar B-and A-scans demonstrate the marked inhomogeneity of the tumor with fluid-filled areas and pulsating echo-movements (amplitude pulsations, in some directions also pulsations of echo-position). Directional Doppler sonography demonstrated strong, pulsating arterial blood flow from the depth of the orbit to the transducer probe at the skin.

This type of Graves' ophthalmopathy can progress to severe compression neuropathy of the optic nerve as well, requiring surgical orbita decompression.

It is helpful to know the degree of fat and muscle fibrosis before decompression surgery; fat fibrosis can be shown best at 10 MHz and a sensitivity of 45 to 50 dB above the standard W 38 test echo; at higher sensitivity levels this would be more difficult to evaluate (Fig. 1).

The echographic differentiation of the numerous other spaceoccupying orbital lesions can be demonstrated here only by using disorders as examples.

Orbital varices usually cause intermittent exophthalmos. The exophthalmos increases with compression of the jugular veins or low head position. The diagnosis can be made clinically. Ultrasonography demonstrates filling of the dilated orbital veins after jugular vein compression. X-ray phlebography would be needed only if the feeding vessels were to be found before surgery, but usually surgery is not indicated (Fig. 2).

Arterio-venous fistulas and hemangiomas in children can be diagnosed with B-scan and Doppler ultrasound. B- and A-scan demonstrate the dilated vessels and their pulsations, sometimes also swirling echoes. Children's hemangiomas, contrary to those in adults, show intensive arterial blood-flow, as a rule directed from the depth to the front, and are evaluated best by directional Doppler sonography (Fig. 3).

Orbital complications in sinusitis may result in an echographically visible subperiostal abscess, its echographic localization is very advisable prior to attempting surgical drainage.

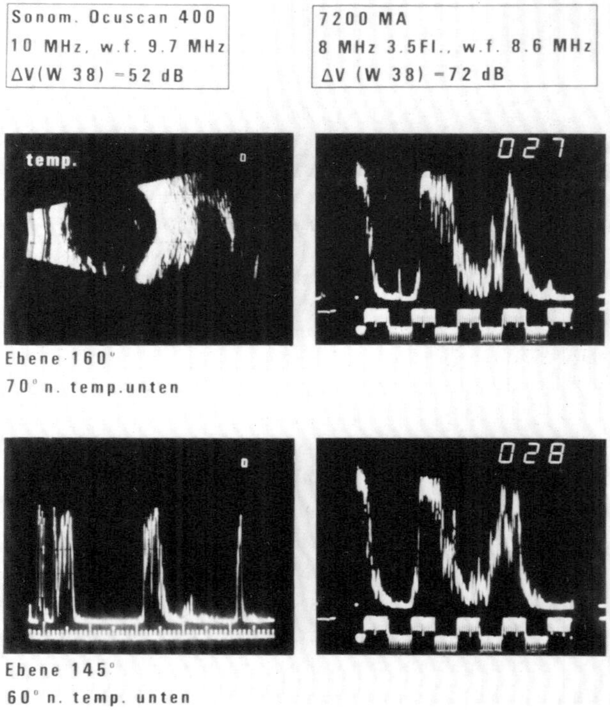

Figure 4: Malignant B-cell lymphoma. Using our Ocuscan 400 with working frequency of 9.7 MHz and a sensitivity of ΔV W38 = 52 dB, a differentiation from an abscess would not be possible echographically (see b-scan and A-scan on the left side and compare with Figure 5). Using higher sensitivity (ΔV W38 = 72 dB, working frequency 8.6 MHz, Kretztechnik 7200 Ma), the solid nature could be demonstrated clearly, and a safe differentiation from a fluid-filled lesion became possible (A-scans on the right side).

The involvement of the sinuses can be demonstrated ultrasonically as well, but the full extent and nature of the underlying disease (e.g., a naso-pharyngeal tumor obstructing sinuses) can be determined better if X-ray computertomography is done in addition.

Measurement-based ultrasonography is indispensable in tumor diagnosis. A malignant B-cell lymphoma may appear like a fluid-filled cyst and its solid nature can be detected only, if an equipment sensitivity of 70 dB is applied at 8 to 9 MHz working frequency (Fig. 4).

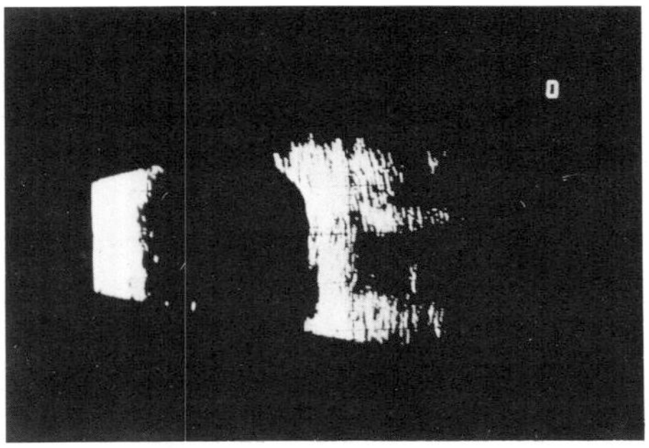

Figure 5: Exudate in the optic nerve sheath. B-scan demonstrating enlargement of the optic nerve diameter adjacent to the sclera, rectangular configuration instead of the normal V-shaped echogram, some exudate in Tenon's space. The cross section of the optic nerve also shows the enlarged diameter (lateral gaze direction, vertical scan from lateral side). Computerized tomography, with the resolution at that time available, showed in the direct corona scan a reduced diameter of the optic nerve - probably the dilated sheath was lost due to the volume - averaging effect.

The echographic structure of tumor metastases is usually very similar to that of the primary tumor. Thus, the echogram of an orbital metastasis of a skin melanoma corresponded to that of a primary choroid melanoma, in view of the internal structure. Otherwise, if one finds in the area of a suspected metastasis echographically a structure which differs considerably from that of the primary tumor, a different origin has to be expected. We found a very homgeneous orbital tumor in a patient who had 1 year before a histologically proven mamma carcinoma. General examination revealed no signs of metastases. Since mamma carcinomas usually reflect intensive structure echoes, we suspected a different origin and removed the tumor via a Kroenlein-Berke operation. Histopathology demonstrated a neurinoma.

Ultrasonography may be more sensitive in detection of increased optic nerve sheath diameter than X-ray computertomography, according to pixel size - especially, if direct corona CT scans would not be possible. This is particularly true for the anterior two thirds of the optic nerve in the orbit (Fig. 5). The posterior third cannot be evaluated safely by ultrasound.

Computerassisted signal analysis may get practical importance in orbital echography as well. Most promising is at present the analysis of back-scattered frequency spectra. Unfortunately, for this purpose it is not sufficient to analyze the rectified (video-) signal. One has to digitize and analyze the high frequency signal, which requires much more storage and computer capacity.

The set of measurement devices for checking the diagnostically important technical parameters of present routine equipment in ophthalmology is commercially available; this means, ophthalmic ultrasonography is in a leading position in this respect.

Summary

The accuracy of diagnostic echography as well as the reproducibility and compatibility of the results could be improved markedly by application of some simple measurement procedures. The diagnostically decisive parameters and adjustments of equipment and transducer probe are checked, the measurement program is based on the recommendations of the International Electrotechnical Commission. The main points are equipment sensitivity, working frequency, lateral and depth resolution, amplifier dynamics, and B-scan distortions. The use of corresponding adjustments in clinical routine and the diagnostic capability of ultrasound in orbital disorders are demonstrated in clinical examples of Graves' Disease with muscle enlargement, with and without fibrosis of the muscle or fat tissue, in orbital varicosis, hemangioma, optic nerve sheath edema, B-cell lymphoma, melanoma metastasis, differentiation of mamma carcinoma metastasis from benign neurinoma, and orbital complications of sinusitis.

Tables

Table I: Echo-detection capability (gain reserve above gain setting for 10 mm echo of W38 interface, positioned 30 μsec apart from transducer in saline) measured in 10 Kretztechnique 7200 apparatuses

Ser.No.	V(W38) in dB	Gain reserve above V (W38) in dB
003	1.0	79
035	8.5	71.5
046	22.0	58
065	8.0	72
076	6.0	74
117	2.0	78
126	0.0	80
145	10.0	70
249	12.0	68
363	10.0	70

Table II: Echo detective capability of 4 equipments Ocuscan 400 at 10 MHz (nominal frequency)

Ocuscan 400 Serial No.	scale readings (dB)	actual DB-reserve above W38 test echo	echo detection capability in DB
328 124	0 - 71	55	≥ 72.4
327 990	0 - 60	52	≥ 69.4
328 025	0 - 62	55	≥ 72.4
328 094	0 - 68	60	≥ 77.4

Table III: Side difference of bulbus center position to temporal orbital bone rim

	Difference of refraction OD/OS (dptr) normal	Difference of bulbus center position between OD/OS (mm) suspected orbital mass
Bilateral emmetropia	0 to 1.5	0 to ± 1.0 ≥ 1.0
Bilateral myopia	(isometropia)	
Bilateral hyperopia		
Unilateral myopia or	1.5 to 15.0	- 3 to + 2 ≥ 2.0
hyperopia	(anisometropia)	

References

[1] Buschmann W, Trier HG: Ophthalmologische Ultraschalldiagnostik (mit Atlas und Einordnung in den augenärztlichen Untersuchungsgang). Springer-Verlag (in preparation)

[2] IEC International Electrotechnical Commission, IEC Report: Methods of measuring the performance of ultrasonic pulse-echo diagnostic equipment, Publication 854; Bureau Central de la Commisssion Electrotechnique Internationale; 3, Rue de Varembe, Geneve, Suisse (1986)

[3] Reuter R, Trier HG, Lepper R-D: Ein elektrisches Prüfgerät für Ultraschalldiagnostik-Anlagen. In: Medizinalmarkt/Acta Mediotechnica, 28. Jg., Nr. 2, p. 58 (1980)

The possible value of Visual Evoked Potentials (VEP) in neurosurgical patients with tumors afflicting the visual pathway (a critical discussion)

H.-E. Nau, M. Foerster, F. Rimbach

Abstract

84 patients with tumors afflicting the visual pathway were examined clinically. Additionally FEP and PREP studies were made. Increase of P1 latency and reduction of amplitude on the involved side were frequently found. A topographic diagnostic was impossible. The type of tumor did not influence the visual responses. A quantitative correlation between visual acuity, field defects and results of conventional perimetry could not be ascertained. The problems of interpreting VEP changes due to check size, state of refractions, pupillary diameter are emphasized. A follow up of tumor growth by means of evoked potentials seems impossible due to the functional organisation of the visual system.

Introduction

Evoked potential monitoring of neurosurgical patients is not a well established method. In recent years, however, it has gained a wider interest. The clinical value of this method depends on several prerequisites: It must be easy to carry out, it must be reproducible and the results must be clear. The visual evoked response (VER, VEP), however, can be altered by a number of factors (Tab. I), which compromise an accurate interpretation. Such factors (4, 5, 9, 17, 17, 30) are e.g. check size, luminescence, visual field, state of refraction, and pupillary diameter and age. Their influence on the various visual evoked responses e.g. PREP (pattern reversal evoked potential), FEP (flash evoked potential), HF (half-field stimulation)), is well known, but difficult to distinguish from other factors e.g. from pathological changes on the VEP.

We tried to evaluate the VEP of patients with tumors in the orbita, the optic nerve, the sellar region and optic radiation in relation to ocular factors, the visual fields and the clinical interpretation of electrophysiological data. The VEP findings in traumatic lesions, during intraoperative monitoring, and their value in neuromonitoring in intensive care units are published elsewhere (25 - 28).

Patients and Methods

153 VEPs (84 FEPs, 69 PREPs) were examined in 84 tumor patients, whose age ranged from 14 to 81 years. 36 patients had supratentorial tumors. 40 patients had space-occupying processes in the sellar region, and 8 processes in the orbita and the optic nerve (Tab. II).

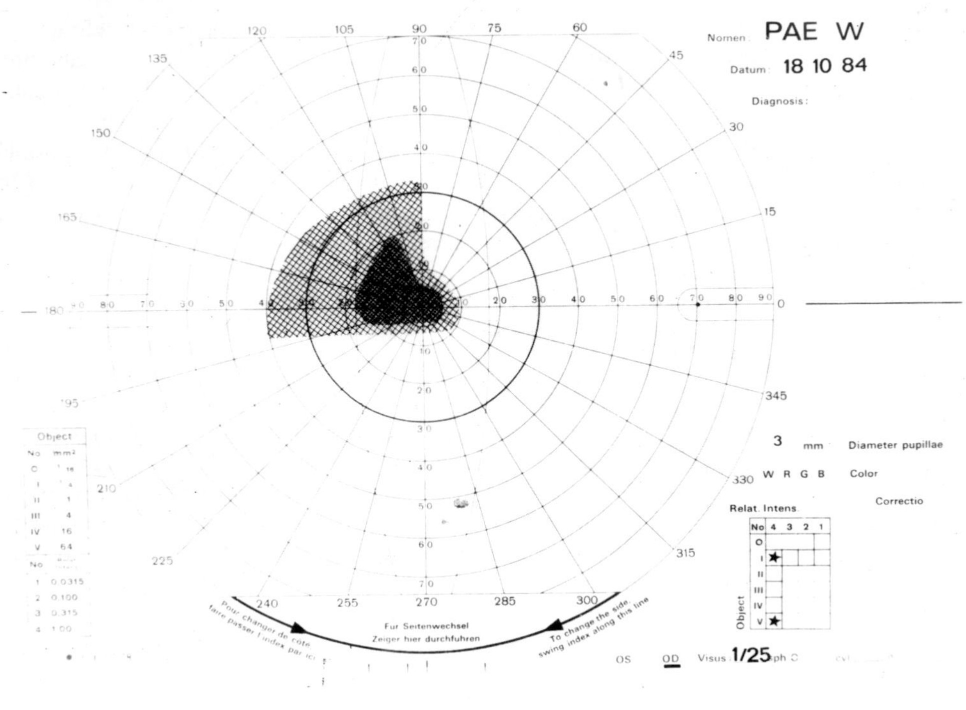

Fig. 1: Corresponding ophthalmological and evoked potential findings in a patient with pituitary adenoma.

All patients underwent surgery after clinical evaluation, which included neurological, radiological, and ophthalmological examinations. The ophthalmological examinations consisted of the state of refraction, visual acuity, fundus examination and visual field testing as well as testing of the ocular motility and sensory motor interaction. Perimetry was done by means of Goldmann perimetry and electrophysiological studies were carried out by Pathfinder II (Nicolet, Madison). Stimulation (PREP as well as FEP) was monocular. The responses were recorded between Oz and CZ. 100 responses were averaged over a period of 300 ms. The stimuli and recording parameters were as follows: repetition rate 1.5/s, high band pass 30 Hz, low band pass 0.5 Hz, sensitivity 100 μV. FEP was done by means of LED with a full field stimulus. PREP was carried out by pattern reversal stimulation with a TV, which had a luminance of 40 cd/m^2 and check sizes of 30'.

Results

General remarks

The investigation of P1 latencies in FEP and PREP in regard to the location of the tumors showed no significant differences between the involved and the normal side (Tab. III).

In 61 cases (Tab. IV) the P1 latency was increased and in 54 cases out of 153 FEP and PREP examinations, the amplitude was reduced on the afflicted side.

The percentage of abnormalities is nearly the same in the three groups. In spide of visual field defects in 17 of 36 cerebral processes there was no pathological FEP; in 15 cases both, the ophthalmological and the electrophysiological findings were normal. 22 patients with perisellar tumors had normal FEP in spite of field defects, but both investigations were normal in 11 patients. Five patients with tumors of the orbita and second brain nerve had normal FEP in spite of visual field defects, but both investigations were normal in 3 patients (Tab. V).

There was no clear connection between PREP and FEP findings on the one hand and the visual acuity and the extension of quadrant defects on the other. Visual acuity differed from 0.01 to 1.0 in cases of pathological FEP and to the same extent in cases of pathological PREP. A pathological VEP latency above 2.5 standard deviations was rare (Tab. VI).

Report of a Special Case

PAE W was an 65-year-old woman with a recurrent chromophobe adenoma and deterioration of vision to 1/25 in the right and .6 in the left eye. The visual field of the right eye was limited to the upper nasal quadrant. The left eye showed a concentric constriction of the visual field (Fig. 1, 2).

FEP had normal amplitude and latency in the left eye and a reduced amplitude in the right eye. The PREP showed normal latencies on both sides and an amplitude reduction of 1/4 on the right side (Fig. 3).

Discussion

General optimism is common, when a new method is inaugurated but today we are looking more for the advantages of this electrophysiological method and the gain for our neurosurgical tumor patients.

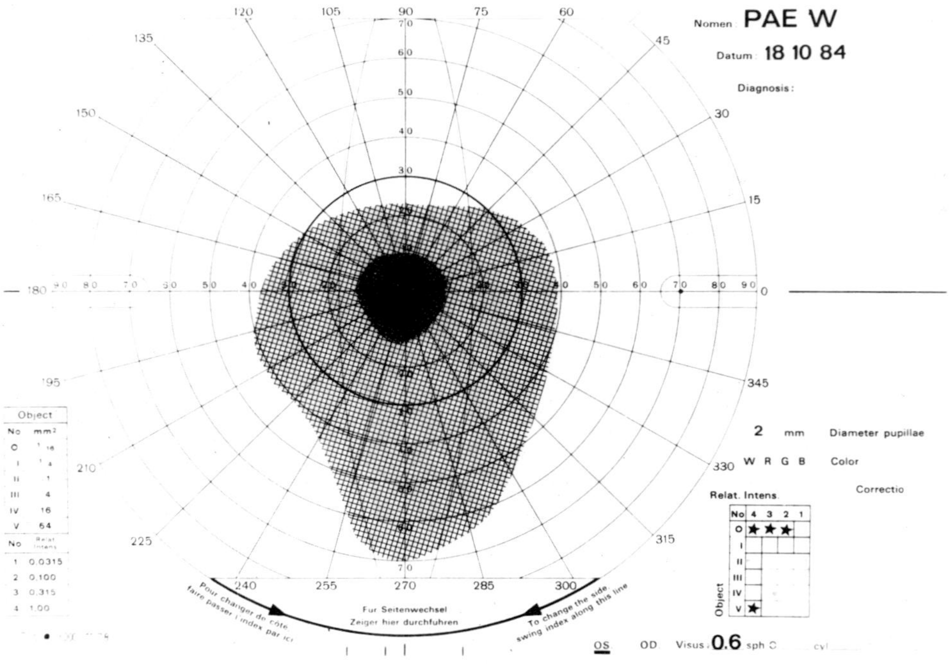

Fig. 2

In VER, the evoked response can be influenced be a number of factors, which can change its form, amplitude, and latency. HARTER and WHITE (15) studied the influence of check size and the function of visual acuity. They found the largest visual evoked response when they projected sharply focused patterns with relatively small check sizes on the retina. COLLINS et al. (7) found a reduction in amplitude of PREP with refractive errors and significant changes in the absolute and relative latencies of the P1 component. Therefore the visual acuity is an important parameter when VER is interpreted.

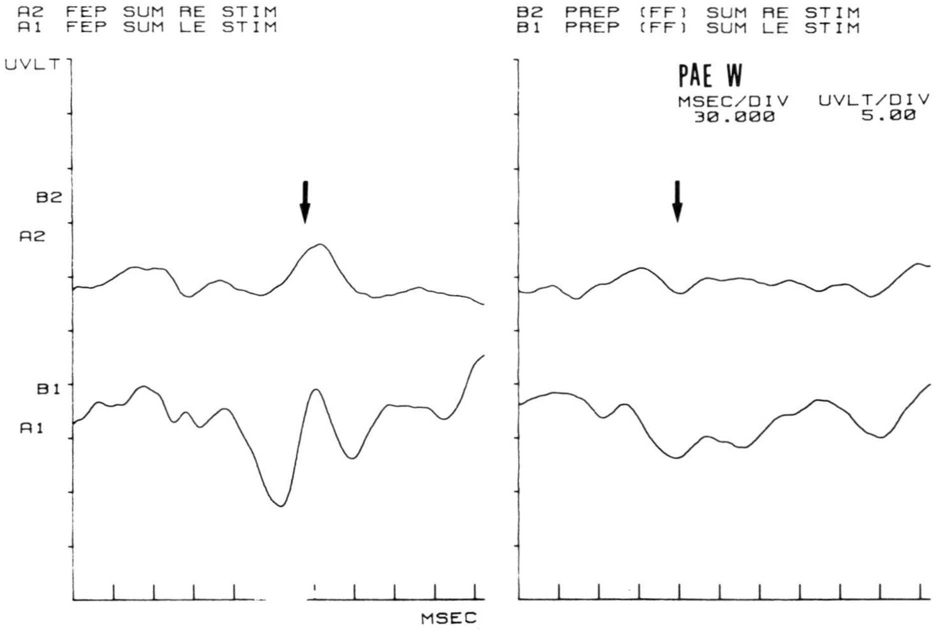

Fig. 3

FEP, however, was not influenced by different refractive lenses according to DUSTMANN and BECK (9). HAWKES and STOW (17) investigated the influence of pupil size on amplitude and latency of PREP. There were no significant changes in amplitude, but a reduction which depended on smaller pupil sizes. KUPERSMITH et al. (21) found in patients with chiasmal glioma and unaltered visual acuity a marked reduction of FEP with latency changes while PREP were absent. The greater sensitivity of PREP was seen by GROSWASSER et al. (11), too. HAIMOVIC and PRETLEY (12) investigated lesions of the chiasm and the posterior visual pathways by HF (half-field) PREP. They compared the results of 21 patients with suprasellar tumors or focal cerebral lesions documented by CT scan and compared visual evoked responses by HF and FF stimulation. Patients with a suprasellar tumor and complete hemianopia had responses after the affected field side was stimulated. Retrochiasmal lesions with homonymous hemianopia had no decernible evoked potentials when stimulating the side ipsilateral to the field defect. HALLIDAY et al. (13) studied the visual pathways extensively. Absent responses were particularly characteristic of patients with intracranial meningeomas. Tumors in the sellar region showed a high incidence of abnormal wave forms of the response. Most, but not all asymmetric cases were found in patients with field defects. MÜLLER-JENSEN et al. (24) analysed chiasmal syndromes and compared the VEP with perimetry. The degree of alterations in both tests correlated fairly well. A slight damage in the nasal hemifield could be detected even earlier by HF stimulation analyses than by conventional perimetry. But such neurophysiological testing needs much time, even more than a perimetry.

Tab. I: Different influences on VEP

Influence on VEP	PREP	FEP
check size/contrast	+	(-)
visual acuity	+	-
refraction	+	-
pupillary diameter	+	(-)
visual field	(+)	+

These above-mentioned factors are apparent in some tests. By doing FEP and PREP and various field stimulations, we could obtain different results. This seems to be the reason for contrary opinions in the literature, esp. concerning mass lesions. Some authors could not find any relation between dispersion pattern, location of tumor and the existence of intracranial hypertension in frontal lobe tumors (8). But a marked latency increase was seen in a tumor of the corpus callosum with bilateral infiltration into the optic radiatio (2). A delay of VER was also found in hemianopic patients (32). STRELETZ et al. (31) found a correlation between unilateral occipital lobe lesion, homonymous visual field loss and the VEP abnormalities. Some authors (13) stressed that there are possible differences in amplitudes depending on the type of the tumor. Recently CLIFFORD-JONES et al. (6) found the mean latency of the major positivity were delayed in different types of stimulation in cases of meningeomas compressing the anterior pathways. Abnormalities of latencies were seen in 69 per cent, those of amplitudes in 73 per cent, abnormalities of either amplitude or latency in 92 per cent.

Tab. II: Histology of the processes affecting the visual pathway

histological findings in the processes afflicting the visual pathway		
supratentorial tumors		36
extracerebral tumors	8	
glioma	15	
metastases	10	
tumor in sellar region		40
pituitary adenomas	18	
tumors in orbit/of n.II		8
total		84

However, even in normal subjects differences in amplitude can amount to 40 per cent (14). These results resemble ours, since both the amplitudes and the latencies are changed. The number of abnormalities is rather small when we consider values which are above the 2.5 standard deviation range. In addition the results are quite different depending on the method of stimulation. ONOFRJ et al. (29) found a great difference in transient and steady-state stimulation. Investigations with half fields (hemi-field and upper and lower fields) were done (1, 19, 22, 23). Some authors (24) thought to get more and earlier information than that given by ophthalmological investigation. Our findings are rather disappointing. But they are confirmed by findings of FLORIS and RIZZO (10). An amplitude reduction can be seen in visual field defects. This is also the most frequent finding in a series of evoked potential in hemianopsia by FLORIS and RIZZO (10). It may correspond to the reduced number of optic fibres. Taking into account the functional organisation of the visual system, we come to the conclusion that these responses must depend on the number and location of the afflicted fibres. A loss of function in some central fibres will not change evoked potentials, neither their amplitude nor their latency. The response decreases in large visual field defects. A discrepancy between PREP and FEP is due to the reduction of visual acuity and the following alteration of the PREP in spite of a normal FEP. In accordance with KOOI et al. (20) we stated frequent asymmetries in patients with field defects, but in our investigations most of them were within the 2.5 standard deviation range. On the other hand even in patients with well defined occipital lobectomy,

HOEPPNER and coworkers (18) recorded normal potentials. They believe this to be supporting the hypothesis of BARRET et al. (3) that the P 100 generator has an equivalent in the calcarine cortex of the contralateral hemisphere. Preliminary conclusions: A pathological process involving the visual pathway can induce a pathological VEP. But it is not possible either to state the location of the process and the quantitative correlations in relation to visual acuity and field defects. Likewise a follow-up of tumor growth in the optic nerve and tract with the VEP is not possible. HF and upper and lower field stimulation may give more information with a largely extended examination time, which is unacceptable considering the small value of information to be expected.

Tables

Tab. III: Average latencies of P1 latency in VEP according to the location

	P1 latency			
location of underlying process	afflicted side FEP	afflicted side PREP	non-afflicted side FEP	non-afflicted side PREP
cerebral hemispher	145.0	114.1	137.8	113.5
sellar region	14.4	124.9	132.5	113.5
orbita/optic n.	130.4	151.2	113.4	106.6

Table IV: Number of side differences in 153 VEP (FEP and PREP) studies in 84 patients

location of underlying process	total amount	reduction of amplitude P1	prolongation of P1 latency
cerebral hemisphere	36	16	28
sellar region	40	33	30
orbita/optic n.	8	5	3
	84	54	61

Table V: Comparison of ophthalmological and FEP findings

location of underlying process	total amount	field defect without alteration of		normal visual field and normal	
		FEP	PREP	FEP	PREP
cerebral hemispher	36	22	8	11	15
sellar region	40	22	8	11	6
orbit/optic n.	8	5	1	3	2

Tab. VI: Differentiation of pathological P1 latency according to the location of the underlying process

location of underlying process	total amount	pathological P1latency 2.5 standard FEP deviation	
		FEP	PREP
cerebral hemisphere	36	3	14
sellar region	40	8	14
orbita/optic n.	8	0	1

References

[1] Arruga J, Feldon SE, Hoyt WF, Aminoff MJ: Monocularly and binocularly evoked visual responses to paterned half-field stimulation. J Neurol Sci 46 (1980) 281 - 290

[2] Ashworth B, Maloney AFJ, Tonsend HRA: Delayed visual evoked potential with bilateral disease of the posterior visual pathway. J Neurol Neurosurg Psychiat 41 (1971) 449 - 451

[3] Barrett G, Blumhardt LD, Halliday AM, Halliday E, Kriss A: A paradox in the lateralization of the visual evoked response. Nature 261 (1976) 253 - 255

[4] Barnett AB, Friedmann SL, Weiss IP, Ohlrich ES, Shanks B, Lodge A: VEP development in infancy and early childhood. A longitudinal study. Electroenceph Clin Neurophysiol 49 (1980) 467 - 489

[5] Blom JL, Barth PG, Visser SL: The visual evoked potential in the first six years of life. Electroenceph Clin Neurophysiol 48 (1980) 395 - 405

[6] Clifford-Jones RE, Cunningham K, Halliday AM, Halliday E, Kriss A, McDonald WI, Peringer E: Visual evoked potential in meningeomas compressing the anterior visual pathways. Electroenceph Clin Neurophysiol 61 (1985) 52

[7] Collins DWK, Carroll WM, Black JL, Walsh M: Effect of refractive error in the visual evoked response. Br Med J 1 (1979) 231 - 232

[8] Crighel E, Arseni C, Matei M: The effect of the maturation and aging on the wave form of visually evoked potentials. Electroenceph Clin Neurophysiol 26 (1969) 2 - 11

[10] Floris V, Rizzo PA: Studio delle risposte evocate visive nelle emianopsie. Riv Pat Nerv ment (1968) 191 - 206

[11] Groswasser Z, Kriss A, Halliday AM, McDonald WI: Optic nerve glioma. A study of pattern and flash evoked potentials. Electroenceph Clin Neurophysiol 61 (1985) S 52

[12] Haimovic IC, Pedley TA: Hemi-field pattern reversal visual evoked potentials. II. Lesions of the chiasm and posterior visual pathways. Electroenceph Clin neurophysiol 54 (1982) 121 - 131

[13] Halliday AM, Halliday E, Kriss A, McDonald WI, Mushin J: The pattern-evoked potential in compression of the anterior visual pathways. Brain 99 (1976) 375 - 347

[14] Harmony T, Ricardo J, Otero G, Fernandez G, Llorento S, Valdes P: Symmetry of the visual evoked potential in normal sujects. Electroenceph Clin Neurophysiol 35 (1973) 237 - 240

[15] Harter MR, Deaton FK, Odom JV: Maturation of evoked potentials and visual preference in 6-45-day-old infants: effects of check size, visual acuity, and refractive error. Electroenc Clin Neurophysiol 42 (1977) 595 - 607

[16] Harter MR, White CT: Effects of contour sharpness and checksize on visually evoked potentials. Vis Res 8 (1968) 701 - 711

[17] Hawkes CH, Stow B: Pupil size and the pattern evoked visual response. J Neurol 44 (1981) 90 - 91

[18] Hoeppner TJ, Bergen D, Morrell F: Hemispheric asymmetry of visual evoked potentials in patients with well-defined occipital lesions. Electroenc Clin Neurophysiol 57 (1984) 310 - 319

[19] Jeffreys DA, Smith AT: The polarity inversion of scalp potentials evoked by upper and lower half-field stimulus patterns: latency or surface distribution differences ? Electroenceph Clin Neurophysiol 46 (1979) 409 - 415

[20] Kooi KA, Güvener AM, Baghi BK: Visual evoked responses in lesions of the higher optic pathways. Neurology 15 (1965) 841 - 854

[21] Kupersmith MJ, Siegel IM, Carr RE, Ransohoff J, Flamm E, Shakin E: Visual evoked potentials in chiasmal gliomas in four adults. Arch Neurol 38 (1981) 362 - 365

[22] Kuroiwa Y, Celesia GG: Visual evoked potentials with hemifield pattern stimulation. Arch Neurol 38 (1981) 86 - 90

[23] Michael WF, Halliday AM: Differences between the occipital distribution of upper and lower field pattern-evoked responses in man. Brain Res 32 (1971) 311 - 324

[24] Müller-Jensen A, Zschocke S, Dannheim F: VER analysis of the chiasmal syndrome. J Neurol 225 (1981) 33 - 40

[25] Nau H-E, Wiedemayer H, Brune-Nau R, Pohlen G, Kilian F: Zur Validität von Elektroenzephalogramm (EEG) und evozierten Potentialen in der Hirntoddiagnostik. Anästhesie Intensivmed Notfalltherapie, im Druck

[26] Nau H-E, Gerhard L, Foerster M, Nahser HC, Reinhardt V, Joka T: Optic nerve trauma: clinica, electrophysiological, and histological remarks. Acta Neurochir, in press

[27] Nau H-E, Hess E, Pohlen G, Marggraf G, Rimpel J: Evozierte Potentiale bei intrakraniellen Eingriffen. Anästhesist 36 (1987)

[28] Nau H-E, Rimpel J: Multimodality evoked potentials and electroencephalography in severe coma cases. Intensive Care Med 13 (1987) 249 - 255

[29] Onofrj M, Bodis-Wollner I, Mylin I: Visual evoked potential diagnosis of field defects in patients with chiasmatic and retrochiasmatic lesions. J Neurol Neurosurg Psychiat 45 (1982) 294 - 302

[30] Sokol S, Moskowitz A, Towle VL: Age-related changes in the latency of the visual evoked potential: Influence of check size. Electroenceph Clin Neurophysiol 51 (1981) 559 - 562

[31] Streletz LJ, Bae SH; Roeshman RM, Schatz NJ, Savino PJ: Visual evoked potentials in occipital lobe lesions. Arch Neurol 38 (1981) 80 - 85

[32] Vaughan HG, Katzman R, Taylor J: Alterations of visual evoked response in the presence of homonymous visual defects. Electroenceph Clin Neurophysiol 15 (1963) 737 - 746

III

TUMORS OF THE ORBIT AND THE VISUAL PATHWAY

Tumours of intracranial visual pathways

F. Gullotta

A short survey of "intrinsic" and "extrinsic" tumours of the intracranial visual pathways is presented. The anterior, "extracerebral" section of the visual pathways (optic nerves, chiasma, optic tracts) is more frequently and directly involved by neoplastic processes than the second one, as tumours arising from the region of the sella turcica may compress or infiltrate the pathway. The posterior, "intracerebral" component (geniculocalcarine tracts, area striata) is less affected directly by tumours, but it is more frequently damaged by every kind of intracranial neoplasm which may produce oedema and compression of posterior cerebral vessels against the edge of tentorium and followed by a calcarine infarction.

Topographically, intracranial visual pathways can be divided into a extracerebral and an intracerebral component. The first part comprises optic nerves, chiasma, optic tracts and ends in the corpora geniculata lateralia. The second one (geniculo-calcarine tract) arises from the lateral geniculate body and forms the optic radiation which ends in the area striata. On account of these anatomical features, the anterior half is much more frequently involved by neoplastic processes than the posterior one. Here, we are dealing not only with "intrinsic" tumours, i.e. tumours arising from the nerve itself or its meningeal coverings, but also with tumours of adjacent structures (hypophysis, sella turcica, etc.), which may damage the visual pathways by compression or infiltration [Table I].

The most common tumours affecting optic nerves and chiasma are: glioma (mostly in children under 10 years of age), meningiomas (in adults), craniopharyngiomas and pituitary adenomas. Optic nerve gliomas may occur mono- or bilaterally; usually they are solitary, i.e. restricted to the nerve(s), but occasionally they may also occur in patients with diffuse neurofibromatosis. They form about 1 % of intracranial tumours; considering only childhood tumours, however, this percentage rises up to 5 % [6]. They are slowly growing gliomas, built up by elongated bipolar cells which according to the recent nomenclature have been defined as "pilocytic astrocytes". According to the WHO-classification these tumours are therefore termed "pilocytic astrocytomas", in correspondence with the definition proposed by Anglo-american authors. In the German literature this tumour is better known as "spongioblastoma" [8], whereas Spanish schools [4, 5] speak of "fusicellular oligodendrogliomas" [for review see 6].

More than 20 years ago our investigations with tissue cultures [3] confirmed that we are in fact dealing with a special kind of glial cell, similar to but not identical with astrocytes and quite different from neoplastic oligodendrocytes. The cells of optic gliomas correspond to the elements of brain stem-, cerebellar and spinal cord-gliomas, and <u>in vitro</u> no signs of differentiation into typical fibrillary or protoplasmic astrocytes could be observed. A clear-cut distinction between this tumour (which we would prefer to call "spongioblastoma") and astrocytomas of cerebral hemispheres is therefore required, also regarding to the different biological behaviour of these two tumour groups (see also 1, 2).

The chiasma may also be involved by hypothalamic hamartomas, i.e. tumours consisting of mixed glial cell populations and neurons. These tumours frequently present the morphological characteristics of a dysplasia rather than those of a neoplasm. Build up by mature, well differentiated cells they are histologically benign, but prognostically unfavourable on account of their localization and the involvement of diencephalic structures.

Occasionally glioblastoma of optic nerves or of chiasma has been described (f.i. by 7). The true nature of such a tumour has been much debated however, because it is known that in optic nerves and chiasma primary, i.e. "intrinsic" glioblastomas do not occur. In my experience, the histological diagnosis "glioblastoma" is frequently made by unexperienced neuropathologists in pilocytic gliomas with degenerative cell changes.

Meningiomas may arise from the sheat of optic nerves, but most commonly they are located in the sphenoid ridge or in the olfactory groove. They grow very slowly and usually appear in adults. Histologically, they are generally benign tumours, endothelial or transitional in type.

The most frequent tumours of the pituitary region which may involve optic nerves and chiasma are craniopharyngiomas (in young people) and pituitary adenomas (in adults). Less common tumours are those of the third ventricle (ependymomas, "ectopic pinealomas" i.e. germinomas, "infundibulomas", etc.), followed those of the base of the skull (chordoma, chondroma, chondroid-chordoma, etc.), by nasopharyngeal carcinomas and metastases.

Isolated, "intrinsic" tumours of optic tracts and corpora geniculata lateralia are rare. These structures are usually involved by tumours which arise from temporal lobe and hippocampus, gliomas occurring as "pilocytic", fibrillary or protoplasmatic astrocytomas, ganglio-gliomas and, in adults, glioblastomas. Extrinsic tumours consist of meningiomas, angiomas, metastases and some large, suprasellarly growing pituitary adenomas.

Tumours of the intracerebral section of visual pathways (geniculo-calcarine tracts, striate cortex) are almost exclusively seen in adults, occurring as different kind of gliomas, which correspond to those seen elsewhere in the brain (Table I). Parasagittal meningiomas have to be mentioned here in particular for they may severely compress the medial surface of occipital lobes, producing therefore mono- or bilateral hemianopsias.

A last point has to be stressed. The anterior part of the optic pathways can also be involved by tumour-like processes as aneurysms or arachnitis cystica ("pseudo-tumours"). The posterior half, particularly the area striata, can be indirectly damaged by all kinds of intracranial tumours. Independent of its localization the tumour is able to produce a herniation of hippocampus with compression of posterior cerebral artery and veins against the free edge of the tentorium and causing a mono- or bilateral calcarine infarction.

Table I: Schematic survey of tumours of intracranial visual pathways on account of their localization.

A - Tumours involving Optic Nerve and Chiasma	
"Intrinsic":	Glioma (mono-, bilat.) Meningioma of Optic nerve Hypothalamic Hamartoma
"Extrinsic":	Meningioma (Sphen. Ridge; Olfact. Groove) "Meningiomatosis" (primary; metast.)
	Pituitary Adenoma Craniopharyngioma a. related tumours "Infundibuloma", Granularcell-Tumour Ependymoma, "Ectopic Pinealoma"
	Chordoma, Chondroma, Osteo-chondroma, Lymphoma, Lipoma, Epiderm.-cyst etc.
	Nasopharyngeal Tumours
	Metastases
Pseudo-Tumours:	Aneurysma; Arachn. adhaesiva cystica
B - Tumours involving Opt. Tract and C. Genic. later.	
"Intrinsic":	Glioma (rare)
"Extrinsic":	Meningioma Pituitary Adenoma Temporobasal Glioma/Ganglioglioma Angioma
	Metastases (see also A)
C - Tumours involving Opt. Radiations and Area striata	
"Intrinsic":	Glioma (Astroc., Oligod., Glioblastoma, Ependymoma, Mixed-Glioma, etc.)
"Extrinsic":	Metastases Meningiomas Meningo-Angiomatosis

References

[1] Gullotta F: Morphological and biological basis for the classification of brain tumours. With a comment on the WHO-classification 1979. In: Krayenbühl U. (Ed.): Advances and Technical Standards in Neurosurgery, vol. 8. Springer-Verlag, Wien-New York 1981

[2] Gullotta F: Zur aktuellen Klassifikation der Hirntumoren. In: Walter W and Krenkel W (Eds.): Jahrbuch der Neurochirurgie, Wissenschaftl. Verlagsgesell., Regenberg & Biermann, Münster 1986

[3] Gullotta F, Kreutzberg GW: Das Gliom des Opticus. Morphologische und histochemische Untersuchungen am Schnittpräparat und der Gewebekultur. Acta Neuropath. (Berlin) 2 (1963) 413 - 424

[4] Polak M: Blastomas del Sistema Nervioso Central y Periferico. Patologia y ordenación histogenética. Lopez Libreros Editores, Buenos Aires 1966

[5] Rio Hortega del P: Estructura y Sistematización de los Gliomas y Paragliomas. Arch. espan. de Oncologia 2 (1932) 411 - 678

[6] Russell D, Rubinstein LJ: Pathology of Tumours of the Nervous System. 4th Ed. Ed. Arnold Publ., London 1977

[7] Saebo J: Primary tumour of optic nerve (glioblastoma multiforme). Brit. J. Ophthalmol. 33 (1949) 701 - 707

[8] Zülch KJ: Biologie und Pathologie der Hirngeschwülste. In: Olivercrona H, Toennis W (Eds.): Handbuch der Neurochirurgie, Band 3. Springer-Verlag, Berlin-Göttingen-Heidelberg 1956

Orbital Invasion by Intraocular Tumours

W. Lieb, A. Nover

Abstract

Secondary orbital tumors can arise from the paranasal sinuses, the intracranial cavity, the ocular adnexa or from the eye itself. The most common intraocular tumor is the choroidal melanoma. Up to 13 % of these tumors penetrate the sclera and may lead to orbital extension or to an orbital recurrence.

The risk factors and types of extrascleral extension are discussed in relation to the literature and on the basis of our experience based on 172 cases of enucleated choroidal melanomas. Besides the choroidal melanoma the retinoblastoma is the most common ocular tumor with tendency for orbital invasion. In contrary to the melanoma however, the retinoblastomas tend to invade the neural tissue of the optic nerve.

Introduction

Out of the great variety of tumors that arise from the ocular structures primarily two malignant tumors tend to invade the orbit: 1. The melanoma of the choroid and the ciliary body 2. the retinoblastoma.

From all secondary orbital tumors, the ocular melanoma is the third most common and ranges behind mucoceles and carcinomas of the paranasal sinuses and meningeomas arising from the sphenoid wings. The secondary orbital melanoma accounts for about 5 % of all orbital neoplasms.

The choroidal melanoma is the most common intraocular tumor. The incidence is about 0.02 - 0.05 %, i.e. two to five cases per 10 000 people. The average age is about 60 years. There is no sexpreference. The prognosis of choroidal melanomas depends on several different factors: 1. tumor volume 2. localisation 3. celltype 4. growthpattern 5. age and sex 6. vortex-vein invasion 7. scleral invasion 8. optic nerve invasion.

Material and Method

172 eyes were enucleated, for intraocular melanoma, during 1973 and 1987. During the same time 15 eyes harbouring a retinoblastoma came to histologic examination.

The eyes were cut in serial section in order to evaluate scleral invasion or extraocular extension. For the present study representative sections and the pathology reports are reviewed.

Case review and Discussion

SHAMMAS and BLODI [89] analysed in a clinico-pathologic study over 432 enucleated melanoma eyes the risk factors for developing orbital growth.

Statistically significant were 1. greatest tumor diameter more than 10 mm 2. ruptured Bruch's membrane 3. a mixed- or epithelioid-cell melanoma 4. a densly pigmented tumor.

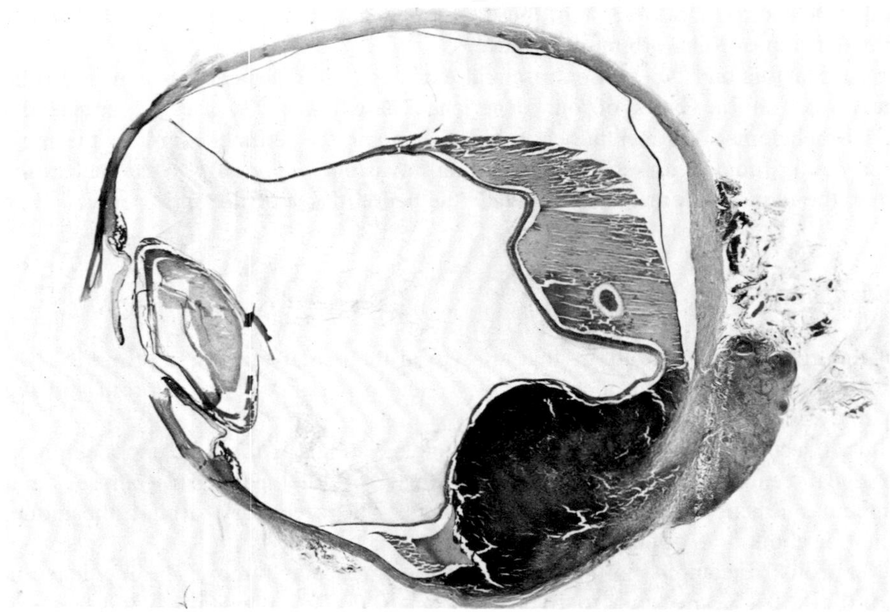

Fig. 1: Histological section of a globe containing a mixed cell choroidal melanoma, with large extrascleral extension. The sclera is almost replaced by tumor cells.

Choroidal melanomas tend to infiltrate the sclera and proceed to extrascleral growth in about 10 % of cases. In contrary to the extrascleral growth of anteriorly located melanomas, in which epibulbar pigment can be seen, posterior melanomas may lead to unnoticed extrascleral growth until the patient develops exophthalmus or signs of endophthalmitis (Fig. 1). In these cases ultrasonography is a very sensitive and specific measure to correctly determine scleral invasion and scleral penetration by intraocular melanoma [5, 6].

Usually the sclera is a natural barrier, preventing extrascleral extension. However the tumors grow along the ciliary vessels and nerves, which lie in defined channels within the sclera (Fig. 2), or through the lumen of the vortex veins. Even clinically stationary melanomas may eventually disseminate through these channels [2].

In contrast to the retinoblastoma, which has a tendency to neural invasion, choroidal melanomas only rarely invade the optic nerve [9]. The rare cases of peripapillary melanomas, with optic nerve infiltration have a extremely poor prognosis. Several authors [1, 4, 11] have shown that the prognosis for survival of melanomas with extraocular growth is rather dismal. KRESTEN et al. [4] have shown that 40 months after the diagnosis 50 % of the patients have died from metastatic disease. In the past the exenteration of the orbit has been proposed as the therapy of choice, in any case of uveal melanoma with extrascleral extension. SHIELDS and WOLTER [10, 12] however have postulated alternatives to exenteration. They use exenteration only in cases of large extraocular tumor volume and no systemic metastases, or in a large orbital recurrence without systemic metastases.

In case there is only a localized small extension, the globe should be enucleated with a localized tenonectomy, or in small tumors the extension can even been shaved off and a radioactive plaque can be applied to the tumor base.

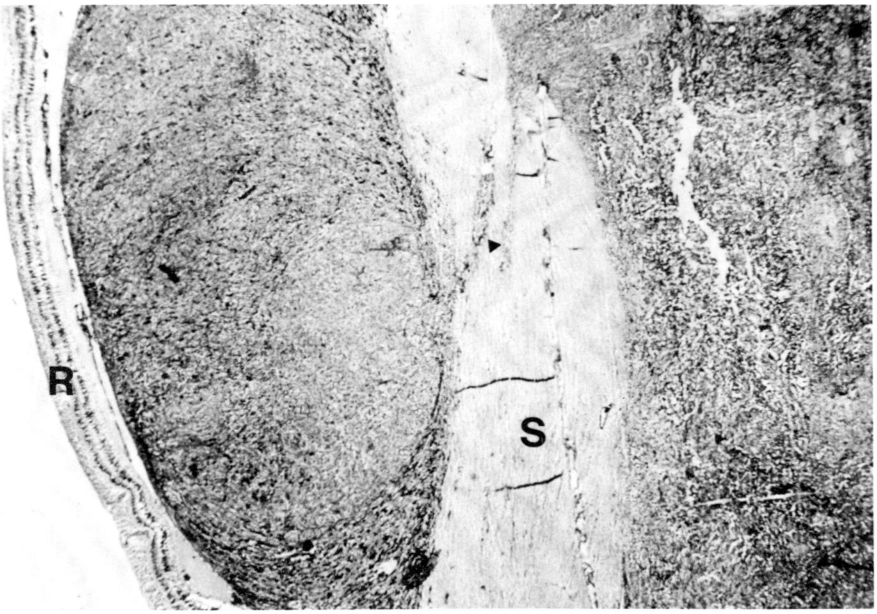

Fig. 2: Histological section of a small melanoma, which lead to extension. The tumor is infiltrating along the scleral channels (arrow). R (retina) S (sclera)

In cases of vortex-vein involvement, metastatic disease is very likely and local orbital radiation and probably chemotherapy are indicated.

Table I demonstrates some histopathologic features of the 172 eyes harbouring a intraocular melanoma, which were enucleated between 1973 and 1987.

18 % had extrascleral growth of the tumor. The higher risk of orbital invasion in the more malignant cell types can be supported by our data.

The retinoblastoma is the most important primary tumor of the retina.

It is a tumor of early childhood and it's prevalence is between 1 : 34 000 to 1 : 15 000 live births [9].

Two major growth types can be distinguished: The endophytic form growing from the retina into the vitreous cavity, and the exophytic growing towards the choroid. The latter form tends to invade the orbit through the scleral canals like the choroidal melanoma [3].

All retinoblastomas independent of their growth patterns have a tendency to invade the optic nerve (Fig. 3). From there the tumor reaches through the meninges into the liquor and the orbit. Besides the bilateral occurrence in genetically determined tumors, optic nerve invasion plays the dominant role in determining prognosis. Retinoblastomas with optic nerve involvement and extrascleral extension still have even today a rather poor survival [3, 7].

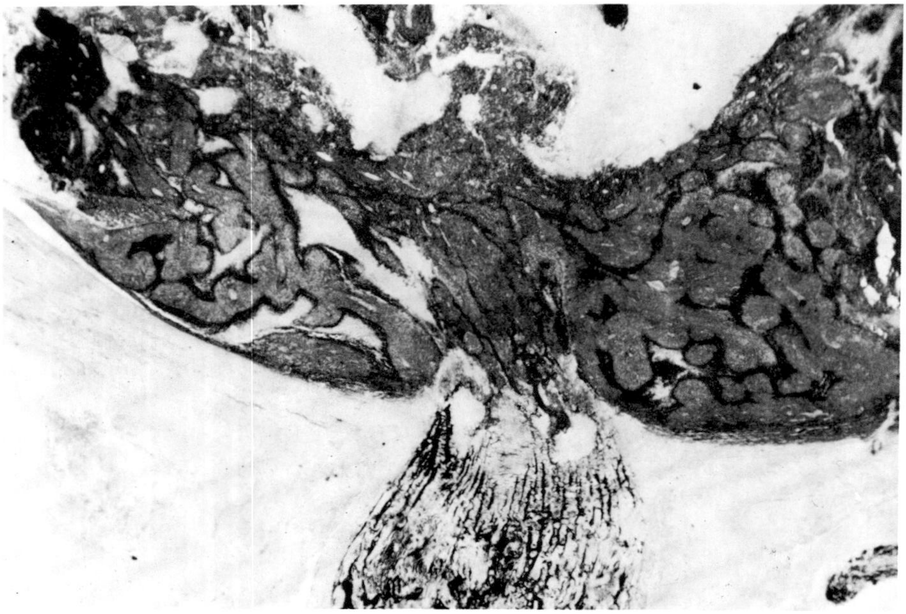

Fig. 3: Retinoblastoma infiltrating the choroid and the optic nerve. The resection line is free of tumor.

In unilateral large tumors enucleation is the therapy of choice. Extrascleral tumor tissue or nerve involvement behind the resection line is treated with adjuvant radiotherapy using 3500 - 40 000 rad. fractioned over three weeks. In addition these patients are often treated with a combined chemotherapy of cyclophosphamid and adriamycin.

Exenteration like in melanoma cases is not indicated.

Despite better therapeutic modalities and earlier detection the prognosis is rather poor, once the tumor has reached the orbit. ROOTMANN et al. [7] have shown that from this group only about 9.4 % survived more than two years after diagnosis. Like in melanomas ultrasonography and computerized tomography are sensitive methods to detect extraocular tumor growth.

In rare cases a orbital tumor can by compressing the globe simulate an intraocular neoplasm. A- and B-scan ultrasonography and CT-scan are helpful in these cases (Fig. 4).

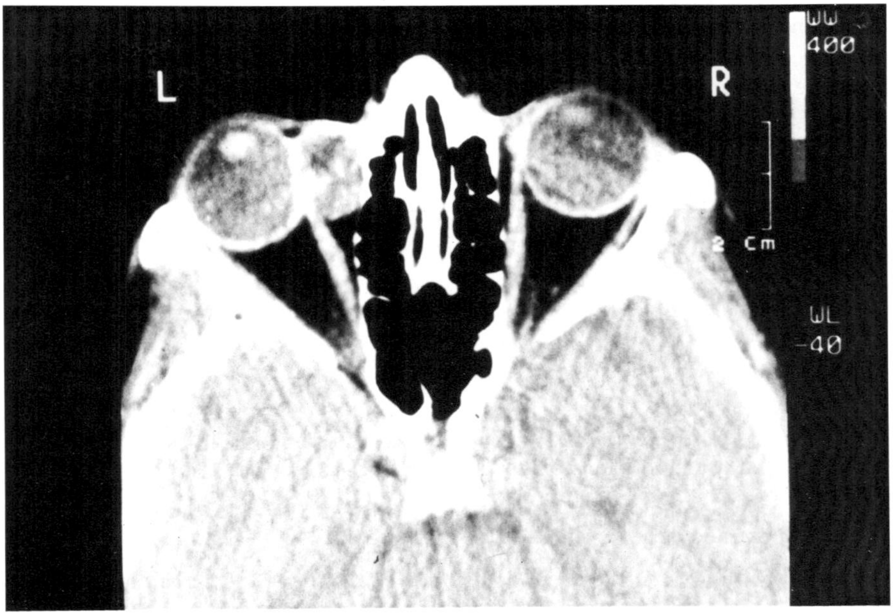

Fig. 4: Axial orbital CT scan of a patient with a dark appearing mass in the nasal fundus. Pathology revealed a cyst impressing the left globe.

In all cases of an orbital mass, an intraocular tumor must be ruled out. For this reason besides the modern imaging techniques, a thorough ophthalmoscopic examination is mandatory.

Table I: Histology of 172 choroidal and ciliary body melanomas

classification	n	SCLERA, % intact	infiltrated	penetrated
spindelcell	116	35	45	16
mixedcell melanomas	38	26	52	22
epitheloidcell melanomas	18	17	55	28
	172	31	51	18

M : F = 1 : 1
Means age: 59 y

References

[1] Affeldt JC, Minckler DS, Azen SP, Yeh L: Prognosis in uveal melanoma with extrascleral extension. Arch. Ophthalmol. 98 (1979) 1975 - 1979

[2] Canny CL, Shields JA, Kay ML: Clinically stationary choroidal melanoma with extraocular extension. Arch. Ophthalmol. 96 (1987) 436 - 439

[3] Ellsworth RM: Orbital retinoblastoma. Trans. Amer. Ophthalmol. Soc. 72 (1974) 79 - 88

[4] Kersten RC, Tse DT, Anderson RL, Blodi FC: Orbital extension of choroidal and ciliary body melanomas. Ophthalmology 92 (1985) 436 -443

[5] Rochels R, Nover A, Neuhann TH, Adam F: Echographic examinations on 110 histologically proven intraocular melanomas; in Lommatzsch, Blodi, Intraocular tumors, pp. 176 - 182 Akademie Verlag, Berlin 1983

[6] Rochels R, Nover A: Small choroidal melanoma with diffuse orbital involvement. Detected and differentiated with standardized echography - with special reference to the reliability of sonography in predicting scleral tumor infiltration. Ophthalmologica, Basel 192 (1986) 39 - 45

[7] Rootmann J, Ellsworth RM, Hofbauer J et al.: Orbital extension of retinoblastoma: a clinicopathological study. Can. J. Ophthalmol. 13 (1987) 72 - 80

[8] Shammas HF, Blodi FC: Orbital extension of choroidal and ciliary body melanomas. Arch. Ophthalmol. 95 (1977) 2002 - 2005

[9] Shields JA: Diagnosis and management of intraocular tumors. C.V. Mosby, St. Louis 1983

[10] Shields JA, Augsburger JJ, Corwin S, Donoso L, Di Santis M: The management of uveal melanomas with extrascleral extension. Orbit 5 (1986) 31- 37

[11] Starr HJ, Zimmermann LE: Extrascleral extension and orbital recurrence of malignant melanomas of the choroid and ciliary body. Int. Ophthalmol. Clin. 2 (1962) 369 - 385

[12] Wolter JR: Tenonectomy. Arch. Ophthal. 86 (1971) 529 - 533

Reconstructive surgery of the Orbital Region

H. v. Domarus

Abstract

Trauma, malformations and particularly defects after resection of benign or malignant tumours pose a multitude of reconstructive problems. To restore body surface, aesthetic appearance and function are the goals of modern surgery which go beyond the aims of curative resection of malignancies. A number of typical operative restorations in the orbital region are demonstrated and discussed.

Introduction

The structures of the orbit and its immediate vicinity are so manyfold that defects in these various regions (socket, eyelids, eyebrows and forehead, medial and lateral canthal region, upper cheek) pose many problems and offer an even greater multitude of reconstructive facilities. Tumour surgery leaves defects of body surface, of aesthetic appearance and function which are the subject of this article. Until recently tumour surgery contented itself with curative resection alone and reconstructive possibilities were few and applied only by a rare number of outstanding surgeons. During the last decades, however, the need to offer the patient more than ablative tumour surgery has been widely recognized in most surgical fields [1, 2, 4 - 8, 11 - 14], a number of old methods have gone through a rejuvenation and an ever growing amount of well defined procedures have replaced the "Cut and Try". For most of a particular area of the body we now have a variety of possibilities to close a defect changing with growing size of the deficiency. Thus resection of a malignancy can be performed more generously and the "Wait and See" attitude can be more and more abandoned in favour of primary reconstruction.

Cases

Reconstruction of the orbital fractures and bony defects have been dealt with in other contributions. Therefore the examples are mainly confined to defects due to resections of malignancies. The majority of malignant tumours in the area are basal cell carcinomas which metastasize only very rarely [9] and inner canthus and lower eyelid are the regions which are involved most commonly. All other premalignant or malignant lesions as squamous cell carcinoma, malignant melanoma or Merkel cell carcinoma are significantly less frequent [8, 11].

Squamous cell carcinomas from the oral and nasal cavity or the nasal sinuses or intracranial malignancies may invade the orbit and leave large defects.

When covering a facial defect there are a few general principles we have to follow to gain an unobtrusive result. For aesthetic purposes the skin around the defect offers the best match in colour and texture. Therefore local flaps are the first choice in facial reconstruction. Meticulous surgical techniques alone are not a guarantee for a fine scar and the lines of elective incisions or of minimal scaring have to be observed carefully when planing flaps [3]. A good blood supply is essential for a flap and knowledge of skin arteries [10], good planing and cautious handling of a flap to avoid kinking or pressure of a pedicle and tension of the tissue during and after the operation are one of the aims when teaching reconstructive surgery. Dressings are thus avoided when possible to allow constant postoperative monitoring of blood perfusion. The following cases can only demonstrate more commonly used techniques as almost every defects shows an individual size and location which alter the considerations for reconstructive methods.

Case 1:

A basal cell carcinoma of the left upper cheek (Fig. 1a) was excised with a 7 to 8 mm margin. The defect was closed with a subcutaneous pedicle flap with an axis taken along the lines of minimal scaring (Fig. 1b). The secondary defect at the lower end of the flap is closed in a V-Y-manner. Figure 1c shows the result almost a year later. Direct closure of the defect would probably have resulted in an ectropium of the lower eyelid or in a compromise with a narrower margin of excision. Free skin grafts, split or full thickness, would have been less of a match for colour and texture and resulted in greater shrinkage. While an Imré's rotation [6] would have been a satisfactory alternative in all respects, Esser's rotation would run perpendicular to the lines of minimal scaring. Finally, transposition flaps from various directions around the defect can leave a temporary dog ear and have to be planned as a compromise concerning the lines of elective incisions as donor site and defect leave scars which run approximately at 90° to each other. Similar reflections of differential therapy as in this simple case can be made for all the following cases.

Case 2:

A larger basal cell carcinoma than in case No 1 and closer to the lower eyelid is excised under local anaesthesia (Fig. 2a). An additional triangular excision below the primary defect to avoid a dog ear and an Esser's cheek rotation flap are marked. The flap is raised with an even layer of subcutaneous fat (Fig. 2b) and rotated into the defect (Fig. 2c). Figure 2d showed the patient five months postoperatively. If necessary the incision for the flap can be taken down into the neck yielding a large amount of skin with which more than the total lower eyelid and all of the medial cheek can be covered if necessary [7].

Cases 3 and 4:

Full thickness postauricular skin grafts are particularly suitable to replace thin skin and give a fairly good colour match in the face.

Case 5:

An alternative method to that in case 3 and preferred for larger defects that reach into areas of thicker skin is a median forehead transposition flap (Fig. 4).

Case 6:

A wedge excision of an eyelid up to a quarter of the total length of a lid margin can be closed directly with a good functional result. This is true for both upper and lower eyelid. While the lower eyelid can be reconstructed as a static tissue the mobility of the upper eyelid is essential for opening and closing. Luckely, tumours of the upper eyelid are rare when compared with those of the lower lid and so a total loss of an upper eyelid is even more of a rarity and functional reconstruction is difficult. The Mustardé procedure for total upper lid reconstruction [2, 13] is the method of choice and figures 5a and b give such an example. A recurrent basal cell carcinoma of the upper lid probably due to inadequate excision which in itself may well have originated from a lack of knowledge how to repair a larger defect made a total excision of the upper lid necessary. A pedicled flap of the lower eyelid restores the whole of the upper lid with the end of the levator muscle carefully reinserted (Fig. 5). The lower lid is reconstructed with nasal mucosa, septal cartilage and an Esser's cheek rotation. Function is already restored seven days after the second phase of the operation still with considerable lid oedema.

Case 7:

To create a socket for an eye prothesis is a special problem as the lining transplanted to form a cavity is suspended in very soft tissue, mainly orbital fat, and considerable contraction results after surgery is well recognized. Ceratinising epithelium as gained from a flap or a split skin graft, can cause such offensive foetor that a patient sometimes becomes socially unacceptable. A mucosa transplant is therefore the method of choice. The patient in figure 6 a had lost his right eye and conjunctiva through a chemical burn in early childhood. A free full thickness cheek mucosa transplant was sutured around a fairly large prothesis and buried in a wound with the eyelids stitched together. The palpebral fissure was reopened a week later giving a moist mucosa lining of the cavity. The final result still showed some scaring of the eyelid skin from the original injury which the patient refused to have corrected.

Case 8:

Occasionally a prothesis is the appropriate way to give acceptable aesthetic appearance. A large recurrent basal cell carcinoma had invaded the orbit and upper cheek. The wound was covered with a cranially pedicled transposition flap from the neck (Fig. 6a and b). The healed surface allowed a prothesis to be fixed which replaced eye, lids, zygoma and upper cheek (Fig. 6c).

Case 9:

A squamos cell carcinoma invading the eye socket necessitated a block resection including right maxilla and hard palate, zygoma and lateral nasal wall, ethmoidal complex and orbital contents (Fig. 7a and b). The temporalis muscle (Fig. 7c) which receives its nerve and blood supply from the region of the coronoid process can be used as a flap hinged on this pedicle and in the case illustrated filled the orbital and sinoidal defect creating a lateral wall of the right nose and seperating the oral cavity from the defects. The patient preferred to wear an eye patch to an external prothesis.

Case 10:

Resection of a liposarcoma of the right forehead left a defect of temple, forehead and eyebrow of which the external layer as further removed for reasons of a safer oncological margin. The defect was too large for a none hair bearing local flap and a scalp rotation flap was used (Fig. 8a) with a split skin graft for the secondary defect. During the years after the operation the patient never consented to have the hair bearing area replaced by a split skin graft but shaved daily instead and used hair style and cover mark (Fig. 8b).

Conclusion

Reconstructive plastic surgery offers possibilities for our patients which go beyond curative tumour surgery only. The defects we are confronted with are individual in size and location and restorations have to be planned for each case. The examples allowed to show some general principles which can be modified for each particular problem.

Figures

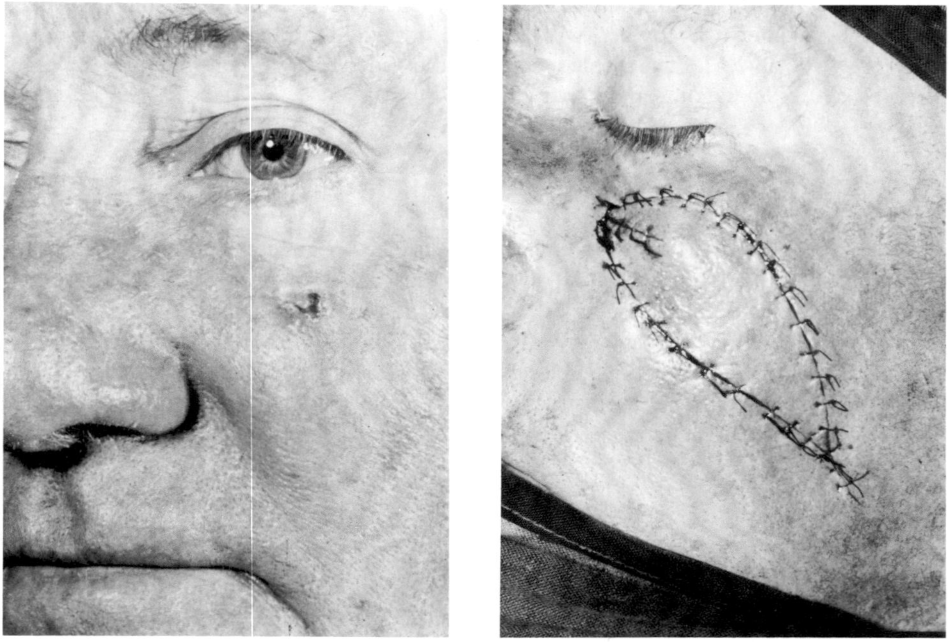

a) b)

Fig. 1: A basal cell carcinoma of the upper cheek (a) is excised and the defect reconstructed with subcutaneous pedicle flap (b).

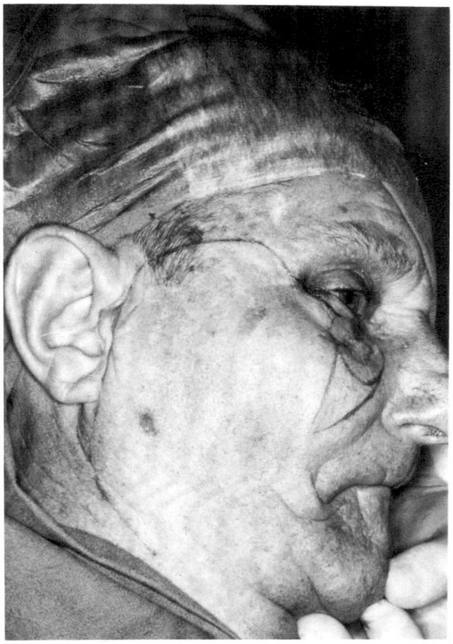

a)

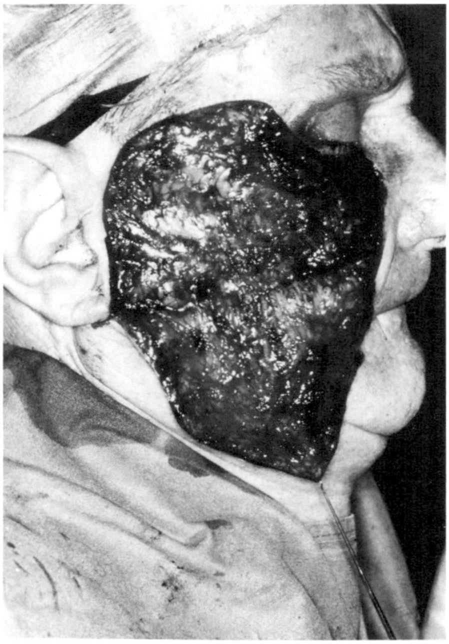

b)

Fig. 2: Excision of a basal cell carcinoma just below the right lower eyelid under local anaesthesia (a). Reconstruction with an Esser's cheek rotation (b), (c) and the patient five months after the operation (d).

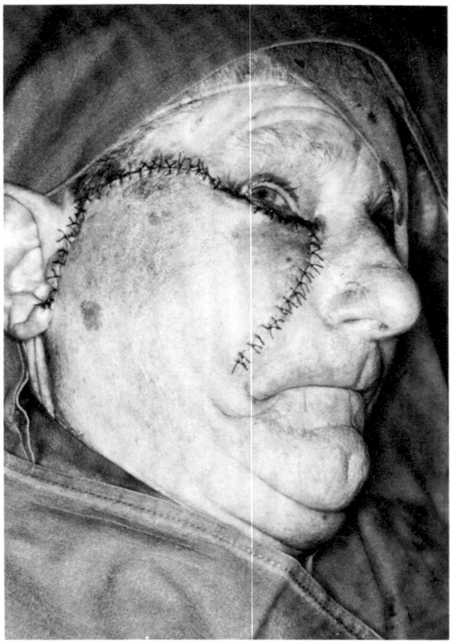

c)

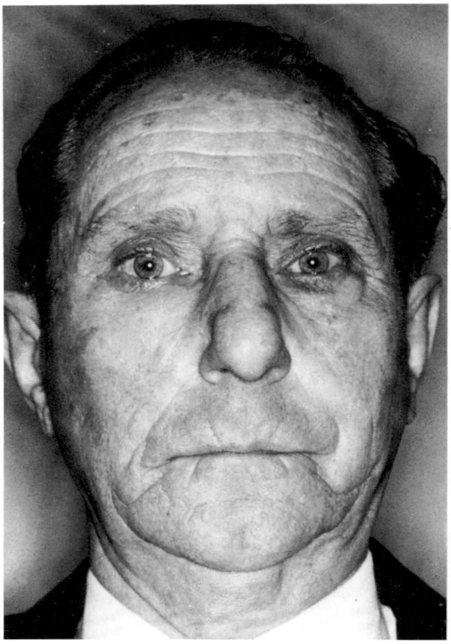

d)

Fig. 2

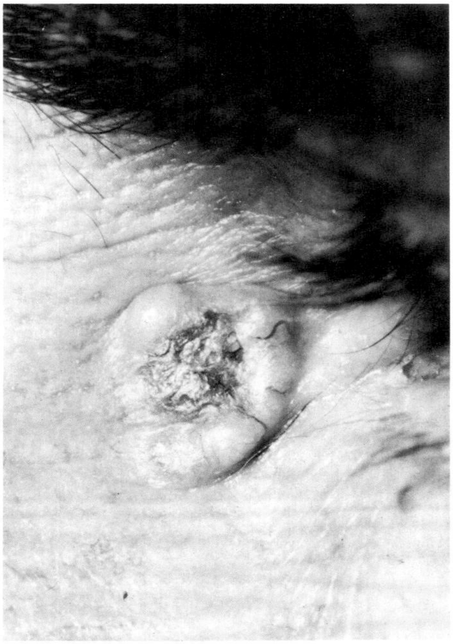

Fig. 3: A typical basal cell carcinoma of the left inner canthus (a).

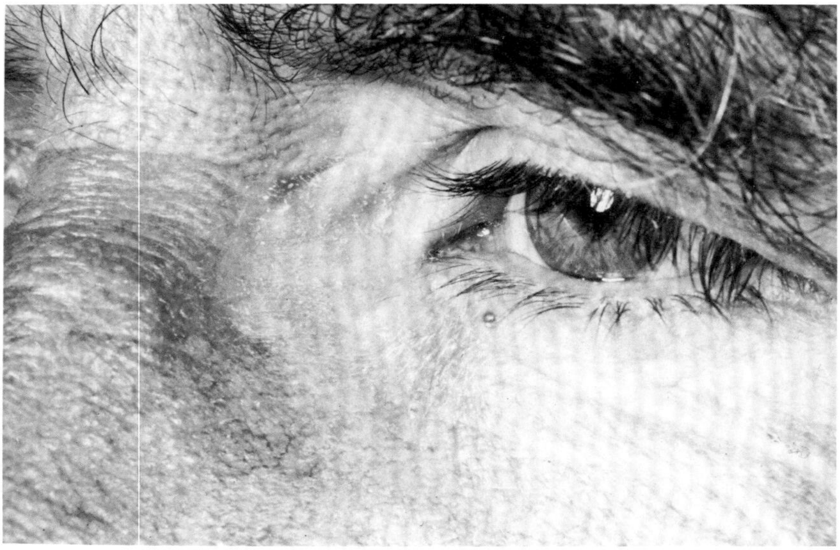

b

Fig. 3b: A full thickness postauricular skin graft showing a fairly good colour match seven months after primary surgery.

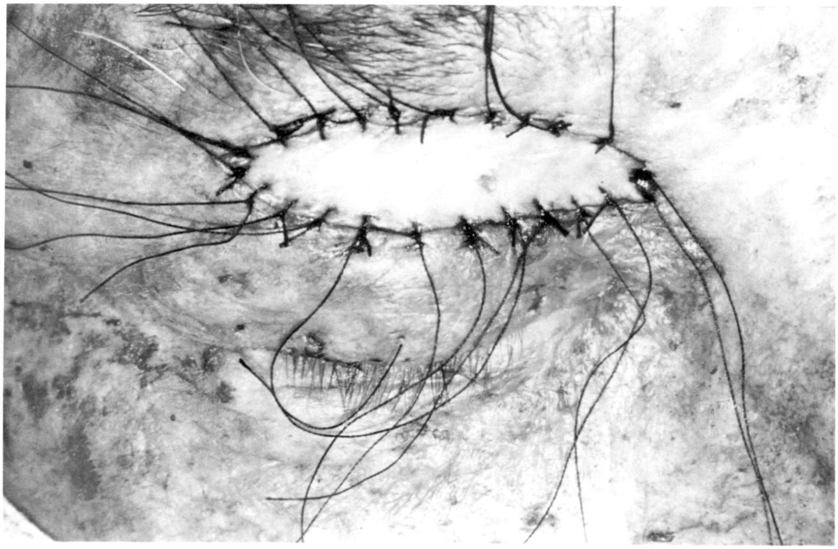

Fig. 4: The rare location of a basal cell carcinoma of the upper lid with the defect covered with a postauricular full thickness skin graft already allowing good motility at the stage four week after the procedure.

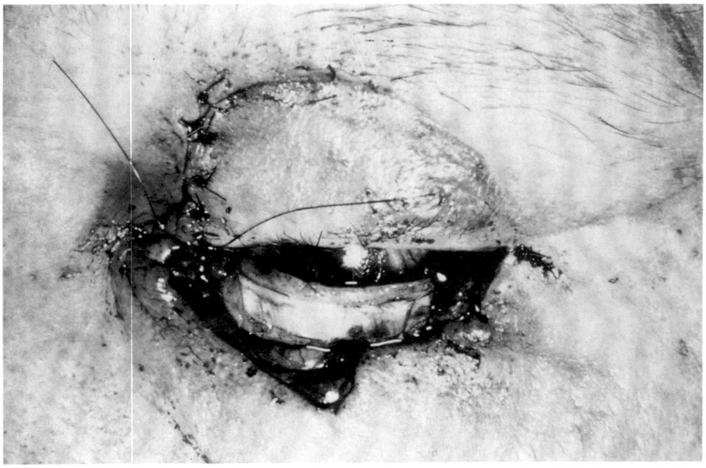

a)

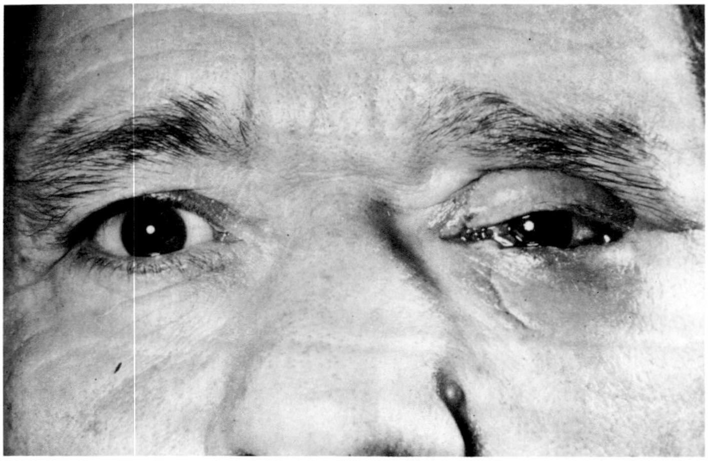

b)

Fig. 5: A radiation scar and a recurrent basal cell carcinoma (a) are replaced with a median forehead transposition flap. Result three years after the operation (b).

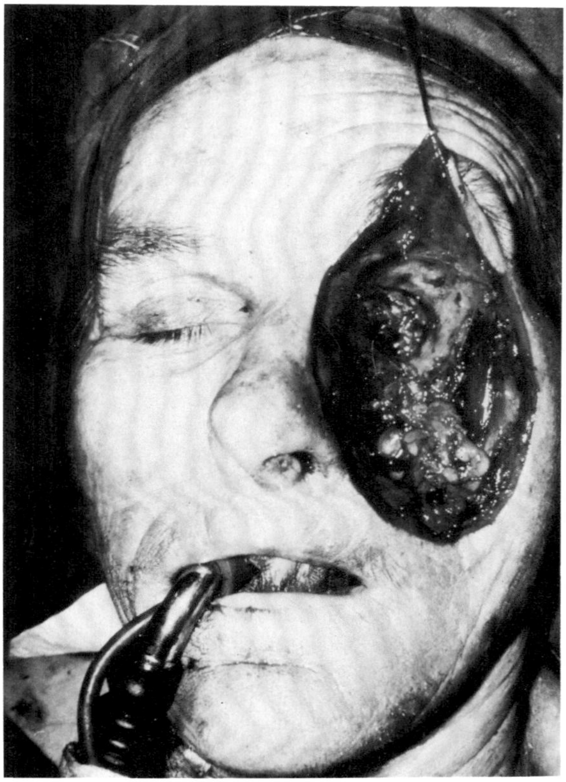

Fig. 6: A recurrent basal cell carcinoma necessitated orbital exenteration and removal of upper cheek (a). A transposition flap from the neck covered the wound (b) to allow an outer prothesis (c).

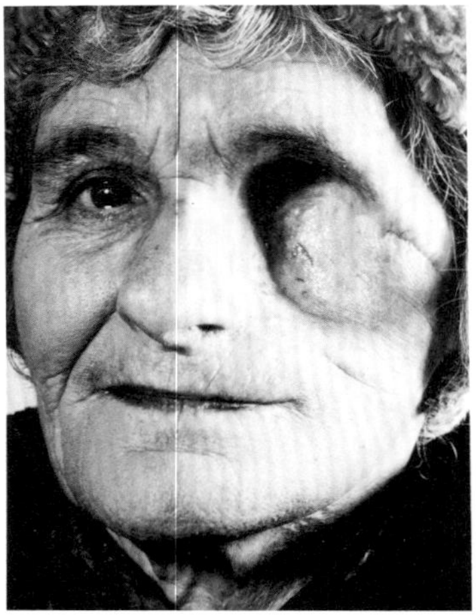

b)

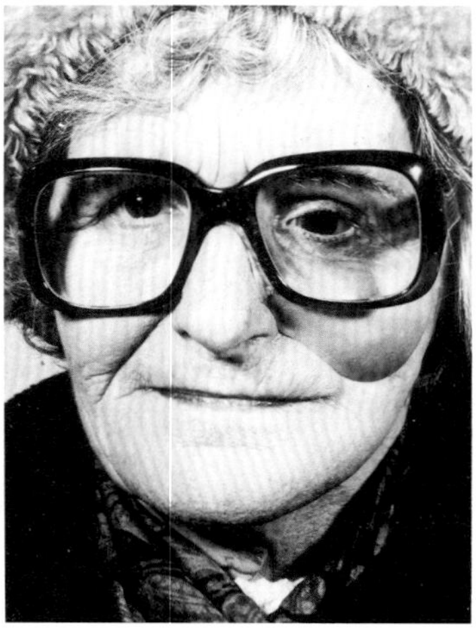

c)

Fig. 6: A recurrent basal cell carcinoma necessitated orbital exenteration and removal of upper cheek (a). A transposition flap from the neck covered the wound (b) to allow an outer prothesis (c).

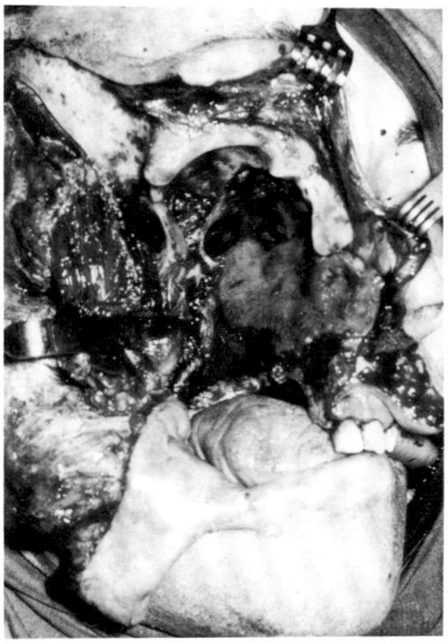

a)

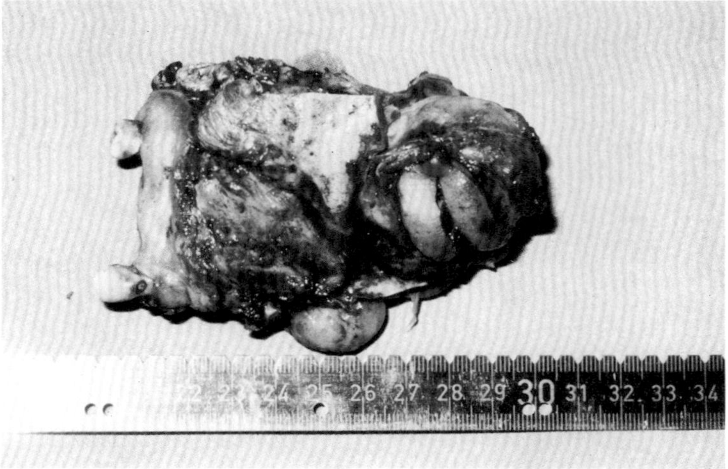

b)

Fig. 7: A squamous cell carcinoma invading the orbit left a defect of maxilla, zygoma, lateral nose and orbit (a and b). A temporalis muscle flap (c) filled the orbital and sinoidal defect separating the oral cavity from the resection wound.

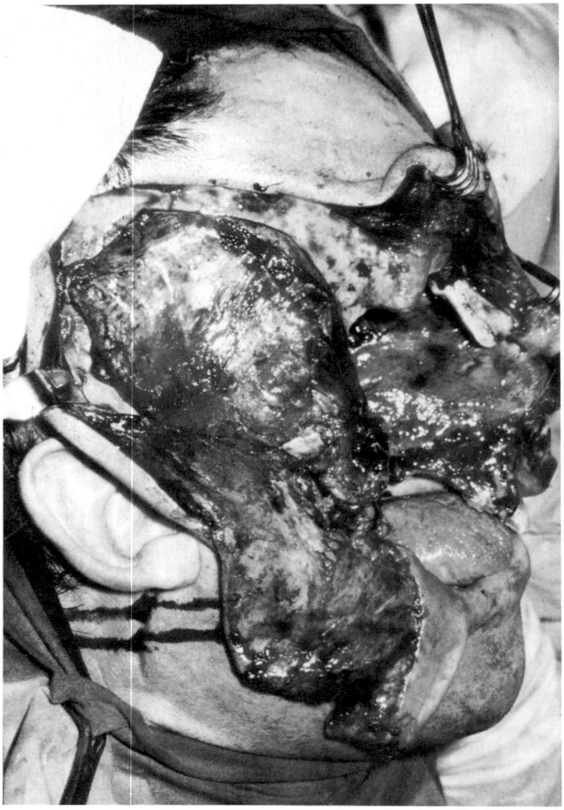

Fig. 7c

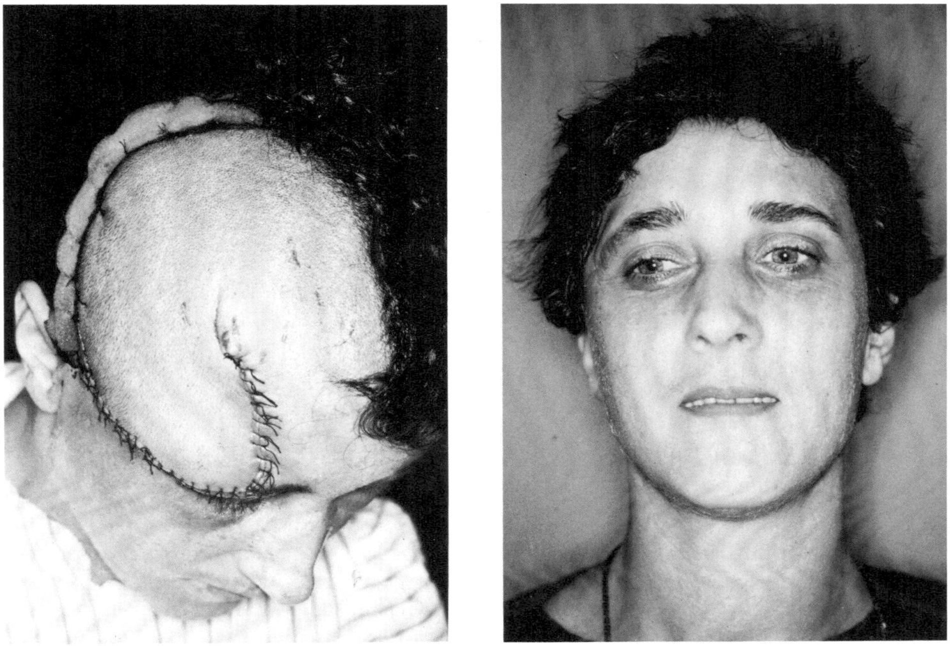

a) b)

Fig. 8: A widely liposarcoma with a defect of eyebrow, temple and forehead. A scalp rotation flap (a) was later shaved by the patient (b) and hidden by a cover mark (see text for details).

References

[1] Barclay TL, Kernahan DA: Rob & Smith's Operative surgery. Plastic surgery. 4th edition, Butterworths, London, Boston, Durban, Singapore, Sydney, Toronto, Wellington 1986

[3] Borges AF: Elective incisions and scar revision. Little, Brown and Company, Boston 1973

[4] Bull TR, Myers E: Plastic reconstruction in the head and neck. Butterworths, London, Boston, Durban, Singapore, Sydney, Toronto, Wellington 1986

[5] Collin JRO: A manual of systematic eyelid surgery. Churchill Livingstone, Edinburgh, London, Melbourne, New York 1983

[6] Convers JM: Reconstructive plastic surgery, Vol 2 and 5, Saunders, Philadelphia, London, Toronto 1977

[7] v. Domarus H: Defektdeckung mit der Esserschen Wangenrotation Dtsch. Z. Mund Kiefer Gesichtschir. 11 (1987) 217 - 222

[8] v. Domarus H, Johannisson R, Schmauz R: Merkel cell carcinoma of the face. Case report and review of the literature. J. Maxillofac. Surg. 13 (1985) 39 - 43

[9] v. Domarus H, Stevens PJ: Metastatic basal cell carcinoma. Report of five cases and review of 170 cases in the literature. J. Am. Acad. Dermatol. 10 (1984) 1043 - 1060

[10] v. Domarus H, Weimer J, Friedrich H-J: Die Hautarterie des Gesichtes. Variationen und mittlerer Verlauf, dargestellt mit der Ultraschall-Doppler-Sonographie Dtsch. Z. Mund Kiefer Gesichtschir. 8 (1984) 112 - 121

[11] Emmett AJJ, O'Rourke MGE: Malignant skin tumours. Churchill Livingstone, Edinburgh, London, Melbourne, New York 1982

[12] Jackson IT: Local flaps in head and neck reconstruction. Mosby, St. Louis, Toronto, Princeton 1985

[13] Mustardé JC: Repair and reconstruction in the orbital region. Churchill Livingstone, Edinburgh, London, New York 1980

[14] Smith BC: Ophthalmic plastic and reconstructive surgery, Vol. 1 and 2, Mosby, St. Louis, Washington, Toronto 1987

Hemangiomas in the periorbital region of infants and children

H. Scheunemann

Introduction

Opinions regarding the best possible therapeutical method for hemangiomas diverge widely. While some authors favour a policy of non-interference, others advocate surgical intervention or radiotherapy [3]. The tendency for spontaneous involution exhibited by capillary and cavernous hemangiomas in a zone of transition to hyperplasia or hamartia as described by BREDT [2] causing many physicians to wait and see [1, 4].

At one month of life 90 % of all hemangiomas are discovered by the mother and more than 99 % are detected by the end of the first year. Frequency of occurrence following the first year of life is negligible [6]. PROPPE and HAUSS (1963) have attempted an exact description of size and number, growth and regression of hemangiomas. The statement that in the great majority of cases hemangiomas in 6-months-old infants measure from 1 - 2 cm^2 is of particular interest to us.

The possibilities of surgical management for hemangiomas in exposed regions of the face have been discussed by SCHEUNEMANN (1975).

Case Reports:

Case 1: Spontaneous Involution

A 4-months-old baby with an extended congenital cavernous hemangioma in the right periorbital region was first admitted to our hospital in January 1980. We did not take primary surgical management into consideration due to the involment of the entire inferior eyelid and extensive expansion into the adjacent soft tissue (Fig. 1 a).

Bases on the observation of frequent spontaneous involution with cavernous hemangiomas, we recommend a policy of non-interference for lesions at this particular site. In accordance to the wishes of the child's parents, another hemangioma in the region of the upper lip was not surgically excised at that time.

In November 1981, 10 months following the first examination, signs of involution were observed; the periorbital hemangioma and the lesion on the upper lip both had regressed (Fig. 1 b).

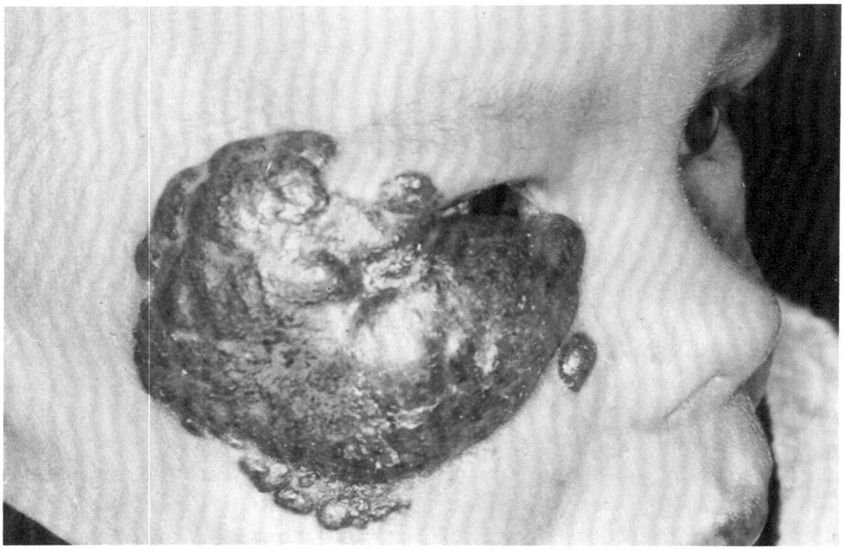

Fig. 1a

In the affected regions progressive cicatrization was noted, reaching its final stage five years later, in 1986. An area of surplus skin remained in the right periorbital regions; the lower lid retained its shape and function completely (Fig. 1 c).

Case 2: Embolization and secondary partial excision of a lesion with a capillary hemangioma of the inferior eyelid-region and of the right cheek.

In a 15-months-old girl a vascular swelling had first appeared in the region of the right cheek and the right lid when the child was approximately 6 weeks old. Both, proptosis and squint vision developed (Fig. 2 a).

Cortisone therapy at the Pediatric Hospital of the university did not result in improvement.

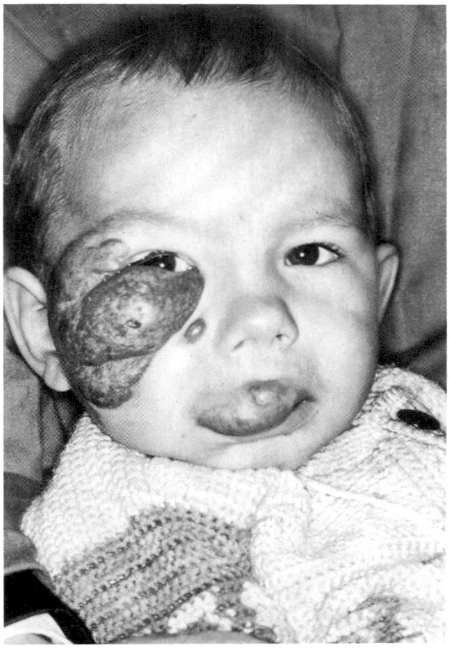

Fig. 1b

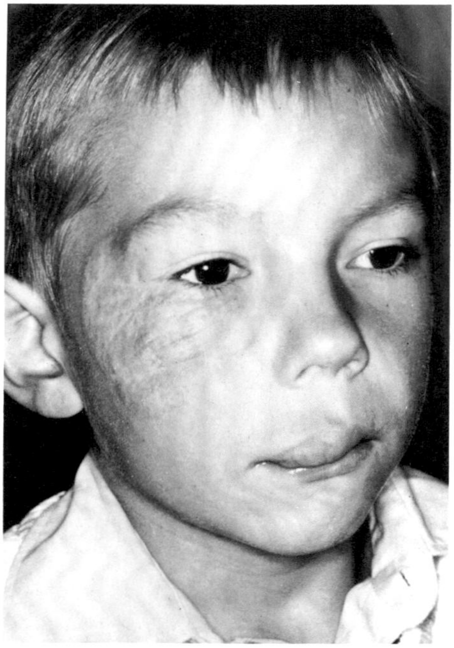

Fig. 1c

In January 1977, when the infant was 5 months old, the hemangioma was embolized by Prof. DJINDIJAN in Paris. Angiography revealed that the capillary hemangioma was supplied by all branches of the external carotid artery with the exception of the occipital artery. Embolization via the external carotid did not result in an improvement. In June 1977, we therefore decided on a partial excision of the hemangioma by infraorbital-transconjunctivcal incision (consult SCHÜRMANN and VOTH (1972)). The ectropium of the inferior lid was eliminated. Although a cone of the tumor remained in the orbit, we observed a steady regression and subsequently a return to normality. The cutaneous hemangioma of the skin above the right zygoma was reduced by serial excisions.

Case 3: Total extirpation of a hemangioma of the parotid gland.

The parents of the child St. C. first detected a swelling in the region of the right parotid when the infant was 3 months old. The swelling was diagnosed as a capillary hemangioma which rapidly increased in size (Fig. 3 a). The infant was operated in 1974, when she was 7 months old (Fig. 3 b). Progressive displacement of the adjacent auditory meatus had occurred. After tracing the trunk of the facial nerve, the hemangioma could be isolated from the peripheral branches thus permitting total extirpation (Fig. 3 b).

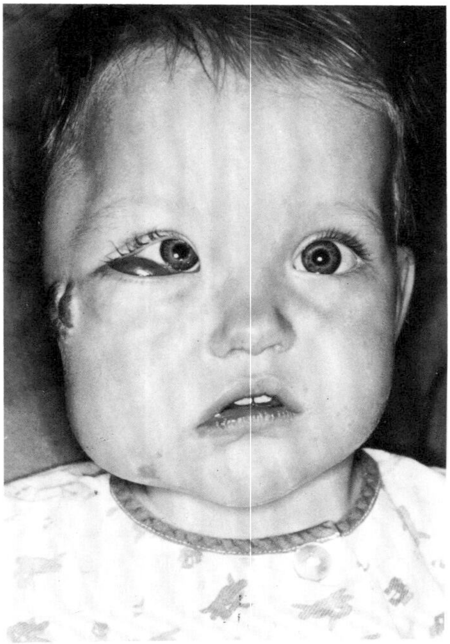

Fig.2a

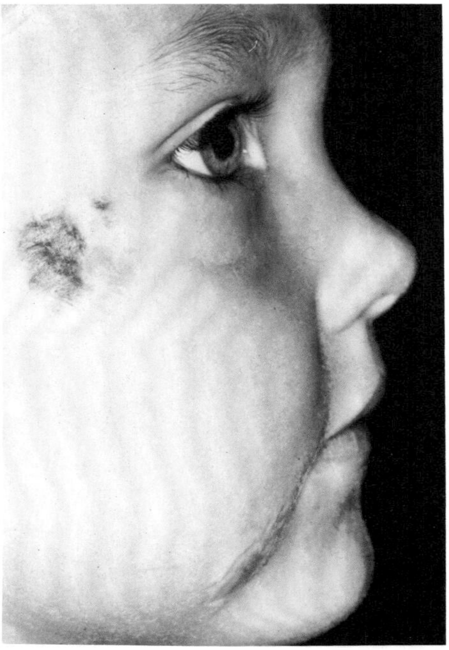

Fig.2b

Fig. 3c shows the final result in the four year old child, demonstrating unrestricted function of the facial nerve.

Case 4: Intraosseous hemangioma of the mandible - An example of a 2-phase therapeutic approach

Osseous hemangiomas can be the cause for life-threatening hemorrhages if a tooth is extracted when the presence of such a lesion is unknown. In this situation, following an attempted tooth extraction at another site, we were forced to use mandibular resection with exarticulation, in order to prevent exsanguination. The mandible was cystically expanded and lined by endothelium (Fig. 4 a).

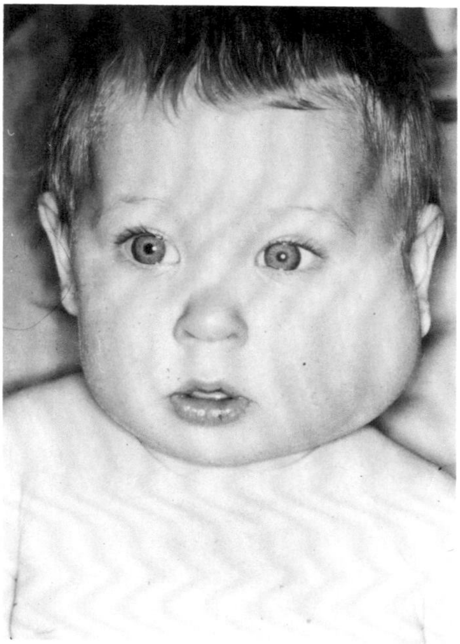

Fig.3a

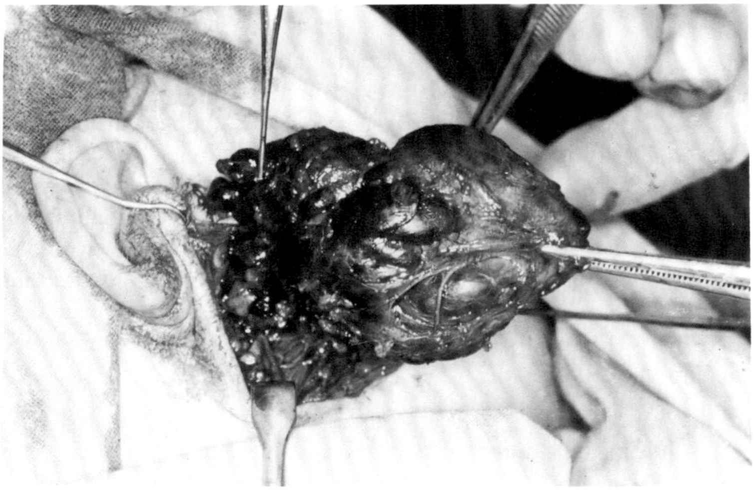

Fig.3b

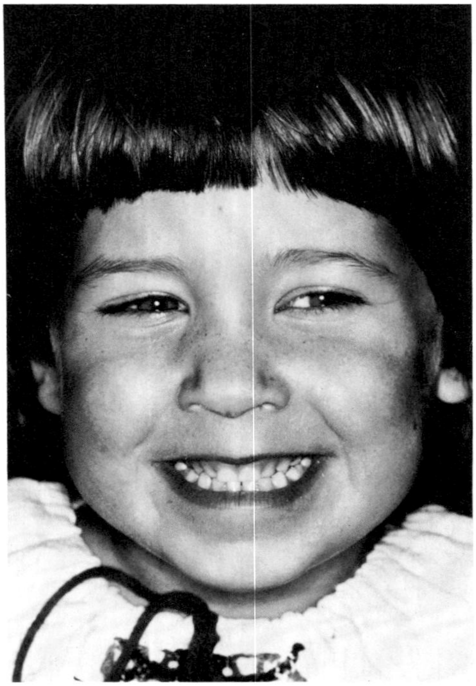

Fig. 3c

Arterial pressure was high in the considerable enlarged blood channel. Later clinical experiences have shown that the extraction site or any other osseous cavity in the region of a hemangioma of bone can be secured by bone cement. Application of this method provides time for planning the subsequent surgical procedure. Depending upon the site, it may be attempted to cut off the supply from the vessels to the respective bone. Bleeding continuing from Haversian canals in spite of this measure can be controlled by application of bone wax. A case from our clinical practice showed that this type of management can result in thrombosis in the hemangioma and thus permit removal of thrombus and endothelium using curettage in the course of follow-up surgery (Fig. 4 b). Some of the bony structure can be preserved and will regenerate (Fig. 4 c).

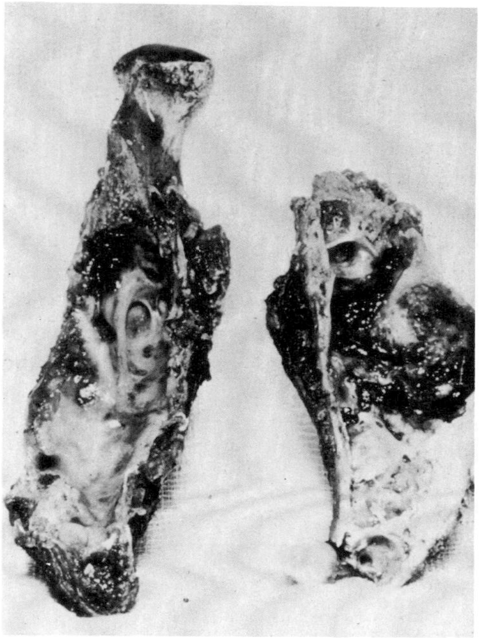

Fig. 4a

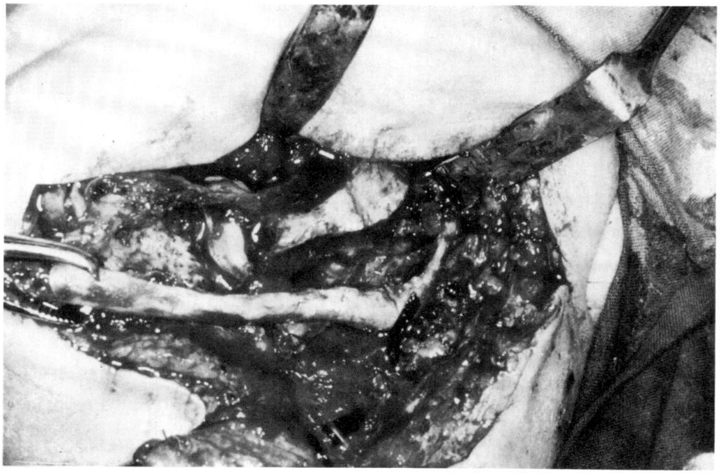

Fig. 4b

Discussion and Conclusion

As demonstrated by the case reports, every individual case requires that consideration be given to the possibility of spontaneous involution of hemangiomas when deciding upon the mode of management, especially if the lesions occur in the exposed regions of the face. Primary excision of very large cavernous and capillary vascular tumors in the periorbital region are accompanied by tissue loss and results obtained following plastic surgery with tissue taken from adjacent regions are still unsatisfactory. Our experiences have shown that partial reduction frequently produces further involution. It appears that processes conducive to the emergence of thrombosis are set in motion which will eventually generate cicatrization. Parents of children suffering from hemangiomas may be acquainted with the possibility of spontaneous involution and, if necessary, with suitable methods of surgery by presenting photographs documenting other case histories. Involution is unlikely to occur with nevus flammeus and is never seen in arterio-venous fistulas.

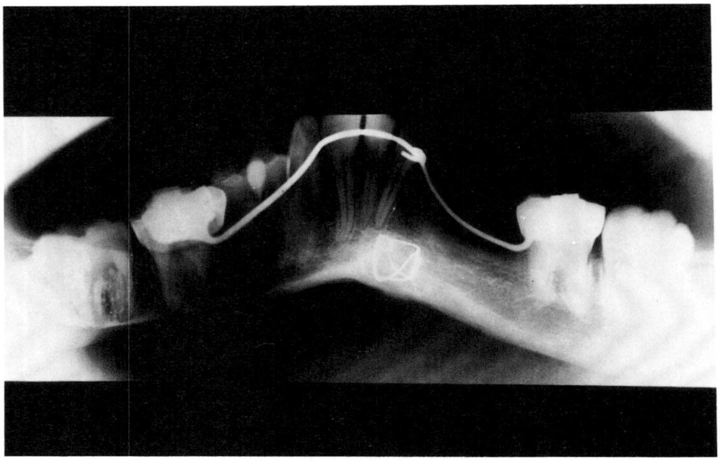

Fig. 4c

The intraosseous hemangioma must be considered as an entity of its own. Using the example of a mandibular hemangioma, we reported on a 2-phase surgical procedure resulting from special circumstances. A 10-year-old boy had been operated on before at another hospital. The vessels supplying the intraosseous lesion, branches of the carotid artery, had already been ligated. As a consequence of this procedure intraosseous thrombosis accompanied by a coagulum was observed. The central coagulum was readily removable and bone resection could be avoided.

References

[1] Batsakis JG: Tumors of the Head and Neck. Williams & Wilkins Baltimore/London, Repring 1980

[2] Bredt H: Formen der Angiome. Deutscher Röntgenkongreß 1963, Teil B. Urban & Schwarzenberg, München-Berlin 1964

[3] Gauwerky F: Diskussionsbemerkungen zum Thema Strahlentherapie der Hämangiome. Deutscher Röntgenkongreß 1963, Teil B. Urban & Schwarzenberg, München-Berlin 1964

[4] Korting GW, Denk R: Dermatologische Differentialdiagnose. Schattauer, Stuttgart-New York 1974

[5] Proppe A: Das klinische Bild der Hämangiome und die Aussichten ihrer Behandlung. Deutscher Röntgenkongreß 1976, Teil B. Urban & Schwarzenberg , München-Berlin 1964

[6] Proppe A, Hauss H: Pathogenese und nosologische Stellung der Blutschwämme. Arch.klin.exp.Derm. (1963) 194 - 216

[7] Scheunemann H: Conservative Parotidectomy in Infancy and Childhood. Journal of maxillo-facial surgery 3 (1975) 37 - 40

[8] Schürmann K, Voth D: Die Bedeutung der transfrontalen Orbitotomie für die operative Behandlung der intraorbitalen raumfordernden Prozesse. Adv. Ophthal., 22 (1972) 188 - 239

Transconjunctival excision of retrobulbar cavernous hemangiomas

G. Kommerell

Abstract

Five large cavernous hemangiomas located in the muscle cone behind the eye were removed through a transconjunctival approach. The traditional lateral orbitotomy was avoided by reducing the tumor size with bipolar diathermy. This technique requires the use of a microscope with coaxial illumination and coaxial observation of both the surgeon and his assistent.

Introduction

Cavernous hemangioma is the most common tumor in the orbit [1], most often localized in the muscle cone behind the eye. It can be diagnosed clinically using the following criteria: (1) An axial exophthalmos that has slowly progressed over years, (2) a globular or oval mass seen in CT scanning, well delineated from muscles and optic nerve [4], (3) high amplitude internal echos throughout the tumor in the ultrasonogram [1], and (4) a moderate visual impairment due to optic nerve compression and/or distorsion of the back of the eye [1].

Table I: Cavernous hemangiomas

case	age	visual acuity before surgery	visual acuity after surgery	complication
1	50	0.03	0.1	-
2	39	1.0	1.0	-
3	61	0.5	0.5	pupil sector paresis
4	63	0.3	0.3	-
5	33	0.5	0.8	lateral rectus palsy (transitory)

Surgery is performed to prevent visual loss, or to relieve headache. The traditional approach to remove the tumor is through a lateral orbitotomy [3]. We have stopped using this technique [2], however, as we have found that cavernous hemangiomas can be shrunk considerably with bipolar diathermy. After reducing their size, they can be removed transconjunctivally. The technique requires the use of a microscope with coaxial illumination and coaxial observation of both the surgeon and his assistent.

Methods

Five patients presented with a cavernous hemangioma (Tab. I). In all cases, the tumor was approximately half the size of the eye ball, located in the retrobulbar muscle cone (Fig. 1). Visual acuity and fields were only moderately affected, except for case 1 with a visual acuity of 0.03. There was only a slight limitation of eye motility in some of the patients.

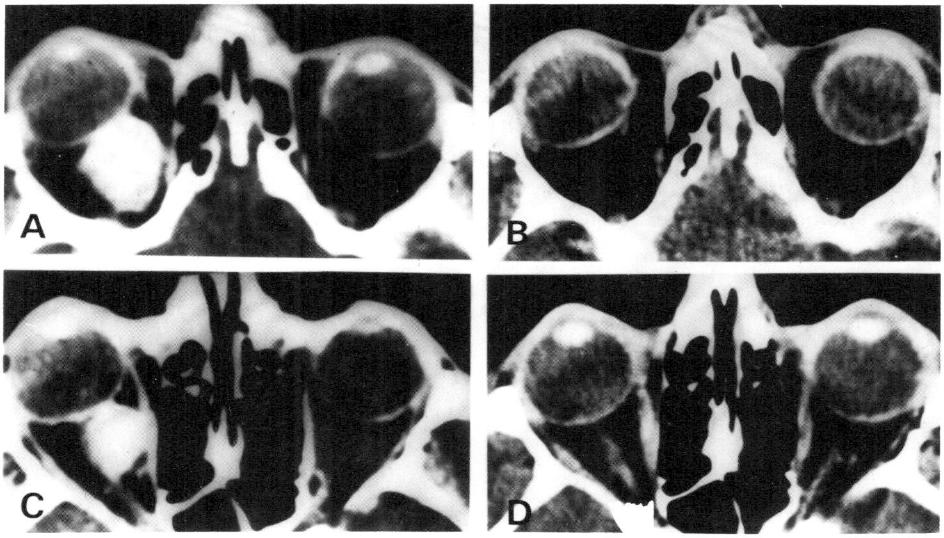

Fig. 1: Computed tomogram of a cavernous hemangioma. Comparable sections before (A, C) and after (B, D) surgery. There was still a slight globe indentation two years after removal of the tumor (B).

The conjunctiva was incised at the limbus of the cornea, in the quadrant where the tumor appeared nearest to the globe in the CT scan. Tenon's capsule was entered by blunt seperation of the connective tissues. The posterior aspect of Tenon's capsule could be reached without turning the globe and without detaching an eye muscle. Two spatulas were introduced; one of them was held against the sclera, the other against the soft orbital tissues. These spatulas were then used to "palpate" the dome of the tumor by gently pressing their tips against retrobulbar tissue, moving the tips in parallel with a constant distance of about 5 mm between them (Fig. 2). This procedure requires some experience because a cavernous hemangioma tends to slosh around in the soft retrobulbar fat. Hence, it is not always easy to locate the tumor. Once the vertex of the tumor had been "felt", the spatulas were handed over to the assistent, and Tenon's capsule was opened between the spatulas using scissors. Retrobulbar fat obscuring the tumor was severed by blunt separation, carefully avoiding nerves and vessels. As soon as the bluish surface of the hemangioma appeared, the capsule was grasped with a very small hook, and the tumor was pulled upwards. This allowed the surrounding fat to fall back, so that a few square millimeters of the tumor surface appeared. This area was then coagulated with bipolar diathermy and grasped with a forceps. The tumor was rotated so as to expose an other part of its surface for repeated bipolar diathermy. Hence, the tumor gradually lost turgor. Eventually, folds could be pulled up with the bipolar forceps, applying diathermy to the interior of the tumor (Fig. 3). This was much more effective in reducing the tumor than surface diathermy. As the hemangioma shrunk, the posterior surface of the tumor could be visualized. in contrast to other vascular tumors, large feeding vessels were not found. small feeding vessels, however, had to be coagulated, The tumor was dissected free directly along its capsule to avoid cutting motor or sensory nerves that traverse the retrobulbar space. A curved spatula facilitated the "delivery" by rendering support from below. The tumor, reduced to a slack bag, could be removed in toto in four of the five cases. Only in case 5, a piecemeal reduction of the tumor was required to cut unusually strong strands of connective tissue between the posterior pole of the tumor and the anulus tendineus of the orbital apex.

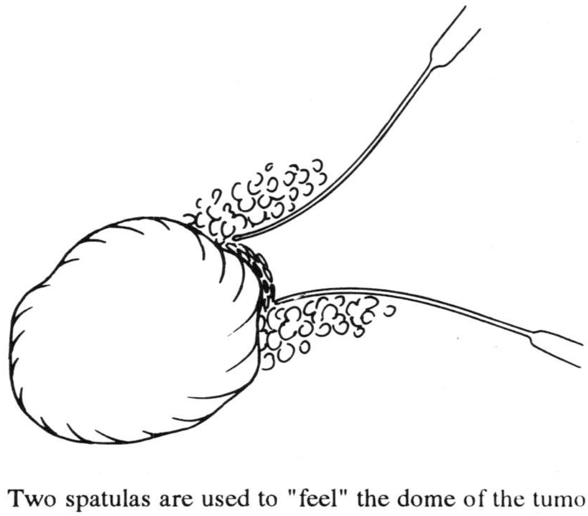

Fig. 2: Two spatulas are used to "feel" the dome of the tumor in the depth of the orbit.

Results

The retrobulbar cavernous hemangioma was completely removed in all cases. In accordance with the literature [1], tumor regrowth was not observed. A postoperative CT scan is generally not indicated after removal of a cavernous hemangioma. However, in one case a postoperative CT scan was made when the patient developed a third nerve palsy two years after surgery, probably due to a microvascular insufficiency. Interestingly, the curvature of the globe was still slightly flattened in the area where the tumor had been pressing on the eye (Fig. 1).

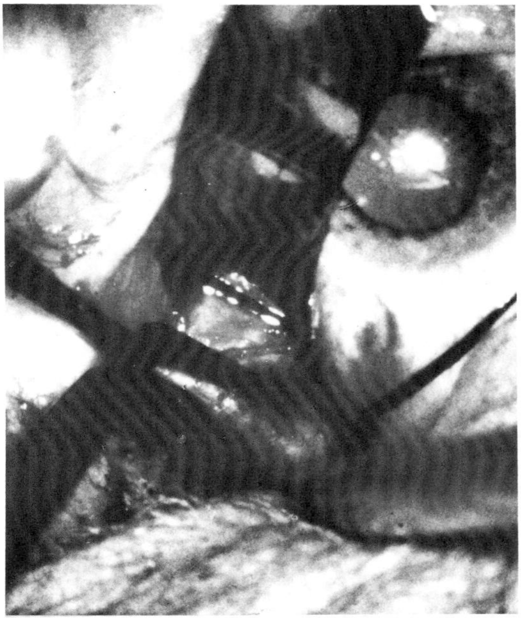

Fig. 3: When the cavernous hemangioma has lost turgor after surface diathermy, folds can be pulled up with the bipolar forceps and diathermy applied to the interior of the tumor.

Visual acuity improved slightly in two, and remained the same in 3 cases (Tab. I). Complete recovery was not expected because chronic pressure of the tumor had led to optic atrophy and/or to choroidal changes. Papilledema, present in four of the five cases before surgery, resolved. There were no serious complications. One patients (case 5) had a lateral rectus palsy postoperatively, but he regained normal motility of the eye within weeks. Another patient had a permanent sector palsy of the sphincter pupillae indicating damage to a posterior ciliary nerve.

References

[1] Harries GF, Jacobiec FA: Cavernous hemangioma in the orbit: a clinicopathologic analysis of sixty-six cases. In: Jacobiec FA (ed): Ocular and Adnexal Tumors. Aesculapius Publishing Company, Alabama, USA, (1978) 741 - 781

[2] Kommerell G, Witschel H: Plädoyer für vordere und laterale Orbitotomie. Fortschr Ophthalmol 79 (1982) 300 - 302

[3] Wright JE: Surgical exploration of the orbit. Trans Ophthalmol Soc UK 99 (1979) 238 - 240

[4] Unsöld R, Hoyt WF, Newton TH: Die computertomographischen Merkmale des kavernösen Hämangioms und ihre Bedeutung für die Differentialdiagnose im Muskeltrichter gelegener Tumoren der Orbita. Klin Mbl Augenheilk 175 (1979) 773 - 785

Primary Non-Hodgkin's Lymphomas of the Orbit

R. Hohle, K. Merkel, D. Dienemann, H. Stein, H.-H. Goebel

Abstract

Nine primary non-Hodgkin's lymphomas (NHL) of the orbit were examined in a retrospective study and classified according to the Kiel classification [13].

The tumors derived from 6 men and 3 women with ages ranging from 42 to 75 years. All tumors were low-grade malignant B-cell NHL with the following distribution:

5 lymphocytic lymphomas, 2 immunocytic lymphomas, 1 centrocytic lymphoma and 1 centroblastic-centrocytic lymphoma. This study demonstrates the importance of immunhistological examination.

Introduction

Reactive hyperplasia as well as neoplasms of the lymphatic tissue of the orbit only rarely occur. The reported incidence of lymphoid neoplasms varies from 4 to 9 % of all orbital biopsies [3, 5, 6, 7, 8, 14, 18]. Whereas Hodgkin's disease is extremely rare [1, 15] and when seen it is mostly part of a known systemic disease. The frequency of pseudolymphoma and primary NHL differs widely in the literature. This may be due to the difficulty in distinguishing a neoplastic process from a reactive hyperplasia seen in small biopsies.

New immunhistological methods are helpful and necessary for the diagnosis of NHL [20].

Material and Methods

In a retrospective study 9 primary orbital NHL were analysed.

They were collected between 1979 and 1986 at the Department of Neuropathology of the University of Mainz. These lymphomas were classified according to the Kiel classification. The tissue was fixed in formalin and embedded in paraffin. Sections were stained with hematoxylin and eosin (H + E), Giemsa, and periodic acid Schiff (PAS). For demonstration of B - or T- cell nature of the tumor cells, as well as membrane or intracytoplasmic immunoglobulins, the APAAP - method [4] was used.

Results

The clinical features of the 9 patients are summarized in Table II.

Most often a protrusio bulbi with diplopia was the leading finding.

Table I: List of used antibodies

Antibody	Specifity	Source
4KB5	Pan-B	D.Y.Mason, Oxford
Ki-B3	Pan-B	A.Feller, Kiel
IgM	my-Kette	D.Y.Mason, Oxford
Kappa	kappy-Kette	Dianova, Hamburg
Lambda	lambda-Kette	Dianova, Hamburg
UCHL-1	Pan-T	P.Beverly, London
LC	Cd 45	Dakopatts, Glostrup
Ra-Lysozym	Muramidase	Dakopatts, Glostrup
Ber-H2	CD 30	H.Stein, Berlin
2G7	CD 21	Th.Schulz, Innsbruck

As expected, none of the tumors reacted with antibodies against Hodgkin cells (Ber- H2). The reaction with common-leucocytic antigen (C11) was positive. The results of conventional and immunohistological examination are presented in Table III. All malignant lymphomas belong to the B-cell system because of its positive or partly positive reaction with the B-cell marker and KB5 or KiB3 and its negative reaction with the T-cell marker UCHL-1. Five of the 9 cases showed a proliferation of small lymphoid cells which displace preserved germinal centers. We proved this phenomenon by using the 2G7 antibody against follicular dendritic reticulum cells. In none of these cases intracytoplasmic immunoglobulins or light chains could be demonstrated. Only in case 3, we could show a discrete expression of immunoglobulin M at the cell surface. Case 5 demonstrated a focal change into an immunoblastic lymphoma. Because of the absence of intracytoplasmic immunoglobulins we had to classify these tumors as malignant lymphocytic lymphoma.

The cases 6 and 7 presented the morphological features of a lymphoplasmocytoid malignant lymphoma. This is proven by a monoclonal expression of intracytoplasmic light chains of immunoglobulins, kappa in case 6 and lambda in case 7. In some cells so called "Dutcher bodies" (intranuclear inclusion of immunoglobulins) were demonstrated.

Case 8 showed the morphological signs of a centrocytic lymphoma. Case 9 presents a typical centroblastic-centrocytic lymphoma with the presence of pseudofollicels.

Discussion

The NHL of the orbit included in our study could all be classified according to the Kiel classification [13].

Table II: Sex, Age and Clinical features

Case	Sex : Age	Clinical features
1	m 68	protrusio bulbi since 1 year
2	m 71	orbital mass
3	m 75	protrusio bulbi 1 year diplopia
4	m 42	protrusio bulbi since 9 years
5	m 79	orbital mass
6	f 59	protrusion bulbi
7	m 75	reccurance/ 1th op 2 years ago
8	f 57	protrusio bulbi
9	f 44	recurrancy/ 1th op 6 years ago protrusio bulbi

The tumors showed no significant histological or cytological differences from NHL occurring in lymphnodes. There was a remarkable difference, however, in the distribution of the various NHL subtypes in the orbit relative to their distribution in the lymph nodes. The comparison with other studies or primary NHL of the orbit is

Table III: Antigen profile of tumor cells

Case	Diagnosis	LC	UCHL-1	4 KB5	KI-B3	Immunoglobulins
1	ml, lymphocytic	pos.	neg.	p/n	p/n	neg.
2	ml, lymphocytic	pos.	neg.	p/n	p/n	neg.
3	ml, lymphocytic	pos	neg.	p/n	p/n	IGM
4	ml, lymphocytic	pos.	neg.	pos.	p/n	neg.
5	ml, lymphocytic with change into an immunoblastoma	pos.	neg.	pos.	p/n	neg.
6	ml, cyotid immunocytoma	pos.	neg.	pos.	pos.	IGM, KAPPA
7	ml, lympho-plasmocyotid, immunocytoma	pos.	neg.	pos.	p/n	IGM, Lambda
8	ml, centrocytic	pos.	neg.	pos.	pos.	IGM, KAPPA
9	ml, centroblastic centrocytic	pos.	neg.	pos.	p/n	neg.

p/n = partly positive

difficult because of the use of different classification which is not comparable with the Kiel classification without the knowledge of further details. In Table IV the results of recent publications are summarized using either the Kiel classification or the American Working Formulation [16].

Table IVa: Results of different authors

	own cases	Schwarze et. al (1975)	Wessel et. al (1983)
	n = 9	n = 4	n = 11
Medium age (range)	63(44 - 79)		64(38 - 82)
Sex ratio m/f	6/3		10/1
ml, lymphomatic	5		
ml, immunocytoma	2	4	6
ml, centricytic	1		
ml, centroblastic centrocytic	1		2
plasmocytoma			1
ml, immunoblastom		1	
ml, lymphoblastic unclassified		1	1
ml, lymphoblastic Burkitt - type			1

We were able to collect 45 NHL of the orbit using the data from the literature. Most tumors occured in the 6th and 7th decade-ranging from 38 to 82 years. Males were more often affected than females. SCHWARZE [17], LAZZARINO [12], HARRIES [9] and we could only find low grade malignant NHL. WESSEL [22] and

BENNET [2], reported 5 cases of high grade malignant NHL: 2 immunoblastic NHL, 2 unclassified NHL and 1 lymphoblastic NHL of Burkitt type. The immunohistological well definable immunocytic lymphoma is reported in 19 of the 45 cases (42 %).

Table IVb: Results of different authors

	Lazzarino et. al (1985) n = 4	Bennet et. al (1986) n = 10	Harries et. al (1984) n = 7
Medium age (range)	65(42 - 78)	63(46 - 71)	
Sex ratio m/f	1/3	1/3	5/5
ml, lymphomatic			
ml, immunocytoma	3	1	3
ml, centricytic	1	1	
ml, centroblastic centrocytic		5	
plasmocytoma			
ml, immunoblastom		1	
ml, lymphoblastic unclassified		1	
ml, lymphoblastic Burkitt - type		1	

Eleven cases of centroblastic-centrocytic lymphoma are mainly reported by American authors corresponding to a more frequent incidence of the lymphomas in the western hemisphere in general.

In our investigation the high number of lymphocytic lymphomas is remarkable. This type of NHL is not reported by the other authors and is not regarded as a separate entity in the Kiel classification. We want to point out this group and distinguish it from immunocytic lymphoma and the chronic lymphocytic leukemia of B-cell type. The diagnosis is based upon immunohistological techniques as well as clinical findings.

We believe that the present immunohistological staining methods are sensible enough and reliable to demonstrate intracytoplasmic immunoglobulins and their light chains.

If there is no reaction of antibodies with immunoglobulins an immunocytic lymphoma cannot be diagnosed. On the other hand a B-cell lymphocytic leukemia can be excluded clinically. None of our patients had a leukemia or an infiltration of the bone marrow at the time of diagnosis. This fact corresponds to the data in the literature. In the literature we could only find one case of B-cell lymphocytic leukemia with bilateral orbital deposits but uninvolved lymphnodes [19].

In comparison to the results of other authors, our findings lead to the following conclusions: Primary NHL of the orbit are rare and are found mainly in the 6th and 7th decade of life. Most frequently these tumors are low-grade malignant NHL.

New immunohistological methods allow a reliable diagnosis of a lymphocytic lymphoma. Only immunohistological investigations separate a T-cell lymphoma from the B-cell type.

Our results support the view, that there may be a lymphocytic lymphoma which is derived from the B-cell population.

References

[1] Azar HA, Espinoza CG, Richman AV, Saba SR, Wang T: "Undifferentiated" large cell malignancies. Hum Pathol 13 (1982) 323 - 333

[2] Bennett CL, Putterman A, Bitran JD, Recant W, Shapiro CM, Karesh J, Kaokhe U: Staging and therapy of orbital lymphomas. Cancer 57 (1986) 1204 - 1208

[3] Berard CW, Dorfman RF, Kaufman N (eds): Malignant Lymphoma. Williams and Wilkins, Baltimore-London-Los Angeles- Sydney 1987

[4] Cordell JL, Falini B, Erber WN, Ghosh AK, Abdulaziz Z, MacDonald S, Pulford KAF, Stein H, Mason DY: Immunoenzymaticlabelling of monoclonal antibodies using immune complexes of alkaline phosphatase and monoklonal antialkaline phospatase (APAAP). J Histochem Cytochem 32 (1984) 219 - 229

[5] Dolman PJ, Rootman J, Quenville NF: Signet-ring cell lymphoma in the orbit. A case report and review. Can J Ophthalm 21 (1986) 242 - 245

[6] Font LR, Shields J: Large cell lymphoma of the orbit with microvillours projections ("Porcupine Lymphoma"): Arch Ophthalm 103 (1985) 1715 - 1719

[7] Gordon PS, Juillard GJF, Selch MT, Parker RG, Fu YS: Orbital lymphomas and pseudolymphomas: Treatment with radiation therapy. Radiology 159 (1986) 797 - 799

[8] Grove AS: Evaluation of exophthalmos. New Engl J Med 292 (1979) 1005 - 1012

[9] Harris NL, Harmon DC, Pilch BZ, Goodman ML, Bhan AK: Immunhistologic diagnosis of orbital lymphoid infiltrates. Am J Surg Pathol 8 (1984) 83 - 91

[10] Knowles DM, Jakobiec FA: Orbital lymphoid neoplasms. A clinico-pathological study of 60 patients. Cancer 46 (1980) 576 - 589

[11] Knowles DM, Jakobiec FA: Ocular adnexal lymphoid neoplasma. Clinical, histopathologic, electron microscopic and immunologic characteristics. Hum Pathol 13 (1982) 148 - 162

[12] Lazzarino M, Morra E, Rosso R, Brusamolino E, Pagnucco G, Castello A, Ghisolfi A, Tafi A, Zennaro G, Bernasconi C: Clinicopathologic and immunologic characteristics of non-Hodgkin's lymphomas presenting in the orbit. A report of 8 cases. Cancer 55 (1985) 1907 - 1912

[13] Lennert K: Malignant Lymphomas other than Hodgkin's disease. In: Uelinger E: Handbuch der speziellen pathologischen Anatomie und Histologie, Bd. 1, Teil 3. Springer Verlag, Berlin-Heidelberg-New York 1978

[14] Mittal BB, Deutsch M, Kennerdell J, Johnson B: Paraocular lymphoid tumors. Radiology 159 (1986) 793 - 796

[15] Patel S, Rootman J: Nodular sclerosing Hodgkin's disease of the orbit. Ophthalmol 90 (1983) 1433 - 1436

[16] Rosenberg SA, Berard CW, Brown BW: National Cancer Institute sponsored study of classifications of non-Hodkin's lymphomas. Summary and description of a "Working Formulation" for clinical usage. Cancer 49 (1982) 2112 - 2135

[17] Schwarze EW, Radaszkiewicz T, Pülhorn G, Goos M, Lennert K: Maligne and benigne Lymphome des Auges, der Lid- und Orbitalregion. Virchows Arch Abt A: Pathol Anat 370 (1976) 85 - 96

[18] Shields JA, Bakewell B, Augsburger JJ, Flanagan JC: Classification and incidence of space occupying lesions of the orbit. A survey of 644 biopsies. Arch ophthalmol 102 (1984) 1606 - 1611

[19] Skinnider LF, Romanchuk KG: Orbital involvement in chronic lymphocytic lymphoma. Can J Ophthalmol 19 (1984) 142 - 144

[20] Stein H, Gerdes J: Phänotypische und genotypische Marker bei malignen Lymphomen: Ein Beitrag zum zellulären Ursprung des Morbus Hodgkin und der malignen Histiozytose sowie Implikationen für die Klassifikation

der T-Cell und B-CellLymphome. Verh Dtsch Ges Path 70 (1986) 127 - 151

[21] Vogiatzis KV: Lymphoid tumors of the orbit and ocular adnexa. A long-term follow up. Ann Ophthalmol 16 (1984) 1046 - 1055

[22] Wessel H, Stiller D, Bahn H, Herde J, Trost M: Maligne Nicht-Hodgkin-Lymphome des Augenbereiches. Histologische KJlassifizierung und immunhistologische Untersuchungen. Zbl allg Path u pathol Anat 128 (1983) 339 - 350

Radiation Therapy of Malignant Lymphoma of the Eye and Orbit

S. Zapf, J. Kutzner

Introduction

Lymphoreticular tumors of the eye and the orbit, including adnexal structures, are known to be rare disorders. According to the literature, the frequency of occurrence lies within the range of 0.5 - 2 % of all malignant lymphomas. Freemen [6] reported only 32 orbital involvements out of 12447 lymphomas collected from 1954 to 1960. The greatest number reported was 115 cases, observed between 1970 and 1980. Due to its rarity, knowledge and understanding of the disease still remain limited. This report attempts to present our data on lymphomas of the eye and its orbit, collected over a period of seven years between 1980 and 1987. A review of the literature is included.

Materials and Methods

From 1980 to 1987 ten patients out of 403 were treated with radiation therapy for primary or secondary malignant lymphoma of the orbit, the eyelid or the lacrimal gland. Prior to irradiation, a complete staging was performed to exclude tumor generalisation. The diagnosis was confirmed histologically. Follow-up was performed by clinical examination, by computed tomography (CT), and ophthalmologically. The youngest patient was 15 years, the oldest 78 years, the mean age being 41.7 years. Clinical signs at initial presentation were exophthalmus, lid swelling, diplopia, and disturbances of ocular movement. In 8 patients the tumor involved one (stage I) or both (stage II) orbits, other sites were both eyelids or the lacrimal gland. Primary tumor occurrence was noted in 6 cases, 4 were secondary. All tumors underwent histological confirmation, 1 case being M. Hodgkin IV, all others were classified as Non Hodgkin Lymphomas (NHL), 4 centrocytic centroblastic, 4 lymphoblastic, 1 immunocytic. Treatment was by radiation therapy alone, in 4 cases following surgical intervention with remaining tumor. Radiation technique was carried out by Co60 using wedge filters with an anterior and lateral field of 6 x 6 cm size with 60 cm SSD. The lens was protected with external blocks, angulation of the lateral field 5° posteriorly to compensate for beam divergence. Each field was treated daily, 5 times per week, with fractions of 2 Gy over a 3 - 4 week period to give a total dose in the range of 30 - 40 Gy. Involvement of both orbits was treated similarly with 2 opposing lateral fields at 60 cm SSD each, the 95 % isodose enveloping the visible tumor entirely. The dosage of one fraction was determined by thermoluminescence dosimeters at the first application. The total dose load to the lens was then evaluated from this determination. Tumors of the eyelid and lacrimal gland were treated with anterior electron fields (5 MeV) with protection of the lens and conjunctiva by a special gold shield.

Results

Complete tumor regression was achieved immediately after end of treatment in all cases. There was no local recurrence up to the last follow-up or time of death, 1 patient died from disseminated lymphoma 2 months after completion of radiotherapy, 2 patients finished radiation just 2 months ago. Thus, with the low number of cases it seems to be of no advantage to determine 5 survival rates. No complications due to radiotherapy were encountered.

Table I: Differential Diagnosis of Orbital Lymphoma

Filiae	mamma BC kidney thyroid
primary carcinoma	lid lacrimal duct
inflammatory disorders of unknown etiology	endocrine ophthalmopathy pseudotumor reactive hyperplasia pseudolymphoma benign lymphoma atypic lymphoid infiltration

Discussion

In contrast to some cases reported [4, 5], local tumor control was obtained in all our cases. This may be attributed, in part, to the technique employed with use of larger fields and wedge filters. Dosage was determined individually for each patient by weighting of fields and improving wedge size leading to a homogenous dose distribution, the 95 % isodose entirely including the tumor and orbit. Similarly, KIM [7] reported of local tumor control in all cases, applying the same field size as described above without use of wedges, the anterior border of the lateral field being the lateral canthus. The medium dose applied was considerable lower than in our case.

AUSTIN-SEYMOUR [1] reported on local tumor control in all of 12 cases with a medium dosage of 36 gy administered similarly to the above. FITZPATRICK [3] recommends different total doses for primary and secondary orbital lymphoma, thus, complete remission is only achieved in 90 % of 35 cases. This distinction is not found elsewhere.

According to the literature, 5 years survival rates vary from 60 - 80 % for stage I and stage II orbital tumors. KIM [7] and FORSTER [4] showed, that the prognosis of bilateral involvement is not worse than for unilateral lymphoma.

Table II: Results of Radiotherapy of Orbital Lymphomas

	n	CR (%)	follow up (Yr)	dose Gy	side effects
Kim, Fayos 1976	18	95	8	30	2/3
Fitzpatrick 1984	35	90	3 - 8	25 - 45	0/3
Austin-Seymour 1985	12	100	6	36	2/0
Mainz 1987	10	100	1.5	37	0/0
Bessell 1987	115	90	1	30 - 40	8/5

The lens is the most radiosensitive part of orbital structures, the maximum tolerated dose being 10 - 12 Gy. Generally, cataract is the main complication that may occur in orbital irradiation. However, side effects of radiation therapy of the orbit are only rarely reported. Data presented by BESSELL [2] show 8 cataracts out of 115 patients. AUSTIN-SEYMOUR [1] and KIM [7] reported 2 radiation induced cataracts. Other side effects such as epiphora and dry eye syndrome are reported in 5 and 3 cases respectively. In our cases we had no severe complication in up to 5 years follow-up. Total absorbed dose of the lens as reported by BESSELL [2] is 15 GyY, well above the generally accepted maximum dose of 12 Gy. Others do not claim the actual dose load of the lens, the percentage of cataracts up to 10 % is similar, however [1, 7]. Therefore, the main goal of radiation therapy of orbital lymphoreticular tumors must be the local destruction of the tumor without the risk of endangering the lens with doses exceeding 10 Gy. Application of exact techniques as described above, which are supported by high resolution computer tomography, will allow administration of high doses to the orbit with homogeneous dose distribution, wedge filters should be used naturally. For curative treatment the resulting maximum absorbed dose of the contralateral lens will be up to 10 % of the applied dose, with ca 20 % ipsilateral. Similar doses are determined, when tumors of the eyelid or lacrimal gland are irradiated, on condition, that conjunctiva and lens are shielded properly.

Summary

Eight patients with orbital lymphoma and one patient each with lymphoma of the lacrimal gland and eyelids were treated with radiation therapy. Local control could be obtained in all cases with a medium dose of 37 Gy. As shown from the literature and from our own data the therapy of choice for orbital and eye lymphomas is irradiation, because curative treatment is possible in almost all cases with total doses of 40 Gy. True 5 years survival rate is up to 80 %, patients die from the generalisation of a tumor cured locally. Doses of less than 40 Gy should be administered only under palliative aspects.

References

[1] Austin-Seymour MM, Donaldson S, Egbert PR, McDougall JR, Kriss JP: Radiotherapy of lymphoid diseases of the orbit. Int. J. Rad. Onc. Biol. Phy. 11, 2 (1985) 371 - 379

[2] Bessell EM, Henk JM, Whitelocke RA, Wright JE: Ocular morbidity after radiotherapy of orbital and conjunctival lymphoma. Eye 1, 1 (1987) 90 -96

[3] Fitzpatrick PJ, Macko S: Lymphoreticular tumors of the orbit. Int. J. Rad. Onc. Biol. Phy. 10, 3 (1984) 333 - 340

[4] Foster SC, Wilson CS, Tretter PK: Radiotherapy of primary lymphoma of the orbit. AJR 111 (1971) 343 - 349

[5] Franklin CIV: Primary lymphoreticular tumors of the orbit. Clin. Radiol. 26 (1975) 137 - 140

[6] Freeman C, Berg JW, Cutler SJ: Occurance and prognosis of extranodal lymphomas. Cancer 29 (1972) 252 - 260

[7] Kim YH, Fayos JV: Primary orbital lymphoma: A radiotherapeutic experience. Int. J. Rad. Onc. Biol. Phys. 1, 11 (1976) 1099 - 1105

Acute hemorrhage and ischemic necrosis in pituitary adenomas - Pituitary Apoplexy

H. Seyer, F. Erbguth, D. Kämpf, G. Koniszewski, R. Fahlbusch

Abstract

"Pituitary apoplexy" - a term easily misunderstood - was coined to describe the sudden onset of drowsiness, ophthalmoplegia, and - sometimes - the loss of pituitary function, caused by an abrupt enlargement of a pituitary adenoma. It usually is due to acute hemorrhage, but can also be the result of ischemic necrosis and subsequent edema. Despite differing opinions, pituitary apoplexy seems to be more common in nonfunctional than in hormone-producing adenomas. Hemorrhage has a much poorer prognosis than ischemic necrosis. Acute ophthalmoplegia is the guiding symptom. Its recovery depends on early operation, but a careful clinical, endocrinologic and radiologic investigation should be performed first.

Introduction

"Pituitary apoplexy", first mentioned in 1905 by BLEIBTREU as the "destruction of the hypophysis by hemorrhage" in an acromegalic patient [1], is a historically based clinical description. It can easily be misunderstood as it does no mean a bleeding or infarction of the pituitary gland itself, as is reported by SHEEHAN and SUMMERS in 1949 [9], but characterizes a sudden onset of drowsiness, blurred vision, ophthalmoplegia and, sometimes, failure of the pituitary function, caused by acute hemorrhage or ischemic necrosis in pituitary adenomas.

The incidence of the event varies widely in reports of different authors ranging from 0.6 % [8], 1.5 % [5], 10.0 % [6] to 25.7 % [7]. This wide range in incidence depends on how often mere intraoperative or histological findings of regressive changes in the adenomas without clinical signs and symptoms of an acute event are included. Only a few authors (e.g. WAKAI et al.) found a total of 16.6 % degenerative changes, but only 9.1 % of their patients had clinical signs [10], whereas MOHR and HARDY saw a total of 9.5 % but only 0.6 %, showing a clinical picture [8]. In our opinion, the term "pituitary apoplexy" should be used only, where an acute collaps occurs clinically, as the word "apoplexy" properly implies. We estimate the actual evidence of pituitary apoplexy to be around 1 to 2 %.

Patients

Among 399 patients with pituitary adenomas, who were operated on in our clinic in 3 years, we saw 8 patients with pituitary apoplexy. This is an incidence of 2 %.

Considering 3 other patients, who were included in our series but were not from this period, a total of 11 patients, of whom 6 were female and 5 male, can be recorded. The ages ranged from 24 to 74 years. 8 patients were over 40 years old.

Results

8 patients suffered from an acute hemorrhage, 3 from an ischemic necrosis. In comparison to all 399 patients of which only 35 % showed a nonfunctional pituitary adenoma, our series of pituitary apoplexies included 9 patients with nonfunctional adenomas, i.e. 80 %. Only one was a prolactinoma and one an acromegalic.

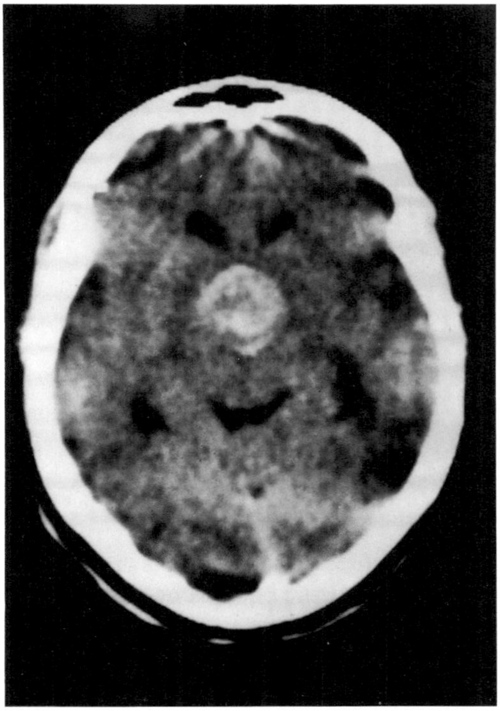

Fig. 1: Hemorrhage into a GH-secreting pituitary adenoma up to the hypothalamic region

An acute onset was the typical presenting symptom in 10 out of 11 patients with a previously unknown adenoma. Only the acromegalic patient was noticed before due to his physiognomical changes.

Ophthalmoplegia was the guiding symptom in 10 of 11 cases. Other symptoms were headache, blurred vision and drowsiness. Severe cases showed unconsciousness and hypothalamic failure, hemiparesis and aphasia. In all the latter cases the cause proved to be an acute hemorrhage. Although ischemic necrosis started dramatically, too, the clinical course turned out to be benign.

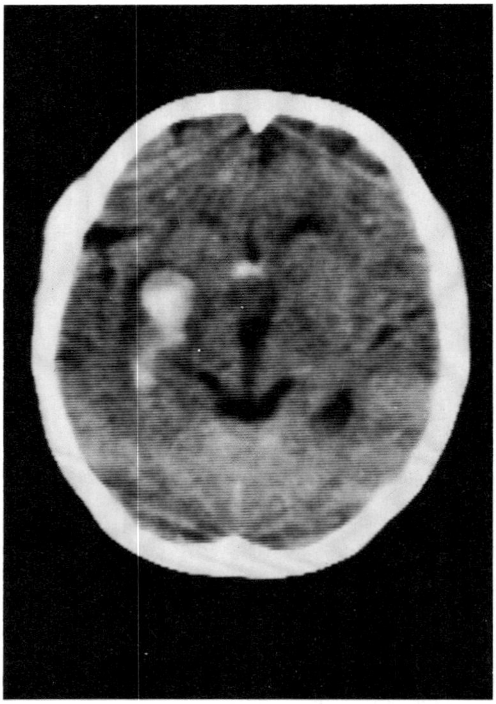

Fig. 2: Hemorrhage into a non-functional pituitary adenoma and to the left hemisphere

Oculomotor palsy was most frequent (6 cases), 2 patients had ophthalmoplegia (fig. 4)of both eyes. 2 other patients suffered from diplopia only for a short while (up to 2 days). Combinations of different optomotoric nerve palsies were seen in 4 patients, in one case a complete ophthalmoplegia of the 3, 4th and 6th nerve. Visual acuity was reduced in 8 patients, partly to light perception with no visual field left. Other field defects were bitemporal hemianopia and concentric field reduction.

All patients showed pathologic X-ray findings with destruction of the sella floor. In many cases the cranial computed tomography was helpful in differentiating between hemorrhage and necrosis. The acromegalic patient had a hemorrhage into the adenoma and up to the hypothalamic region, which caused hydrocephalus and made ventriculo-atrial shunting necessary (see fig. 1). Clinically we saw a nearly total loss of visual acuity, ophthalmoplegia, unconsciousness and hypothalamic dysregulation was observed. The severe diencephalic lesion operation on the adenoma itself precluded any operation on the adenoma itself. The patient survived. The adenoma had been partially destroyed by the hemorrhage, so that the GH levels were reduced to half of the previous value. Three years later, after radiation and pharmacotherapy, the GH levels were normal, and only partial oculomotor palsy on one eye and a light organic brain syndrome persisted.

Another patient had a hemorrhage into the adenoma and into the left hemisphere, which caused a hemiparesis, drowsiness and aphasia in addition to ophthalmologic disorders, i.e. paresis of the 6th nerve and blurred vision (see fig. 2).

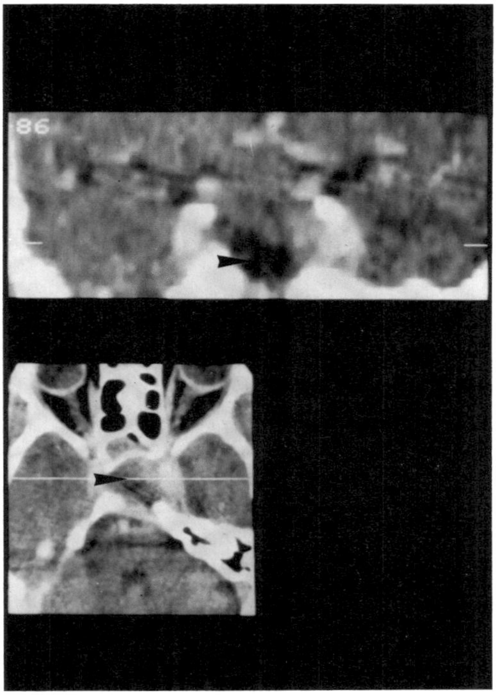

Fig. 3

In a 3rd case suffering from complete ophthalmoplegia and a decrease of the visual acuity of the right eye, combined with severe headache and drowsiness, the CT showed no sign of an intracranial hemorrhage. However a intracranial hemorrhage was present in the sellar region (see fig. 3) At operation we found an ischemic necrosis.

Discussion

Since the introduction of cranial computed tomography parasellar extension of pituitary adenomas are found to occur more often than is clinically assumed. Normally the optomotoric nerves are able to evade the slow growth of pituitary adenomas. However in cases of sudden enlargement of the adenomas caused by acute hemorrhage or ischemic necrosis with edema, ophthalmoplegia is inevitable. This is the crucial factor in pituitary apoplexy.

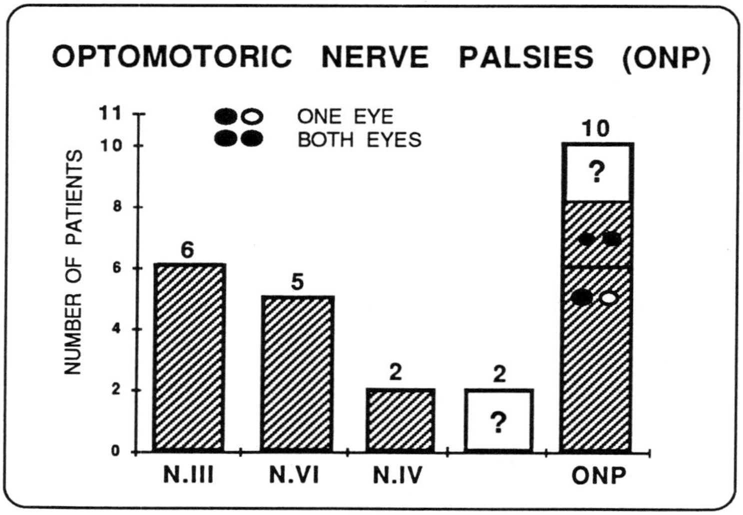

Fig. 4

Nevertheless, optomotoric nerve palsies show good recovery. Only in 2 patients did the partial oculomotor palsies persist for several years. For this reason the operation should take place within 2 weeks time after the event, when oculomotor palsies occur [4]. In all cases is enough time for careful clinical, radiologic and neurendocrinologic investigations. Only acute amaurosis requires an emergency operation.

The expression "pituitary apoplexy" was coined in 1950 by BROUGHAM et al. [2]. It is a clinical description, which may have lost its importance nowadays because of the excellency of modern methods of investigation. Nevertheless it is a useful term and in view of the possible abrupt loss of pituitary function [3], it focusses the clinician's attention to a special clinical course in the disease process of pituitary adenomas.

References

[1] Bleibtreu L: Ein Fall von Akromegalie (Zerstörung der Hypophysis durch Blutung). Münch. med. Wschr. 41 (1905) 2079 - 80

[2] Brougham M, Heusner AP, Adams RS: Acute degenerative changes in adenomas of the pituitary body - with special reference to pituitary apoplexy. J. Neurosurg. 7 (1950) 421 - 439

[3] Fahlbusch R, Marguth F: Klinik und Behandlung der Hypophysen-ademome. Dtsch. Ärztebl. 27 (1973) 1795 - 1804

[4] Hamer J: Incidence and prognosis of oculomotor palsy after subarachnoid hemorrhage due to ruptured aneurysms of the posterior communicating artery. In Samii M, Jannetta PJ (eds.): The cranial nerves. Springer, Berlin 1981 237 - 240

[5] Hollenhorst RW, Younge BR: Ocular manifestations produced by adenomas of the pituitary gland: analysis of 1000 cases. In Kohler PO, Ross GT (eds.), Diagnosis and treatment of pituitary tumors. Excerpta Medica, Amsterdam (1973) 53 - 68

[6] Kaplan B, Day AL, Quisling R, Ballinger W: Hemorrhage into pituitary adenomas. Surg. Neurol. 20 (1983) 280 - 287

[7] Mohanty S, Tandon PN, Banerjii AK, Prakash B: Haemorrhage into pituitary adenomas. J. Neurol. Neurosurg. Psychiat. 40 (1977) 987 - 991

[8] Mohr G, Hardy J: Hemorrhage, necrosis, and apoplexy in pituitary adenomas. Surg. Neurol. 18 (1982) 181 - 189

[9] Sheehan HL, Summers VK: The syndrome of hypopituitarism. Q. J. Med. 18 (1949) 319 - 378

[10] Wakai S, Fukushima T, Teramoto A, Sano K: Pituitary apoplexy: Its incidence and clinical significance. J. Neurosurg. 55 (1981) 187 - 193

Visual Disturbances in Childhood caused by Craniopharyngiomas

K.-E. Richard, P. Sanker, A. Swinka, R.A. Frowein

Introduction

The extraordinarily successful operative results of craniopharyngiomas in children, published by MATSON [9] in 1969, provoked numerous comments on both the operative, the palliative procedures and the postoperative irradiation of the remaining tumor [2 - 6, 10, 12, 13], while some of these authors studied the fate of the visual function in the course of the disease [2 - 5, 8].

Craniopharyngiomas a complex impairment both of the visual and the endocrine system leading to many clinical problems. Under this reason it is still an open question how far microsurgical techniques have brought distinct improvements not only for the survival rate but also for the visual functions, necessary for the quality of life of these patients.

Patient material

Ten percent of children with symptoms of a brain tumor suffered from a craniopharyngioma. During the period 1951 - 86, 54 children between 1 and 14 years old with this type of tumor were operated on and since 1969 with the aid of an operating microscope. The tumor mainly spread suprasellarly in 27 children, mainly retrosellarly in 16 children, and in 11 children, intrasellarly, parasellarly or presellarly.

The main age at time of surgery ranged between 7 and 8 years (Fig. 1)

Results

1. Visual disturbances present at first admission

At the initial examination visual disturbances ranked first. They were present in every child with a supra- or a retrosellar tumor (Fig. 2). Signs and symptoms of intracranial pressure (ICP) increase, such as headache, vomiting or papilledema, and endocrine disturbances followed.

The frequency of preceding false diagnoses resulting from visual disturbances in our children was 22 %.

In 59 % of the children a reduced visual acuity was found particularly frequently in tumors with supra- or with retro-sellar tumor growth (Tab. I).

Only in half of the children were visual field defects detected, just as frequently an optic atrophy, and only in 43 % of the patients a papilledema.

These figures correspond to the data of CARMEL and KENNEDY [2, 8].

2. *Visual disturbances in the course of the disease*

2.1. *Suprasellar craniopharyngiomas*

Most of the children with suprasellar craniopharyngiomas had noticed visual disturbances up to 3 to 6 months before the operation, some of the 1 - 3 years before (Fig. 3a).

Tab. I: Pre-operative visual dysfunction in children with cranio-pharyngiomas

	KENNEDY Glasgow CC.	CARMEL New York (43)	COLOGNE 1951 - 1986 Total (54)	Suprasellar (27)	Retrosellar (16)	Atypical (11)
Diminished Vision	60%	--	59% (32)	70% (19)	63%(10)	27% (11)
Visual Field Defects	50%	54%	50% (27)	48% (13)	63% (10)	36% (4)
Optic Atrophy	60%	--	50% (27)	52% (14)	38% (6)	64% (7)
Papilledema	40%	40%	43% (23)	41% (11)	50% (8)	46% (5)

The significantly longer mean survival time (x) of the children operated on with the aid of the microscope is remarkable.

After 10 years more than 80 % of them were alive, compared to 5 % of those operated on before 1969 (Fig. 4a).

Visual functions, too, were significantly better. If severe visual reduction or amaurosis had developed preoperatively visual function could no longer recover even in patients operated on with the aid of the microscope.

However, recovery of vision was observed in several patients after operation of the relapsed tumor.

Example 1: In an 8-year-old boy in 1975, after development of symptoms of ICP increase, suprasellar calcification was found. Visual functions were normal. On operation a large suprasellar craniopharyngioma was totally removed, except some remnants within the wall of the cavernous sinus.

Post-operative visual functions were normal.

In 1976, headaches, left temporal hemianopia. Reoperation, involution of the visual field disturbance.

Table II: Post-operative Visual Function in Children with Craniopharyngiomas

		TOTAL		SUPRASELLAR		RETROSELLAR		ATYPICAL	
Slight defects:		'51-'69	'70-'86	'51-'69	'70-'86	'51-'69	'70-'86'	51-'69	'70-'86
Total	54	33	21	19	8	8	8	6	5
Survivors	33	16 (48%)	17 (81%)	12 (63%)	8 (100%)	2 (25%)	6 (75%)	2 (33%)	3 (60%)
Vision	6	1	5	1	3	--	1	1	1
No defects í	8	5	2	2	--	1	1	2	1
Visual field defects	17	7	10	6	61	3	--	1	
Slight defects: visual + neurolog.	4	2	2	2	1	--	--	--	1
Severe defects: visual + neurolog.	3	2	3	2	1	--	2	--	--
Diab. insipid. Hormonal Substitution	11 19	2 6	9 13	1 5	4 7	-- --	4 4	1 1	1 2

In 1977, computed tomography of the skull revealed the parasellar remainder of the tumor. In 1978, diagnosis of a temporal hemianopia, now rightsided. After the 2nd tumor operation once again involution of the visual field defect occured.

A temporary hemianopia early in 1979 turned into a quadrantic hemianopia, from which a bitemporal hemianopia finally developed.

After third operation, again improvement of visual fields. Finally the parasellar residual tumor led to the appearance of cerebral fits.

Six months after the 4th operation, concentric cuts of the visual fields and a left temporal hemianopia developed. After shunting a hydrocephalus occlusus, the visual fields improved for a short time

Two months later the patient went blind and died after a disease course of 11 years.

2.2 Retrosellar craniopharyngiomas

The pre-operative symptoms of craniopharyngiomas with mainly retrosellar expansion were mostly visual disturbances over a long period (Fig. 3b).

As far as the survival time is concerned the results of the children operated on after 1960 with the aid of the microscope were also better (Fig. 4b).
After 10 years 75 % of the patients were still alive. The visual acuity of these children after operation was significantly reduced, corresponding to the low preoperative level of visual function.

2.3 Unusually located craniopharyngiomas

The children with unusual location of the tumor, i.e. intrasellar, parasellar or presellar, had relatively good visual functions in the case of survival (Fig. 3 c).
Example 2: An 11-year-old boy with a parasellar craniopharyngioma operated on in 1969 fell ill with symptoms of ICP increase. Pneumencephalographic signs of the mainly parasellarly expanding tumor and occlusion of the right foramen Monro and unilateral ventricular dilation.

After insertion of a VA-shunt the tumor was microscopically extirpated.

In 1979 appearance of a left homonymous hemianopia which spontaneously receded after a temporal increment. In 1986 epileptic seizures. Under anticonvulsive medication the patient became free from attacks. The CT revealed calcific deposits in the para-sellar region.

In 1987, 18 years after tumor resection, outstanding intelligence, unrestricted visual acuity and normal working capacity were noteworthy.

3. Survival rates and visual function

Independent of the direction of tumor growth, the operating microscope, which has been available since 1969, has led to a significant increase in the survival rate. Of the 33 children operated on before 1969 16 (48 %) survived; of the 21 children operated on since 1969 17 (81 %) survived (Tab. II).

The mean duration of survival (x) could be prolonged in many cases (Fig. 2 a - c). Comparing the two operative periods: 1951 - 69, and 1970 - 86, we can state that the number of children with improved vision or the number of patients without postoperative neurological defects in total was about the same.

About the same number of children retained visual field defects, slight visual disturbances with neurological defects or severe visual disturbances with neurological defects (Tab. II).

A temporary diabetes insipidus appeared more frequently in those children who were operated on after 1969.

4. Tumor recurrence

A recurrence of the tumor was mostly recognizable by the appearance of or the increase in visual field defects, by hemipareses or cerebral fits. Tumor recurrence most frequently was detected by perimetric examination.

5. Postoperative pupillary dysfunctions

For a duration of some days bilateral dilated and fixed pupils appeared, postoperatively, in 8 children, unless space-occupying lesions, such as brain edema or hemorrhage were detected. Six of these 8 children recovered.

Conclusions

In children with craniopharyngioma surgery performed with the aid of the operating microscope has led both to a significant reduction in operative/post-operative mortality and to a considerable lengthening of the survival time. The most sensitive clinical parameter of tumor recurrence was visual field findings. The type of visual field disturbances varied greatly.

As KENNEDY pointed out, such "pleomorphisms" of visual field defects are typical of craniopharyngiomas. He found this phenomenon in 22 % of the patients and explained spontaneous improvements by intermittent leaks of cystic fluid into the ventricular system.

For a recovery of the disturbed visual function it was essential that pre-operative visual impairment was detected very early [7, 11].

An advanced decline in visual functions by ischemia of the visual pathways cannot be rectified, not even by using microsurgical operative techniques. Early diagnosis and periodical, careful supervision of visual function have to be combined with operative possibilities in order to lengthen the time of survival and to preserve a sufficient capacity of vision.

Summary

We investigated the fate of the visual function in children with craniopharyngiomas. After development of microsurgical techniques the results both of the survival rate and of the survival time improved significantly. However, an advanced failure of visual functions could not be rectified by modern operative techniques. A recovery of the disturbed visual functions was dependent on an early diagnosis of the tumor and operation.

Figures

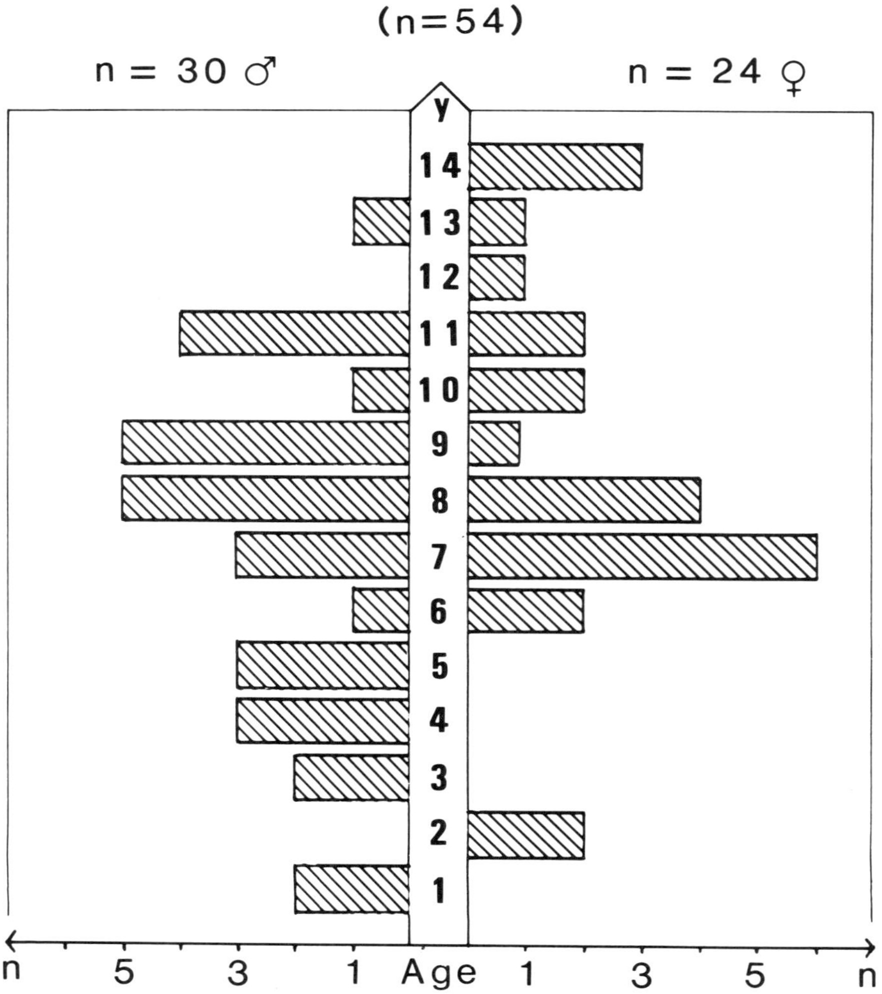

Fig. 1: Age distribution of 54 children with craniopharyngiomas

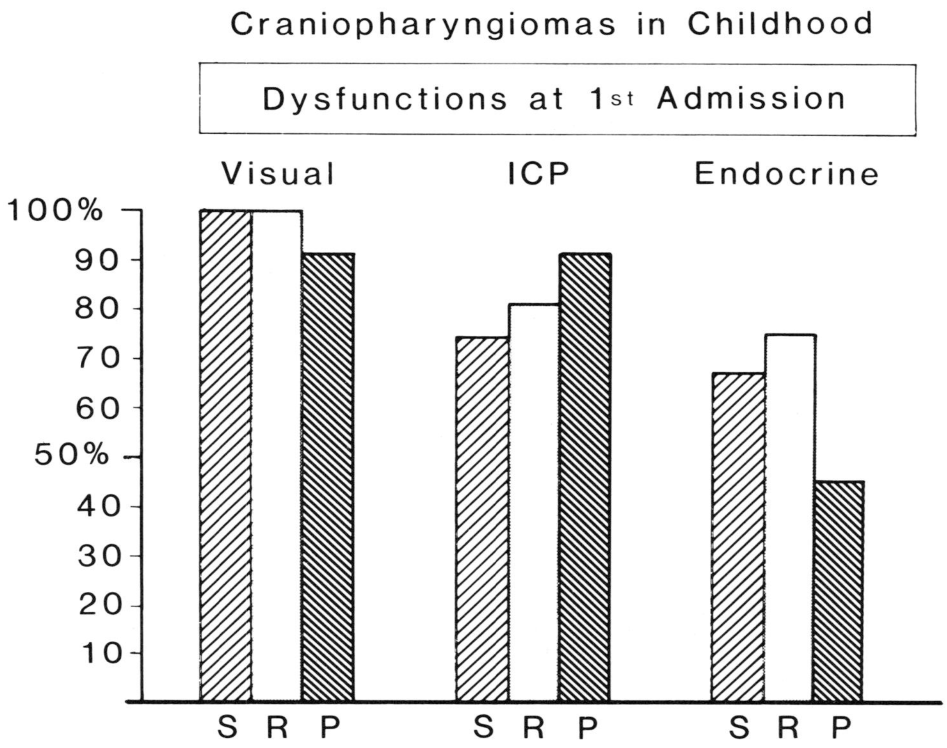

Fig. 2: Dysfunctions at first admission in children with craniopharyngiomas located suprasellarly (S), retrosellarly (R) or parasellarly (P)

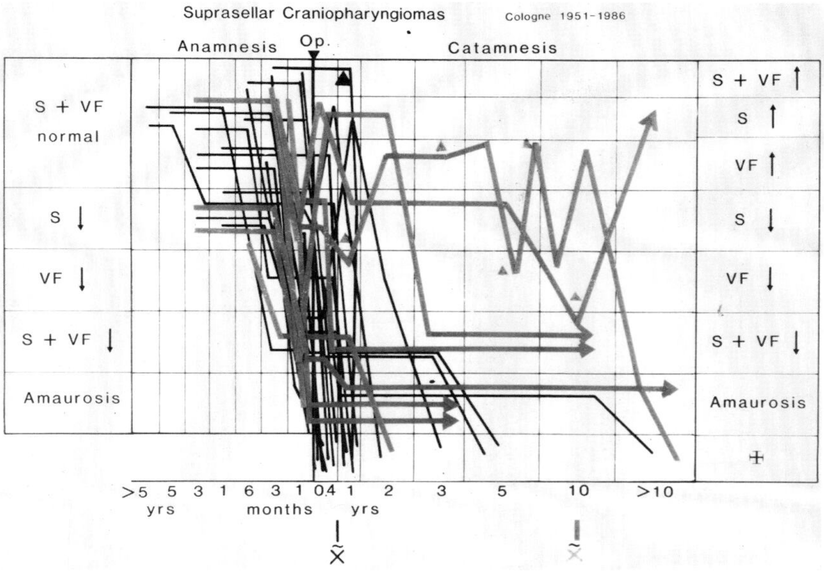

Fig. 3a: Visual function in the disease course of suprasellar craniopharyngiomas. Thick grey lines: course of visual function in children operated on after 1969 with the aid of operating microscope. Thin black lines: course of visual function in children operated before 1969 without the aid of operating microscope. (Abbrev.: S: sight/Vision; VF: Visual Field; ↓: Deterioration; x: mean survival time)

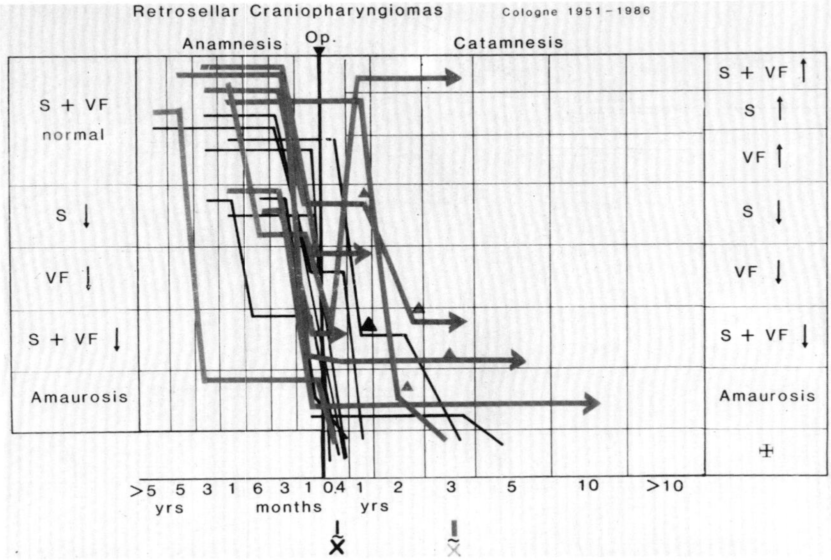

Fig. 3b: Visual function in the disease course of retrosellar craniopharyngiomas

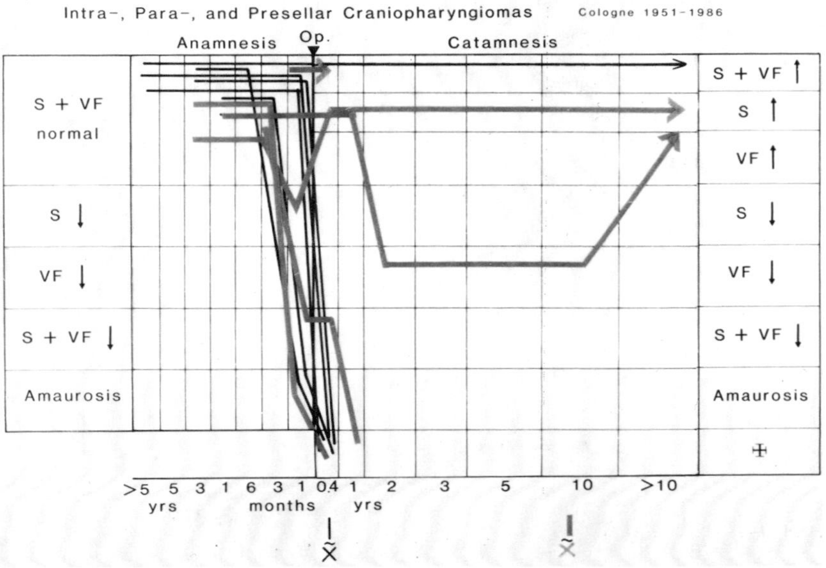

Fig. 3c: Visual function in the disease course of intra-, para- and presellar craniopharyngiomas

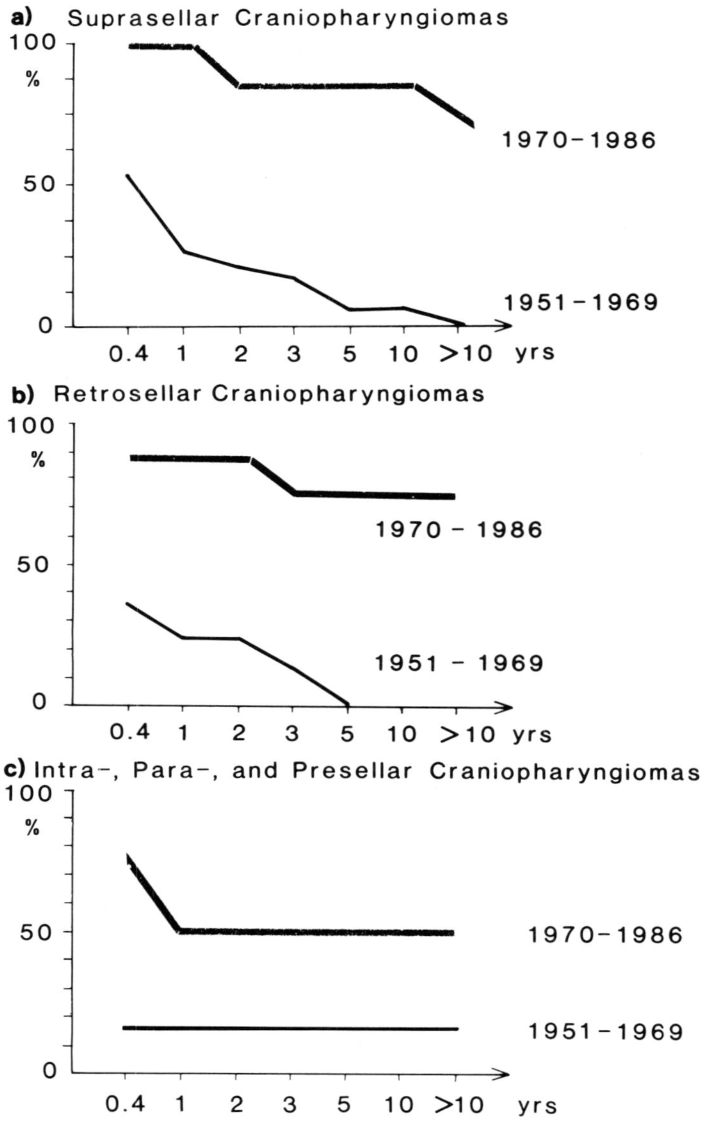

Fig. 4: Comparison of survival times in children operated on 1951 - 69 with those of children operated on 1970 - 86. a) suprasellar craniopharyngiomas b) retrosellar craniopharyngiomas c) intra-, para-, pre-sellar craniopharyngiomas

References

[1] Bergland R, Ray BS: The arterial supply of the human optic chiasm. J. Neurosurg. 31 (1969) 327 - 334

[2] Carmel PW, Antunes JL, Chang CHH: Craniopharyngiomas in children. Neurosurgery 11 (1982) 382 - 389

[3] Cavazzuti V, Fischer EG, Welch K, Bell JA, Winston KR: Neurological and psychophysiological sequelae following different treatments of craniopharyngioma in children. J. Neurosurg. 59 (1983) 409 - 417

[4] Hoff JT, Patterson RH: Craniopharyngiomas in children and adults. J. Neurosurg. 36 (1972) 299 - 302

[5] Hoffman HJ, Hendrick EB, Humphreys RP, Buncic JR, Armstrong DL, Jenkin RDT: Management of craniopharyngioma in Children. J. Neurosurg. 47 (1977) 218 - 227

[6] Katz EL: Late results of radical excision of craniopharyngiomas in children. J. Neurosurg. 42 (1975) 86 - 93

[7] Lods F, Mannassero J, Martin J, Coussement N: Manifestations ophthalmologiques des craniopharyngiomes de l'enfant: A propos de 4 cas. Bull. Soc. Ophthalmol. Fr. 80 (1980) 73 - 77

[8] Kennedy HB, Smith RFS: Eye signs in craniopharyngioma. Brit. J. Ophthal. 59 (1975) 689 - 695

[9] Matson DD, Crigler JF: Managment of craniopharyngioma in childhood. J. Neurosurg. 30 (1969) 377 - 390

[10] Raimondi AJ, Rougerie J: A critical review of personal experiences with craniopharyngioma: Surgical technique and operative results. Concepts in Pediatric Neurosurgery 3 (1983) 1 - 34

[11] Richard KE, Sanker P, Greib N, Nanassis K: Fehldiagnosen beim Hirntumor des Kindesalters. In: Bock WJ, Schirmer M (eds.): Differentialdiagnosen in der Neurochirurgie. Urban und Schwarzenberg, München-Wien-Baltimore 1987

[12] Shapiro K, Till K, Grant DN: Craniopharyngiomas in childhood. A rational approach to treatment. J. Neurosurg. 50 (1979) 617 - 623

[13] Thomsett MJ, Conte FA, Kaplan SL, Grumbach MM: Endocrine and neurologic outcome in childhood craniopharyngioma: Review of effect of treatment in 42 patients. J. Pediatr. 97 (1980) 728 - 735

Optic nerve glioma

M. Mohadjer, A. Etou, E. Millios, R. Baden, F. Mundinger

Summary

Optic nerve gliomas is a rare tumor usually occurring in small children. How these tumors should be treated, especially if they are located in or around the chiasma, is a matter of controversy. Almost all optic gliomas are benign pilocytic astrocytomas which grow diffusely in the optic nerve. Recommended treatment ranges from a wait-and-see policy to radical excision with or without subsequent radiotherapy. Comparative data on these lesions are limited, as there are no randomized investigations and long-term studies reported in the literature. The small number of patients with optic nerve glioma makes it difficult to carry out a reliable comparison.

In 24 patients treated in the Department of Stereotaxy and Neuronuclear Medicine between 1980 and 1987, interstitial irradiation with other modes of therapy are compared based on a 1 - 6 year follow up. Twelve patients in whom iodine-125 was implanted into the center of the lesion following biopsy performed to confirm the histological diagnosis are reported. The results are compared with those of 10 patients who underwent only biopsy for histological confirmation.

CT-stereotaxic biopsy to verify the histological diagnosis with subsequent interstitial irradiation is presented as an alternative therapy for optic gliomas.

Introduction

Optic nerve gliomas are rare tumors accounting for approximately 9 % of all intracranial tumors and 5 % of tumors occurring in the 0 - 20 year age group (6, 7, 10, 20). Incidence is highest among children between 5 and 10 years. In the presence of fohn Recklinghausen`s disease incidence is 15 % higher (19, 5). In 1923 VON VERHOEFF observed a relationship between age and development and the occurrence of optic nerve glioma in a study of 300 patients with optic gliomas (22). The tumors are usually low grade pilocytic astrocytomas located in the optic nerve from the retina to the optic tract. They are nevertheless divided into three groups: intracanalicular, intracranial, and diffusely growing in front of or behind the chiasm (24).

There is controversy in the literature over the management of these tumors. Some authors favour radical excision with or without subsequent irradiation (17, 12, 21); others recomment only radiotherapy (4). Recently, chemotherapy has been suggested (18).

There have been frequent reports on "spontaneous cures" without any therapy (8, 20, 3, 1). Every therapeutic measure was rejected on the grounds of side effects of the various forms of therapy, the rate of disease recurrence in treated and non-treated patients, and the capability of the tumor to regress spontaneously.

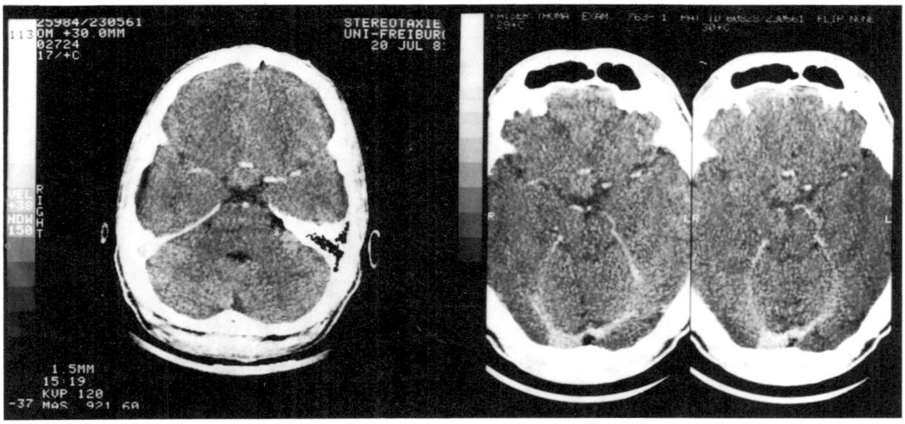

Fig. 1a,b: Patient K.T., aged 26, male. Isodense chiasmatic lesion diagnosed by CT-stereotaxic biopsy as pilocytic astrocytoma in July 1981 (a). No change in findings 6 years later (b)

In the present study we report on our follow up observations in 24 patients with histologically documented chiasmal gliomas.

Material and Methods

From the beginning of 1980 to the end of 1986, a total of 24 chiasmal gliomas with different degrees of tumor extension were diagnosed, stereotactically biospied, and histologically confirmed in the Division of Stereotaxy and Neuronuclear medicine of the University of Freiburg neurosurgical Department. Of the 24 patients 12 were female and 12 were male (Table I).

Table I: Glioma of the optic nerve

n.of cases	no.patients				age
	male	female		(years)	
			1 - 10	10 - 20	20
24	12	12	11	10	3

An average of 9 months lay between the onset of the disease and the diagnosis. The major clinical symptoms were reduced visual field and loss of vision, followed by intracranial pressure symptoms due to occlusion of the foramen of Monro in the presence of hydrocephalus, hypothalamic disturbances with obesity and polyuria, and pareses due to compression or lesioning of the internal capsule (Table II). the diagnosis was made on the basis of clinical and ophthalmological examination, X-ray native scans of the skull, and CT and mR scans. The biopsy for histological confirmation was performed according to the RIECHERT/MUNDINGER CT stereotaxic technique (14, 2).

In 11 patients, interstitital radiotherapy was carried out by the implantation of I-125 seeds in the same operative session following confirmation of the histological diagnosis. Implantation was done in such a way that a homogenous surface dose of 8 - 10 000 cGy was achieved. Two of these patients had already undergone conventional surgery. In 10 patients only biopsy was performed. The site of the biopsy in these cases was marked for later control. In two patients external radiotherapy was carried out with a total of 3 000 cGy administered in 3 weeks. In one patient additional partial resection was performed due to a rapid enlargement of the tumor.

Histological examination revealed pilocytic astrocytomas. The location and extent of the lesion varies; some were in front of the chiasm, some inside it, and some behind it, in the optic tract, on one or both sides. The period of observation after stereotaxic puncture was an average of 2.8 years (maximum 6 years, minimum 1 year). Intraoperative and postoperative complications were not observed in any of the 24 cases during this period. The preoperative neurological deficits did not increase.

Results

Within a follow up period of 1 - 6 years (average 2.8 years) out-patient examinations were performed in all of the patients. These included clinical and neuro-ophthalmological examinations, as well as CT scans.

Table II: Incidence of symptoms in 24 diagnosed chiasmal gliomas

Symptoms	number
Reduced visionand limited field of vision	20
Hydrocephalus and cerebral pressure	12
Hypothalamic disturbance	4
Amaurosis	3
Hemiparesis	3

After the follow up period, subtle tumor regression was observed in only one of the 10 patients who underwent biopsy alone. In this group, the findings in five patients remained largely unchanged with no tumor enlargement or change in shape in CT and with no change in the clinical symptoms (Figs. 1 a + b). In comparison, four patients showed continuous deterioration of the clinical symptoms as well as a slow progression of the CT findings (Table III).

Of the 11 patients who were subsequently treated with I-125, the findings of five patients remained unchanged over the entire observation period. In four patients, definite tumor regression could be seen after one year. Cyst formation can occur around the implant (Figs. 2a + b). Two patients had renewed tumor progression with gradual enlargement.

The patients who underwent biopsy and partial resection or biopsy and external radiotherapy were further treated elsewhere. We have no reports of any changes in the findings in any of the three patients.

Discussion

Optic nerve gliomas occur mainly in children and adolescents (90 % up to the age of 20 years) (20). The most frequent localization is intraorbital (9) . The prognosis in term of the preservation of vision and the general life expectancy is only favourable if just one isolated optic nerve is involved. In this case, close cooperation between the ophthalmologist and the neurossurgeon is required.

PAULUS et al. (16) in 1983 published a report of 33 children with tumors of the optic nerve. All of these children had undergone surgery with total removal of the tumor. Seventeen years later 85 % of the patients were still in good general and neurological condition. Of the 52 patients with tumors that had reached the chiasma, only 44 % were still alive after 19 years, regardless of the therapy.

The opinions as to whether therapeutic intervention has a positive effect on the survival rate begin to diverge as soon as the glioma has reached and involved the chiasm. Generally, a wait-and-see policy is recommended. When progression has been clinically and computer tomographically documented, particularly when additional neurological deficits such as motor paresis occur, resection is considered. Although partial resection does not represent a curative treatment, in some cases clinical improvement can be achieved by palliative decompression of the thalamic and hypothalamic structures.

Table III: Therapy and follow up during 1 - 5 year period in 24 patients undergoing puncture

type of treatment		course		
		unchanged	better	worse
biopsy only	n = 0	5	1	4
biopsy and I - 125	n = 11	5	4	2
biopsy and external radiotherapy	n = 2	1	-	1
biopsy and partial resection	n = 1	1	-	-

Judgement as to whether external radiotherapy has an effect on the visual function and the survival rate can only be made in about half of the cases. Randomized long-term studies with regard to this point are lacking (15). In general, a total dose of 50 Gy is recommended (13, 23). Lower doses are usually not sufficient to prevent further growth or recurrence of the disease. What is not lacking, however, are warnings about the side effects of external therapy, which can include vasculopathy, vessel occlusion, hypothalamic disturbances and residual visual deterioration, and ultimately lead to necrosis with tissue destruction (1, 11).

Surgical partial resection in our opinion is justified only if there is evidence of progression or if there is increased compression, especially on the hypothalamus.

The CT-stereotaxic method is indispensable for confirming the histological diagnosis and for planning further therapy. The implantation of radionuclides in the center of the tumor in the same operative session offers a real alternative to the methods of managing intracranial optic gliomas available thus far.

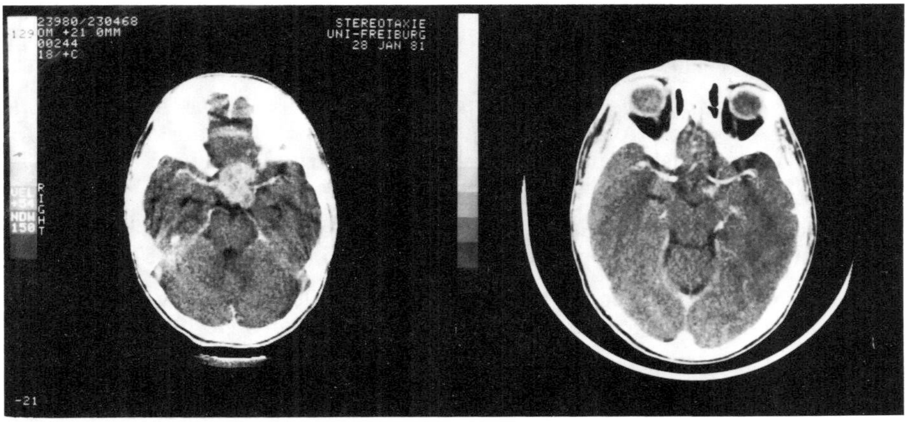

Fig. 2a,b: Patient Z.A., aged 13, male. Hypersense irregular chiasmatic lesion with prechiasmatic and retrochiasmatic extension. Diagnosis by Ct-stereotaxic biopsy and therapy with I-125 in January 1981 (a). CT follow up 6 years later reveals slight scar formation with no visible residual tumor (b).

In a follow up of 1 - 6 years, we found - in a total of 11 patients who underwent biopsy and implantation - unchanged findings in five cases, marked improvement of the disease in four cases, and slight tumor shrinkage in two cases. These results are far better than those of the 10 patients who underwent biopsy with no irradiation therapy. And they correlate well with the outcome following external radiotherapy with, as reported in the literature, a maximum of 50 % showing improvement (13). None of the patients who received implantation treatment developed additional neurological deficits. The seeds were placed and the isodoses calculated such that additional impared vision or progressive visual deterioration could be avoided.

The advantages of this method include the guided puncture of the lesion, the short operation time, and, because the operation is usually carried out under local anesthesia, the relatively low surgical risk. Radiation doses are relatively low so that there is no damage to the surrounding tissue. The implantation can be repeated in the case of recurring tumor growth.

References

[1] Beyer RA, Paden P, Sobel DF, Flynn F: Moyamoya pattern of vascular occlusion after radiotherapy for glioma of the optic chiasma. Neurology 36 (1986) 1173 - 1178

[2] Birg W, Mundinger F: Direct target point determination for stereotactic brain operation from CT data and the calculation of setting parameters for polar coordinate stereotactic device. Appl. Neurophysiol. 45 (1982) 387 - 395

[3] Borit A, Richardson EP: The biological and clinical behaviour of pilocytic astrocytomas of the optic pathways. Brain 105 (1982) 161 - 187

[4] Brand WN, Hoover SV: Optic glioma in children. Review of 16 cases given megavoltage radiation therapy. Childs` Brain 5 (1979) 449 - 466

[5] Diebler C, Dulac O (Eds.): Pediatric Neurology and Neuroradiology. Springer-Verlag Berlin-Heidelberg-New York (1987)

[6] Farwell JR, Dohrmann GJ, Flannery JT: Central nervous system tumors in children. Cancer 40 (1977) 3123 - 3132

[7] Fowler FD, Matson DO: Gliomas of the optic pathways in childhood. J. Neurosurgery 14 (1957) 515 - 528

[8] Glaser JS, Hoyt WF, Corbett J: Visual morbidity with chiasmal glioma. Long term studies of visual fields in untreated and irradiated cases. Arch. Ophthalmol 85 (1076) 3 - 12

[9] Grote W, Bettag W: Supratentorielle Tumoren, Tumoren des Nervus opticus und des Chiasmas. IN: Dietz M, Umbach W, Wüllenweber R (eds.): Klinische Neurochirurgie, Band II (1984) 120 - 123

[10] Harwood-Wash DC:Optic gliomas and pediatric neuroradiology. Radiol. Clin. North. Am. 10 (1972) 83 - 100

[11] Hirata Y, Matsukado Y, Mihara Y, Kocchi M, Sonoda H, Fukumura A: Occlusion of the internal carotid artery after radiation therapy for the chiasmal lesion. Acta Neurochirurgica 74 (1985) 141 - 147

[12] Housepian EM: Surgical Treatment of unlateral optic nerve gliomas. J. Neurol 31 (1969) 604 - 607

[13] Montgomery AB, Griffin T, Parker RG, Cerdes AS: Optic nerve glioma: The Role of radiation therapy. Cancer 40 (1977) 2079 - 2080

[14] Mundinger F: CT-stereotactic biopsy of brain tumours. In: Voth D, Gutjahr P, Langmaid C (eds.): Tumors in infancy and childhood. Springer-Verlag, Berlin (1982) 234 - 246

[15] Packer RJ, Sarino PJ, Bilaniuk LT, Zimmermann A, Schatz NJ, Rosenstock JG, nelson DS, Jarret PD, Bruce DA, Schut L: Chiasmatic gliomas of childhood. Childs` Brain 10 (1983) 393 - 403

[16] Paulus WM, Brandt TH, Kuhne D, Leopold HC, Möbius E: Therapie orbitaler und retroorbitaler raumfordernder Prozesse mit Sehnervkompression. Nervenarzt 50 (1983) 519 - 534

[17] Richards RD, Lynn JR. The surgical management of gliomas of the optic nerve. Am J Opthalmol 62 (1966) 60 - 65

[18] Rosenstock JG, Packer RJ, Bilaniuk LT, Bruce DA, Radclifte JL, Savino P (1985): Chiasmatic optic glioma treated with chemotherapy. A preliminary report. J. Neurosurg 63 (1985) 862 - 866

[19] Slamovits TL: Von Recklinghausen neurofibromatosis. Incidence of optic gliomas (letter). Ophthalmology 92 (1985) 984

[20] Tym R: Piloid gliomas of the anterior optic pathways. Br J Surg 49 (1961) 322 - 331

[21] Tanny RT, Laws ER, Yound BR, Rush JA: The neurosurgical management of optic glioma. Results in 104 patients. J. neurosurg. 57 (1982)425 - 458

[22] Verhoeff FH: Primary intraneural tumors (gliomas) of the optic nerve. Arch Ophthalmol 51 (1922) 239 - 254

[23] Weiss L, Sagerman RH, King GA, Chung CT, Dubowy RL: Controversy in the management of optic nerve glioma. Cancer 59 (1987) 1000 - 1004

[24] Zülch KJ: Brain Tumors. Their Biology and Pathology. Third, completely revised edition. Springer Verlag Berlin-Heidelberg-New York (1986)

IV

GRAVE'S OPHTHALMOPATHY

CT-diagnosis in Grave's disease

W. Müller-Forell

The clinical diagnosis of Grave's disease is independent of cranial computerized tomography. But this investigation allows to delineate the grading of the disease (7, 15, 22) and a follow up-study (23).

The orbit nearly looks like a foursided pyramid, the axis going from the ventral basis to the dorsal apex. Therefore, the intraorbital structures are only shown partially by the scanning axias. The coronal imaging should go nearly vertical to the skull base, it allows a better examination of the Mm. recti inferiores and superiores, the last ones cannot always be separated from the M. levator palpebrae (15, 16, 21).

The most important diagnostic criteria in CT of Grave's disease are:

1. Enlargement of the extraocular muscles, sparing the tendinous insertion,
2. slight bowing of medial orbital wall, caused by the enlarged extraocular muscles,
3. the compression of the optic nerve in the apex of the orbit.

It should be mentioned that all these CT signs could be seen in patients without a clinical or laboratory abnormality as well as in patients with thyroid disease such as thyreotoxicosis as in patients without any known abnormalities of the thyroid (7, 15, 22).

Ad 1):

The most common and best seen sign of Grave's disease is, besides the exophthalmus, the enlargement of the extraocular muscles, seen in 85 % of all cases (7, 10). Some authors say that the spindle-like enlargement of the muscle, sparing the tendines, should be pathognomonic (15, 19, 23, Fig. 1).

Nearly all authors show (in various frequency) that the M. rectus inferior is the first (Fig. 2) followed by the M. rectus medialis and M. rectus superior (7, 15, 23) which is enlarged. Normally it is bilateral (3), in 3 quarters of the cases the enlargment is symmetrical, in 1 quarter asymmetrical. In about 40 % of the patients without any clinical sign of exophthalmus the enlargment of the muscles is shown in CT (7, 9, 15). In rare cases it is only unilateral (3, 15, Fig. 3). If there is an enlargment of only one muscle, especially the M. rectus inferior, differential diagnosis has to exclude a tumor (3, 7).

Histologically, in the acute stage there is an evidence of numerous lymphocytes, plasmacells and mucopolysaccharid-infiltrations, macrophages and an edema in the extraocular muscle (14, 18, 22). Some authors show a vacuolization of the sarcoplasms (22) or fatty infiltration. Late in the course of thyroid disease you can see a fibrotic and shrunken muscle. (3, 4).

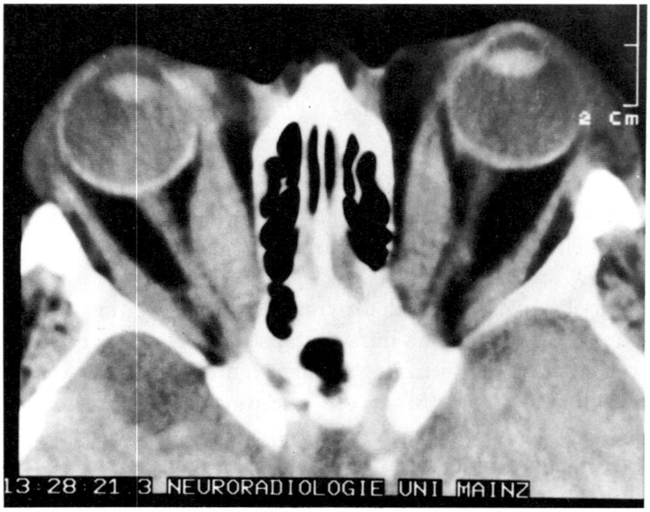

Fig. 1: 51 year old female patient with Grave's disease. Bilateral spindle-like enlargement of the Mm. recti mediales sparing the tendons.

Ad 2):

The impression of bony walls of the orbit is not as often, FORBES (11) described it in 7 %, but it is a very remarkable sign of the increase of the intraorbital contents. The lamina papyracea , as it is the thinnest wall, is impressed, as a spontaneous decompression. If there is a symmetrical enlargement, especially of the Mm. recti mediales, it shows a typical form ("Coca-Cola"-sign) (3, 15, 23, Fig. 4, 5, 6). One case report shows the impression of the roof of the orbit because of an enlarged M. rectus superior (11).

Ad 3)

The most severe complication of Grave's disease in rare cases (5 %, CHAR (3)) is the visual loss (13). Not only the extension of the optic nerve because of the exophthalmus (Fig. 5), but the direct compression of the optic nerve in the apex of the orbit by the enlarged muscles is responsible for this visual loss (Fig. 6), because of a deminution of the blood and liquor circulation in the neurilemma (13). It results an edematous swelling (papillary edema), followed by a degeneration and therefore irreversible atrophic damage of the optic nerve (3, 12, 22, 23).

Table 1: The most important diagnostic finding in CT in patients with Grave's disease:

1. Enlargement of the extraocular muscles sparing the tendons.
2. Impression of the orbital walls, especially medially, because of the enlarged muscles ("Coca-Cola-sign").
3. Compression of the optic nerve in the apex of the orbit.

The literature does not mention additional intraorbital masses in Grave's disease, therefore CHAR (3) mentions it as an additional diagnostic sign.

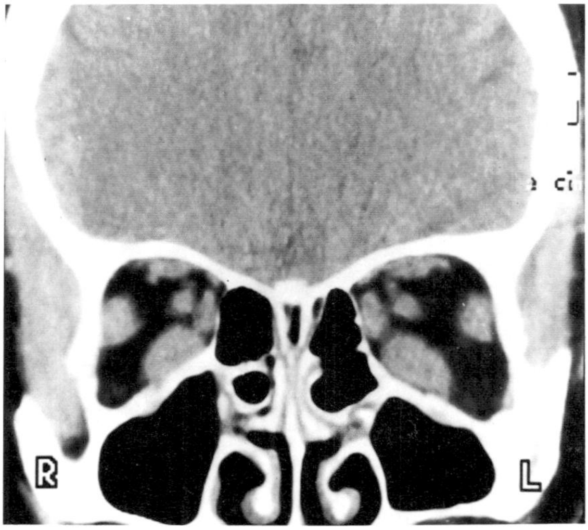

Fig. 2: 49 year old female patient with Grave's disease. In coronary section you see the preponderant enlargement of the Mm. recti inferiores.

The importance of the retrobulbar fat in Grave's disease is contested in literature. Some authors (3, 15, 19) do not see any important changes, some investigators describe an enlargment of the retrobulbar fat (13) because of an extension between the M. rectus medialis and the medial orbital wall (22) (Fig. 7). Some investigators show a different enlargement of muscles or fat in patients with Grave's disease. In about 8 % of the patients with exophthalmus there is only an enlargement of the volume of the fat but normal muscle volumes (9, 10, 16). FELDON (8) describes only a little correlation between the exophthalmus and the enlargement of the muscles, in contrast to the enlargement of the fat (16).

The histological sections show infiltration of lymphocytes and mast-cells as well as an increase of the content of mucopolysaccharides in the tissue resulting in a fibrosis of the retrobulbar fat (3, 17). In summary the histologically investigations of postmortal or bioptic speciment do not show any changes of the fat. Therefore, the changes of the volume should not be caused by an enlargement or increase of the fat cells, but there should be an increased hydration, which might be caused e.g. by the osmotic effect of the mucopolysaccharides of the tissue or the venous congestion in the apex of the orbit, caused by a tissue edema (3, 14, 18).

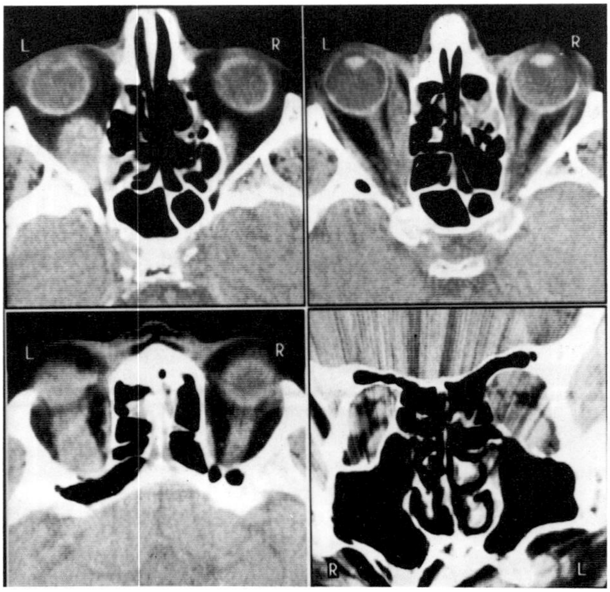

Fig. 3: 68 year old male patient with preponderant unilateral enlargement of the M. rectus inferior and superior of the left orbit.

In differential diagnosis, especially of the unilateral exophthamus, myositis has to take the first place. Besides the different clinical signs with inflammation, the acute beginning of the exophthalmus with pain (24) the CT investigation shows the enlargement of the muscles without sparing the tendons. The acute myositis also prefers the M. rectus inferior, is mostly unilateral (19) but can be extended as well as Grave's disease in more than one muscle (23). But even that finding, as well as the enlargement excluding the tendons do not exclude a myotisis (6).

Vascular diseases, as AVM, with a venous drainage over the sinus petrosus superior and the ophthalmic vein, sinus thrombosis or carotid sinus cavernosus-fistulas (CCF) can show an exophthalmus, conjunctival injections and visual loss (23). The leading sign in CT diagnosis of carotid sinus cavernosus fistula is a native hyperdense, asymmetrically enlarged V. ophthalmica superior (1, 23).

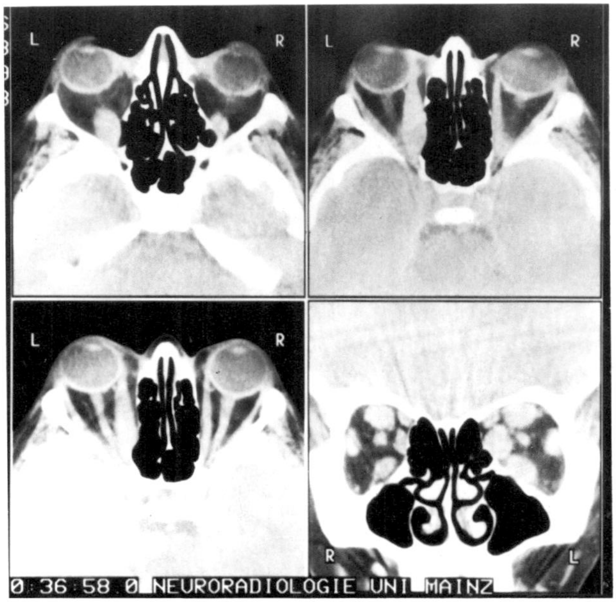

Fig. 4: 48 year old female patient. Impression of the left lamina papyracea because of the enlarged M. rectus medialis.

There are numerous tumor changes as metastases and lymphomas (Fig. 8) which cause exophthalmus because of infiltration of the extraocular muscles. In lympho-, reticulo- or rhabdomyosarcoma additional destructions of the orbital walls are often seen (23, 25). DAL PAZZO (5) and BONNEVILLE (2) describe a bilateral enlargement of the extraocular muscles without exophthalmos in acromegaly.

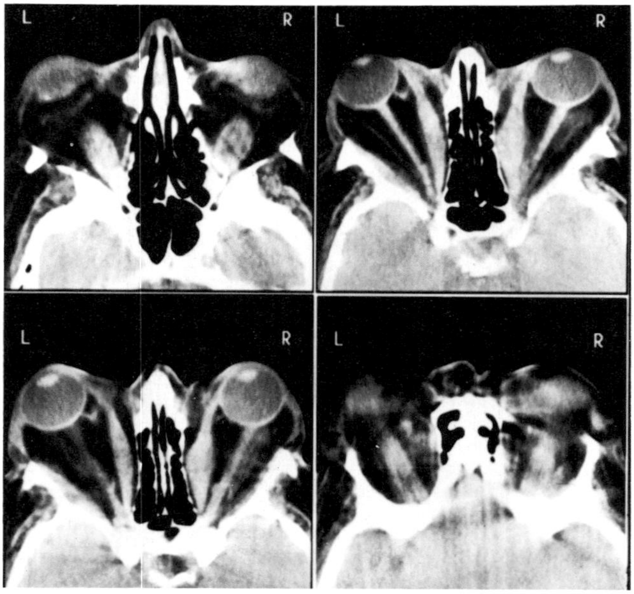

Fig. 5: 51 year old patient with Grave's disease. Extension of both optic nerves because of an extreme exophthalmos. "Coca-Cola"-sign with impressions of the medial orbital walls.

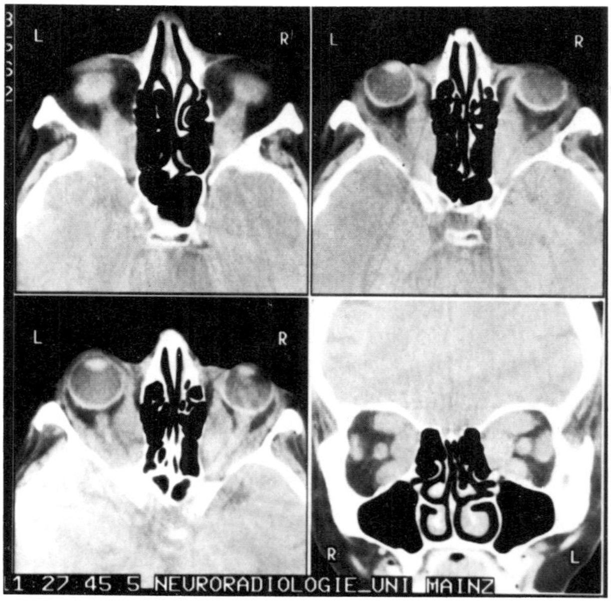

Fig. 6: 71 year old female patient with compression of the optic nerve because of the massive enlargement of the muscles in the apex of the orbit and bilateral impression of the lamina papyracea.

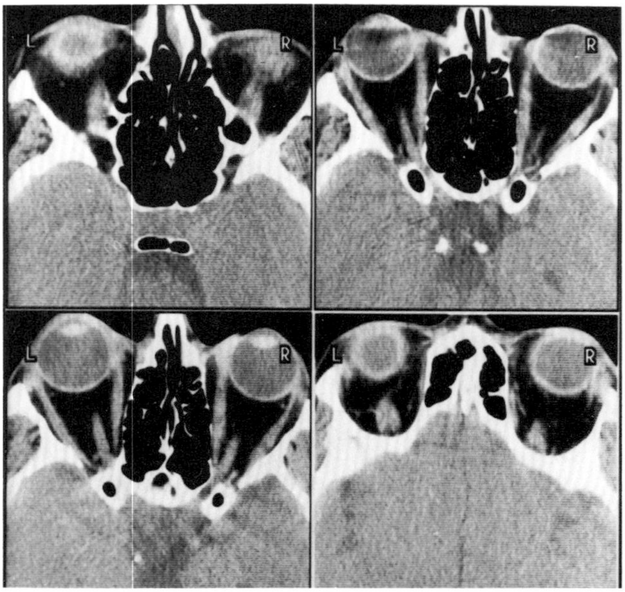

Fig. 7: 69 year old female patient with well-seen exophthalmus but nearly normal extraocular muscles.

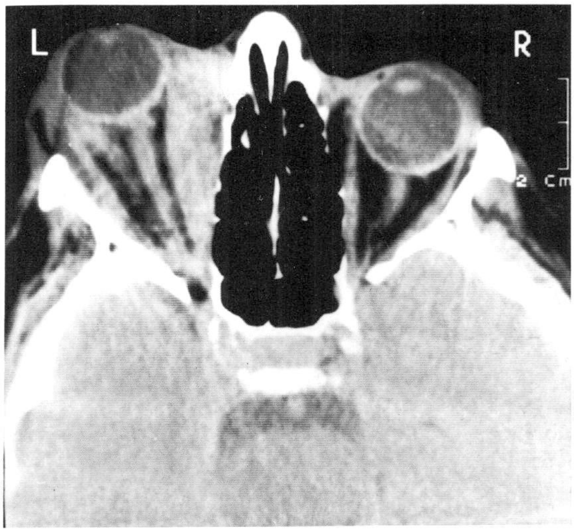

Fig. 8: 57 year old female patient with lymphoma in the left M. rectus medialis

References

[1] Ahamadi J, Teal JS, Segall HD, Zee CS, Han JS, Becker TS: Computed tomography of carotid-cavernous-fistula. AJNR 4 (1983) 131 - 136

[2] Bonneville JF, Cattin F, Dietemann JL: Computed tomography of the pitiutary gland. Springer-Verlag, Berlin, Heidelberg, New-York, Tokyo (1986) 121 ff.

[3] Char DH: Thyroid eye disease. Williams and Wilkins (1985) 65 ff.

[4] Daicker B: Das gewebliche Substrat der verdickten äußeren Augenmuskeln bei der endokrinen Orbitopathie. Klin Monatsbl Augenh 174 (1979) 843 - 847

[5] Dal Pazzo G, Boschi JC: Extraocular muscle enlargement in acromegaly. J Comput Assist Tomogr 6 (1979) 706 - 707

[6] Dresdner SC, Rothfus WE, Slamovits TH, Kennerdell JS, Curtin HC: Computed tomography of orbital myositis. AJNR 5 (1984) 351 - 345

[7] Enzmann DR, Donaldson SS, Kriss JP: Appearance of Grave's disease in orbital computed tomography. J Comput Assist Tomogr Vol 3, No 6 (1979) 815 - 819

[8] Feldon SE, Muramatsu S, Weiner JM: Clinical classification of Grave's ophthalmopathy: identification of risk factors for optic neuropathology. Arch Opthalmol 102 (1984) 1469 - 1472

[9] Forbes G, Gorman CA, Gehring HR, Baker Jr. HR: Computed analysis of orbital fat and muscle volumes in Grave's opthalmopathy. AJNR 4 (1983) 737 - 740

[10] Forbes G, Gorman CA, Brennan MD, Gehring DG, Ilstrup DM, Earnest IV: Opthalmopathy in Grave's disease: Computerised volume measurements of orbital fat and muscle. AJNR 7 (1986) 651 - 656

[11] Healy JF, Metcalf JH, Brahme FJ: Thyroid opthalmopathy. Bony erosion of CT and increased vascularity on angiography. AJNR 2 (1981) 472 - 474

[12] Hilal SK: Computed tomography of the orbit. Opthalmology 86 (1979) 864 - 870

[13] Kennerdell JS, Rosenbaum AE, El Hoshy MH: Apical optic nerve compression of dysthyroid optic neuropathy on computed tomography. Arch Opthalmol. 99 (1981) 807 - 809

[14] Kroll AJ, Kuwabara T: Dysthyroid ocular myopathy: anatomy, histology and electron microsurgery. Arch Opthalmol 76 (1966) 244 - 257

[15] Nowinski TH, Flanagan JC: Evaluation of exophtalmus and thyroid opthalmopathy. In: Gonzales CF, Becker MH, Flanagan JC (eds): Diagnostic imaging in opthalmology. Springer-Verlag, Berlin, Heidelber, New-York, Tokyo (1986) 189 - 199

[16] Peyster RG: Computed tomography of the orbit. In: Gonzales CF, Becker MH, Flanagan JC (eds): Diagnostic imaging in opthalmology. Springer-Verlag (1986) 19 - 37

[17] Riley FC: Orbital pathology in Grave's disease. Mayo Clin Proc 47 (1972) 975 - 979

[18] Tengroth B: Histological studies of orbital tissue in a case of endocrine exophthalmus before and after remission. Acta Ophthalmol 42 (1964) 588 - 591

[20] Trokel SL, Hilal SK: Submillimeter resolution CT scanning of orbital disease Opthalmol (Rochester) 87 (1980) 412 - 417

[21] Uhlenbrock D, Becker W, Appel W, Rohwerder R: Die alte und neu aufgetretene endokrine Opthalmopathie in der Computertomographie. Gemeinsamkeiten - Unterschiede. Fortschr Röntgenst 139, 6 (1983) 644 - 647

[22] Vignaud J, Clay C, Salvolini U, Bilaniuk CT (eds.): Traité de radiodiagnostic, Tome XVI. Radioopthalmologie Masson, Paris (1982) 548 ff

[23] Voidgt B, Kreztschmar K, Wende S: Computertomographische Diagnostik der endokrinen Orbitopathie. Radiologe 24 (1984) 468 - 471

[24] Weinstein G, Dresner ST, Slamovitz TH, Kennerdell JS: Acute and subacute orbital myositis. J Ophthalmol 96 (1983) 209 - 217

[25] Wende S, Kazner E, Grumme TH: The diagnostic value of computed tomography in orbital disease. A cooperative study of 520 cases. Neurosurg Rev 3 (1980) 43 - 49

Orbital Decompression in severe Graves' Ophthalmopathy - Indication and Results in 110 operations

W. Buschmann, W. Richter, W. Kley, Ph. Kruse

Introduction

The members of the interdisciplinary team on orbita problems at Würzburg cooperate in diagnosis and treatment of all kinds of orbital diseases. Diagnosis and medical, surgical, or radiological treatment are resulting from this interdisciplinary approach.

Graves' Disease

Our treatment in severe Graves' ophthalmopathy is as follows:

1: Regulation of thyroid metabolism
2: One course of corticosteroids
3: Orbital decompression (technique of BUSCHMANN and RICHTER, 1984; RICHTER, KLEY and BUSCHMANN, 1984)

Radiation treatment as cyclosporin A or plasmapheresis are no longer recommended by us before surgery.

The majority of the patients included in our report however, do not come from the Würzburg area alone, but from all regions of Western Germany. Most of the hospitals in this country concentrated in the past fully on conservative treatment of the disease , and these patients mostly received more than one course of corticosteroids, often additional radiation treatment of the orbits, and in some cases also Cyclosporin A, but no success was achieved, and therefore they were finally transferred to us for surgery.

Our surgical technique was developed and is performed as an interdisciplinary approach (see contribution of W. RICHTER et al.).

Indications for orbital decompression

Surgical decompression is urgent if compression neuropathy of the optic nerve progresses or persists despite medical therapy; otherwise, a permanent total or partial optic nerve atrophy may develop. The losses in visual acuity and visual field are reversible, if they are not long-standing. Effective surgical decompression, especially near the tip of the orbit, is decisive (see figures 1 and 3).

Surgical decompression is also indicated in grade Vb and Vc of the disease with lagophthalmos problems, recurrent corneal erosions, and marked keratoconjunctivitis sicca, especially if ointment applications at night prover insufficient.

Combined decompression and squint surgery is planned in severe grade IV cases, if motility disturbances and double images would affect practically important directions of gaze (fig. 2). The contractility of the diseased muscles is usually sufficient, but the extensibility is markedly reduced, making recession of the fibrotic muscle the method of choice. Myectomies of the opposite muscle, which only seemingly contracts inadequately, are rarely indicated. Squint surgery without simultaneous orbital decompression is performed by us in exceptional cases only

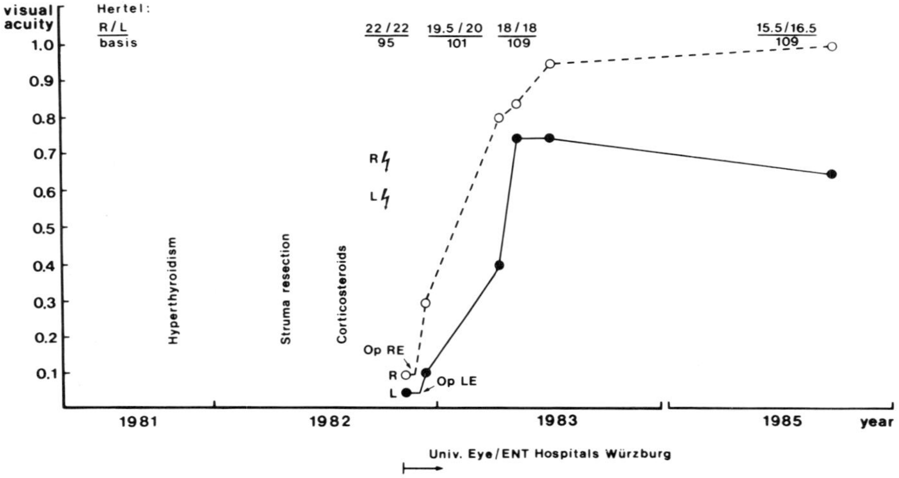

Orbitadecompression (Buschmann and Richter) bilaterally

Fig. 1: Restoration of visual acuity after orbita decompression surgery (technique of BUSCHMANN and RICHTER, 1984) in a patient aged 60 with grade VIc of Graves' ophthalmopathy

The muscle recession would result in some increase of the exophthalmos; it proved superior to combine orbital decompression in the majority of these patients. As results of exophthalmos, all external eye muscles are extended. This reduces motility. Squint surgery could provide parallel position of the eyes, but the area of the gaze directions free from double images remains small. Simultaneous orbital decompression results in restoration of the former bulbus position, the exophthalmos-induced extension of the external eye muscles is removed. The result is a much larger area of binocular vision.

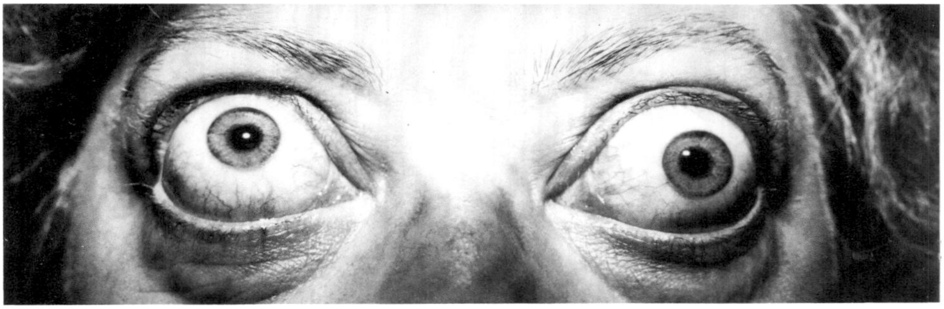

a

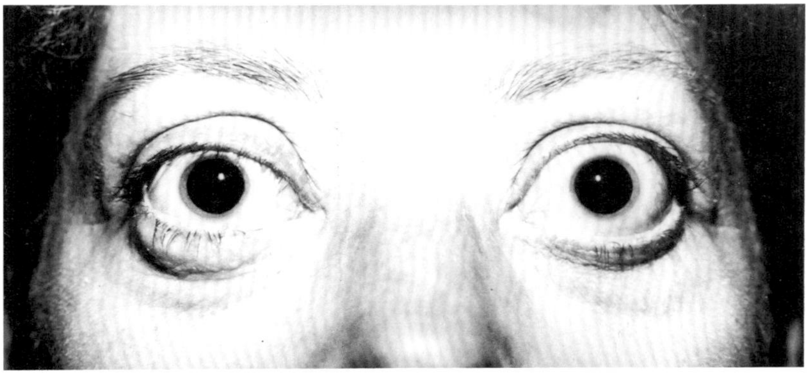

b

Fig. 2: Patient with grade IVc, Vb, and VIa of Graves' ophthalmopathy before (2 a) and after (2 b) orbital decompression. Addition lid surgery was performed on her right eye and is planned for the left eye, too

Our orbita decompression procedure includes practically always a recession of the medial rectus muscle. Effective decompression near the orbita tip can be achieved only if the muscle there becomes displaced medially, thus having a more curved, longer way. Fat tissue is often not any more present in this area. - Marked vertical motility disturbances are corrected as well at the time of decompression surgery. In case of minor vertical motility problems, however, it is better to postpone vertical muscle surgery. Often orbital decompression without vertical muscle recession proved sufficient to get a satisfying binocular field of gaze.

In severe grade III cases of the disease, orbital decompression is indicated especially if severe defacement would cause problems in private or professional life, and if medical treatment did not improve the situation.

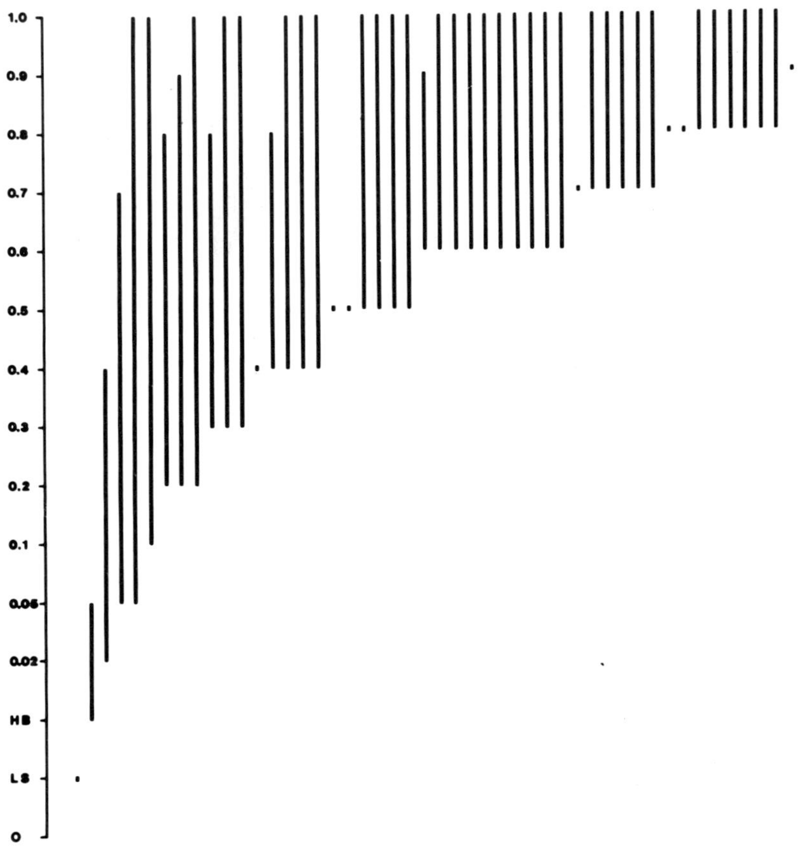

Fig. 3: Pre- and postoperative visual acuity in 48 eyes with compression neuropathy of the optic nerve. The preoperative visual acuity is shown at the lower end of the columns, the postoperative one at the upper end

Number of cases

From October 1982 to April 1987, 110 surgical orbital decompressions (technique of BUSCHMANN and RICHTER) were performed in 64 patients.

Results

Figure 3 demonstrates the pre- and postoperative visual acuity in 48 eyes in which the loss of visual acuity resulted solely from optic nerve compression neuropathy. The lower end of the columns indicates the preoperative visual acuity, the upper end the postoperative visual acuity. Changes of one line only were disregarded. There was no case in which postoperative visual acuity was reduced, compared to the preoperative one. The patients who had preoperatively a visual acuity of .2 and improved, with few exceptions, to normal or nearly normal vision. The extent of this improvement was very surprising for us. The cases at the left margin of this figure demonstrate that one has to be careful not to wait too long before transferring such patients for surgery. The improvement from .02 to .4 visual acuity is yet remarkable, but two other eyes with a vision of hand movements or light projection preoperatively did not improve much.

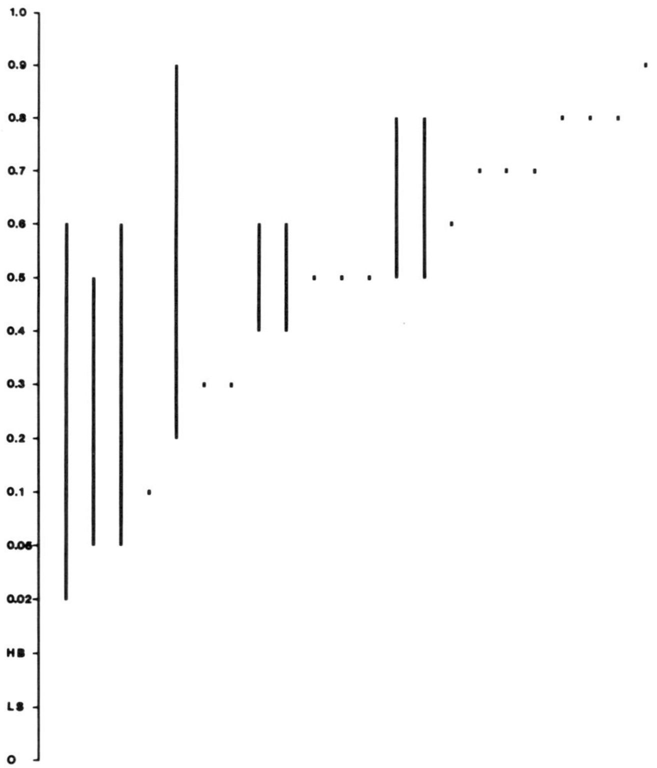

Fig. 4: Pre- and posteroperative visual acuity in 22 eyes, in which the reduction of visual acuity was due to other eye diseases (diabetic retinopathy, cataract, primary glaucoma or corneal scars) alone, or in addition to compression neuropathy of the optic nerve. Pre- and postoperative visual acuity marked as in Fig. 3

Figure 4 shows the pre- and postoperative visual acuity in 22 eyes in which the visual acuity was reduced by other eye diseases, possibly in addition to compression neuropathy, e.g. diabetic retinopathy, cataract, primary glaucoma, or corneal scars. In cases without suspected compression neuropathy, orbita decompression was done to improve severe grade IV or ophthalmopathy, and no improvement of visual acuity was to be expected. These are the cases in which here no change of visual acuity resulted postoperatively.

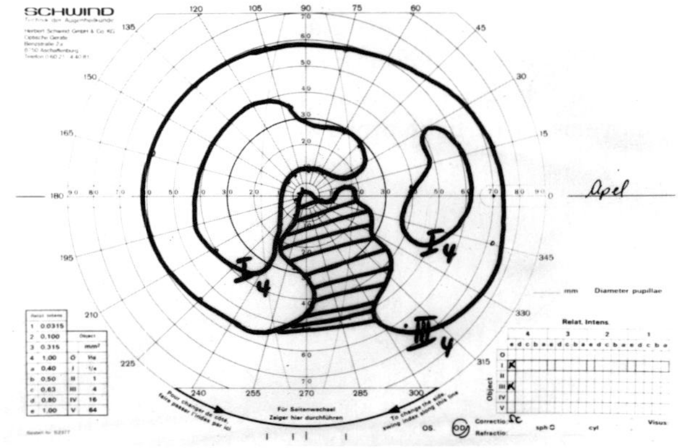

a

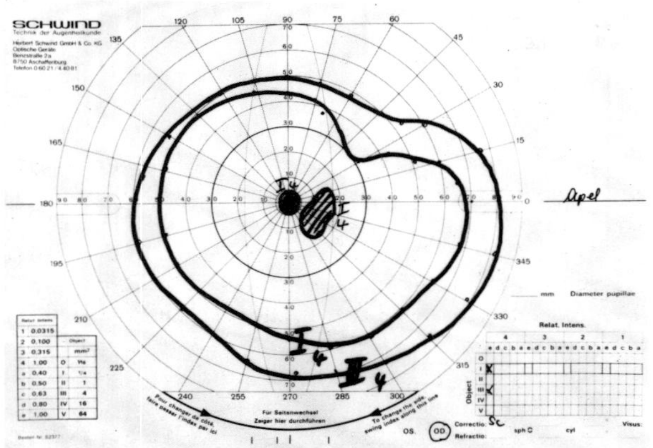

b

Fig. 5

In case of simultaneous cataract in Graves' disease, one has to check carefully whether loss of visual acuity and field defects are due to the cataract alone, or to a beginning optic nerve compression neuropathy as well. In the middle of Figure 4 we have patients with postoperative improvement of visual acuity after orbital decompression. This proves that a noteworthy part of visual acuity reduction was due to compression neuropathy; only the remaining reduction, compared with full visual acuity, is due to the beginning cataract formation. A cataract operation had not yet been carried out.

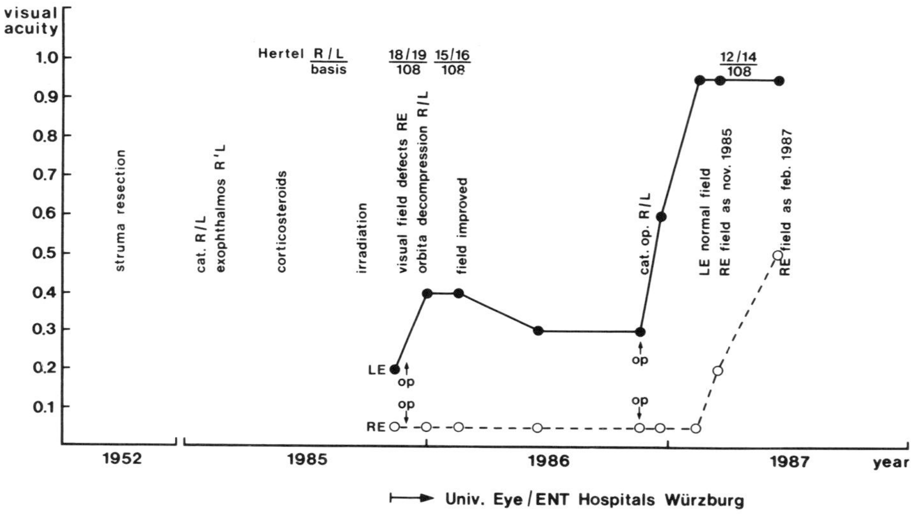

5c

Fig. 5: Visual acuity and visual field in a patient with cataract and compression neuropathy. In another clinic, the functional loss in both eyes was attributed solely to progressive cataract formation in both eyes. However, the degree of cataract was nearly equal in both eyes, but the visual acuity was markedly poorer in the right eye. Ultrasonography and CT scans proved compression neuropathy of the optic nerve of the right eye, due to Graves' ophthalmopathy. The visual field improved markedly after orbital decompression. The preoperative visual field is shown in figure 5a, the improvement after orbita decompression in Fig. 5b. the cataract was not yet operated at this time ! Later on, cataract surgery was performed. the visual acuity of RE (Fig. 5c), however, did not improve thereafter, despite the completely uneventful course and clear optic media. the disc showed partial optic nerve atrophy. About 6 months later, however, marked improvement of the visual acuity was found (Fig. 5c). Apparently, this has to be attributed to a late partial recovery of optic nerve functions, which was really surprising

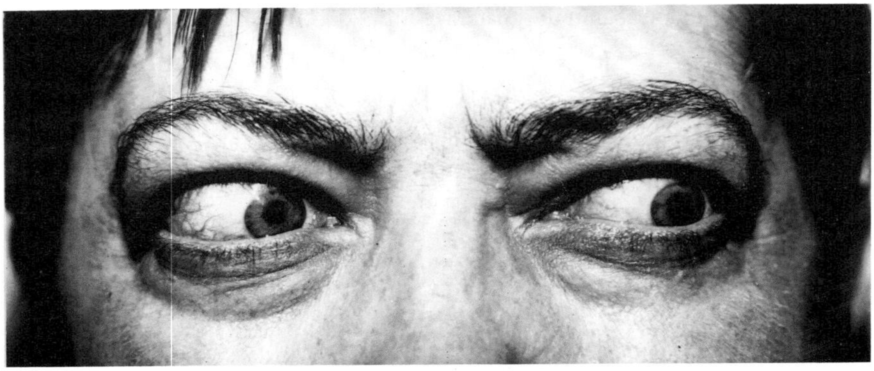

a

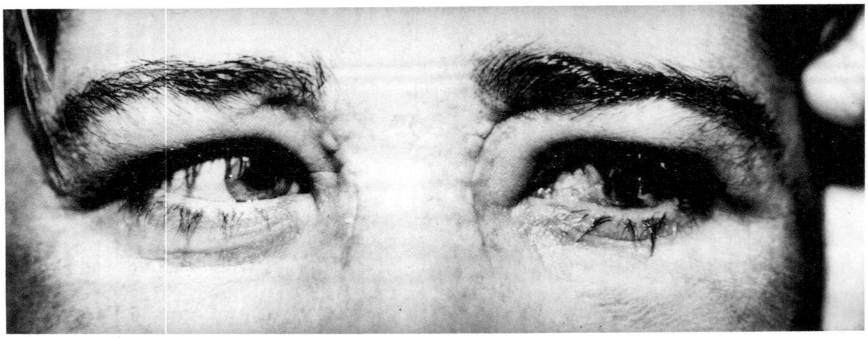

b

Fig. 6: Pre- and postoperative portrait (Figure 6a and 6b) of a patient who received unsuccessful corticosteroid and radiation therapy for grade VI of Graves' ophthalmopathy. pseudoglaucoma was mistaken for glaucoma, and glaucoma surgery performed before she was transferred to our Hospital. The result was marked worsening of the compression neuropathy with severe papilledema and reduction of visual acuity to .1 on both eyes. The preoperative papilledema is shown in figure 6c, its postoperative regression within 4 weeks after orbita decompression in Figure 6d. Fortunately, the visual acuity recovered (as well as the visual field), and improved markedly after orbita decompression (Figure 6e), which was done at once as an emergency operation

On the left side of figure 4, we have patients with considerable postoperative improvement of visual acuity; here, this is the result of orbita decompression surgery and subsequent cataract operation. These patients had advanced cataract. After uncomplicated cataract surgery, the final visual acuity can be determined within 2 to 3 weeks. In our cases here, however, we have seen improvements of visual acuity after months. it is very probable, therefore, that this resulted from optic nerve decompression, because recovery of visual acuity takes much more time and proceeds for months, after compression neuropathy. A remarkable example is shown in Figure 5.

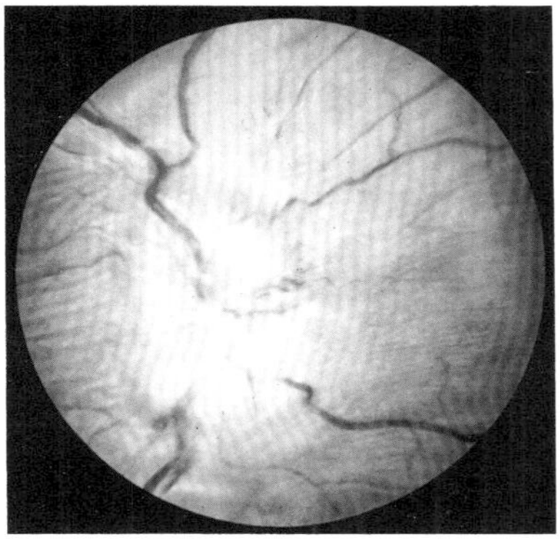

c

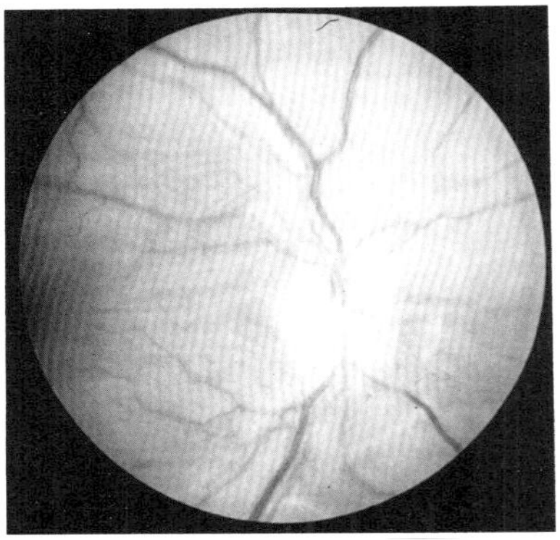

d

Fig. 6

The pre- and postoperative visual acuity found in 12 eyes was not included here, since the postoperative follow-up time was less than 2 months, and this is too short for evaluation of the postoperative vision.

Visual acuity and visual field were normal pre- and postoperatively in the other 30 eyes, the operation was indicated due to severe grades IV and V of Graves' ophthalmopathy.

Visual field defects, found preoperatively in both groups of Figures 3 and 4, improved markedly as well (mostly normalized).

In case of severe Graves' ophthalmopathy and simultaneous primary glaucoma or cataract, orbital decompression has to be done <u>before</u> intraocular surgery. Otherwise, the result of intraocular surgery could be disastrous.

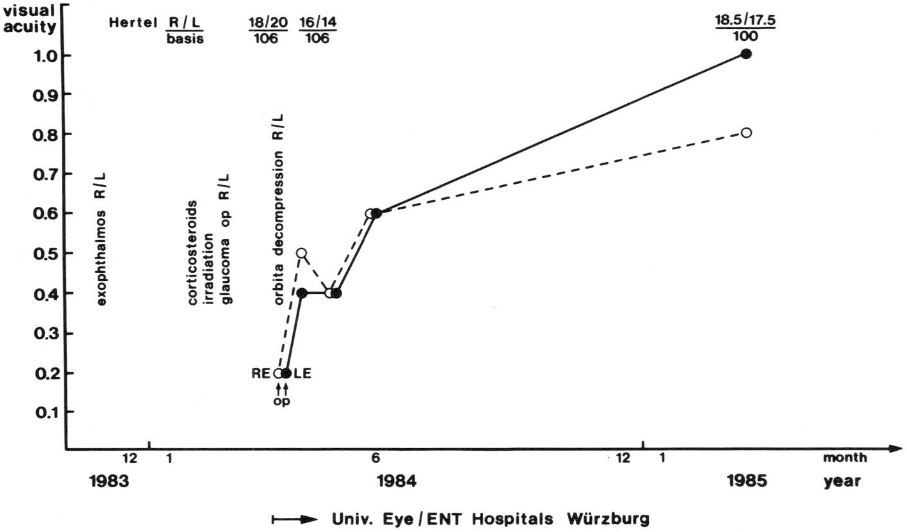

6e

Figure 6 shows an example in which medical and radiation therapy of grade VI Graves' ophthalmopathy were not effectful, glaucoma and pseudoglaucoma were not carefully differentiated, and glaucoma surgery (done elsewhere) resulted in dramatic progression of optic neuropathy with reduction of visual acuity to .1 on both eyes. In this case we did orbital decompression surgery as an emergency, and papilledema, visual acuity and visual field recovered promptly. Afterward, there was no sign of glaucoma left.

Another patient (Figure 7) had a primary glaucoma, which could be controlled by medical therapy for years. More recently, he has developed severe Graves' ophthalmopathy, and the intraocular pressure was raised in all gaze direction in spite of maximum antiglaucomatous therapy. Orbita decompression was performed, and in the further course the intraocular pressure could again be controlled by medical glaucoma therapy, and no glaucoma surgery was required. (BUSCHMANN, 1986).

The pre- and postoperative situation of the optic nerve in another patient is shown in the coronal CT after unilateral operation [2].

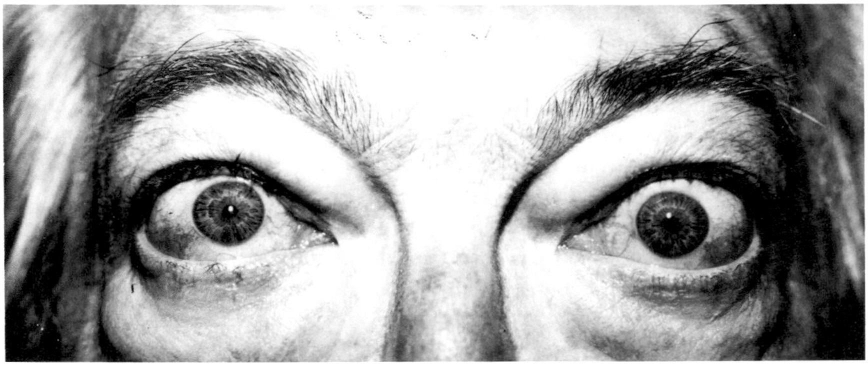

a

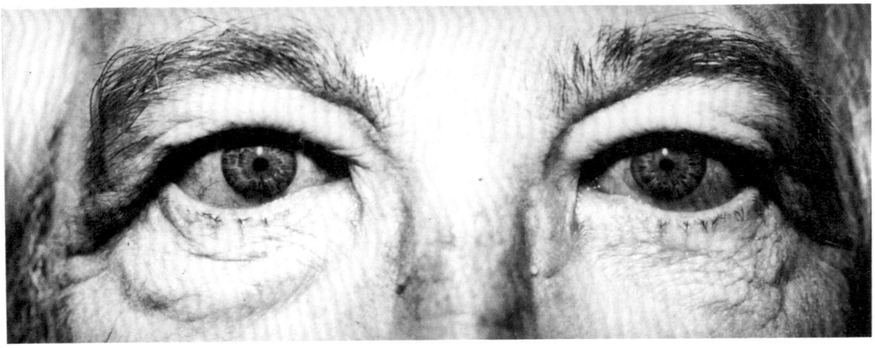

b

Fig. 7: Preoperative (Figure 7a) and postoperative (Figure 7b) portrait of a patient who had had primary glaucoma for years, which was controlled by topical application of miotics. Then, he developed Graves' ophthalmopathy (grade Vb). Medical treatment of his glaucoma now proved insufficient. We decided to postpone glaucoma surgery, and did orbita decompression first. After that, no glaucoma surgery has been required up to now - his glaucoma is again controlled by topical application of miotics

Results and view of exophthalmos and lagophthalmos

The extent of bulbus retroposition can be controlled by the extent of bone-wall resection. Therefore, the differences in the hertel readings before and after orbita decompression are various. The maximum reduction of Hertel readings was 10 to 11 mm in patients with high Hertel readings before surgery. The average reduction in all patients was 4.6 mm.

The resulting bulbus position can be evaluated on the first postoperative day, when the compression bandage has to be changed. As reaction to the surgical trauma, some postoperative edema may develop in the subsequent days, which usually disappears within 1 to 3 weeks of medical therapy. In some cases, however, the postoperative edema persisted longer and regressed slowly during several months. For this reason, we evaluated the postoperative bulbus position here only in those eyes in which the interval between date of surgery and recent examination was at least 6 months (68 eyes). Some of the other orbitas which has been operated were excluded here, because the Hertel readings proved not to be reliabely comparable (measurements performed with different types of exophthalmometers or with different base adjustments).

The lagophthalmos problems were solved in the majority of the 110 eyes after orbita decompression. But in 8 patients, retractions of the upper and/or lower lid persisted due to involvement of the retracting lid muscles (Mueller's muscles), so that additional lid surgery was required. We used the techniques recommended by WALLER, SAMPLES and YEATS (MAYO-Klinik, 1984) - a sclera implant for the lower lid and stepwise desinsertion of the levator aponeurosis at the upper lid. An additional tarsorrhaphy was necessary in one case only.

Motility results

Severe motility restrictions with double images in practically important gaze directions were fund in many patients preoperatively, often combined with lagophthalmos and/or compression neuropathy of the optic nerve. Postoperatively, the majority of these patients had normal binocular vision for the practically important gaze directions in the far and in the near. In 18 eyes only, additional squint surgery proved necessary. In these cases, mostly recessions of the inferior rectus muscle were done. Thereafter, these patients reached binocular vision and a useful field of gaze directions as well. The ability to read without getting double images is much more important than the upwards gaze direction. Thus, we (as well as the patients) were satisfied in cases of limited vertical motility, if the straight-forward gaze direction could be achieved without problems.

One patient was transferred to our Hospital when already complete immobilization of both eyes had developed (corresponding to complete external ophthalmoplegia). Despite effective reduction of the exophthalmos to normal eye position after decompression surgery, the complete immobilization has persisted up to now. A nearly parallel position of both eyes could be achieved, the double images could be avoided using small prism corrections.

Discussion and Conclusion

Orbita decompression surgery [4] proved to be a symptomatic, but very effective way of treatment in severe grades of Graves' ophthalmopathy, which should be applied in time. Cyclosporin A and plasmapheresis were, according to the reports of the other authors, less effective, especially in severe grades of the disease, and there are considerable side-effects. In our opinion, their use seems to be justified if severe recurrences of the disease after decompression surgery require intensive treatment. Until now, however, we have succeeded in these cases with a course of corticosteroid (2 patients), respectively combined corticosteroids and radiation treatment of the orbits (1 patients) - despite the fact that these measures proved ineffective in the same patients before orbita surgery.

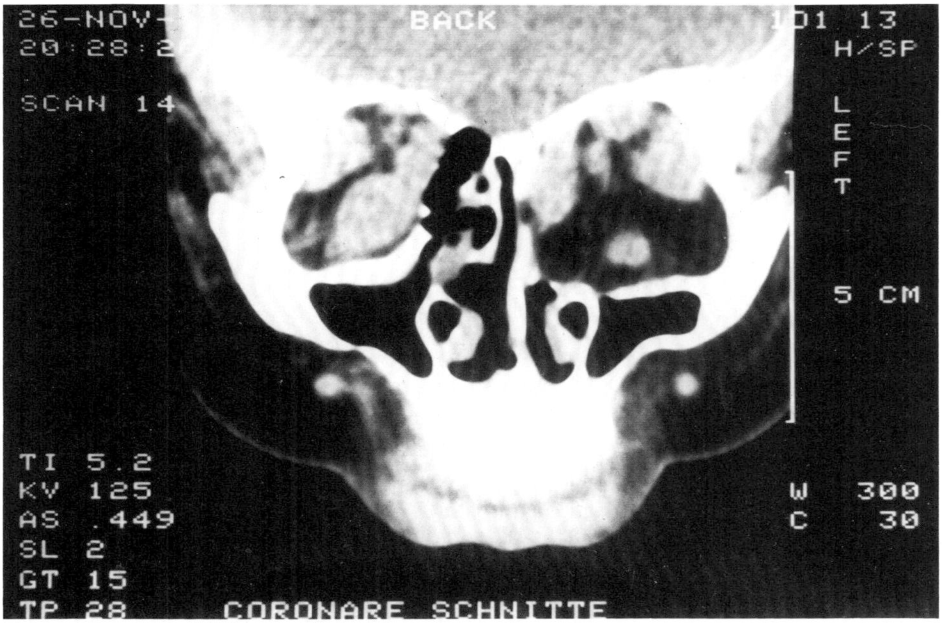

Fig. 8: Coronar computer tomogram of a patient with Graves' ophthalmopathy in both orbits. Decompression surgery was performed on the left side and is planned for the right side. One can see to which extent more space became available for the swollen orbital tissues on the left side, giving room to the optic nerve

Fortunately, up to now we have had no serious ophthalmic complications during or after decompression (only some corneal erosions). But it must be emphasized that the kind and the duration of the previous treatment have a marked influence on the risks of later surgery. Longterm conservative treatment and particularly radiation before decompression results in marked fibrosis of the muscles and orbital fat. Then, one has to cut, in addition to the periosteum, fibrose layers, before the fat tissue can really move into the spaces provided. It may even become necessary to mobilize the fat tissue actively (with blunt instruments). The risk of damaging hereby atypically positioned vessels or nerves is higher.

Orbita tumors

It is not possible to describe at this occasion our techniques and results in orbital tumor surgery as well. The improved interdisciplinary cooperation was found advantageous in this field, too. We use a modified Krönlein-Berke operation for tumors located laterally, above or below in the anterior two thirds of the retrobulbar space. The neurosurgical subfrontal approach is preferred in patients in whom the tumor is located in the orbital tip, and had invaded the optic canal.

For tumors located medially, we chose in cooperation with the rhinosurgeons the removal via an ethmoidectomy. Sometimes, it proved helpful in larger tumors a combination with a Krönlein-Berke operation, allowing the displacement of the whole content of the orbit laterally during tumor resection. In this procedure and even better view into the depth of the orbit [1, 3].

Summary

As a consequence of a new interdisciplinary approach (Orbita Team Wuerzburg), patients with severe Graves' Ophthalmopathy were sent to our Hospital from all parts of West Germany. A report is given on the results achieved in the first consecutive series of 110 orbita decompression operations. The decompression technique resulted in dramatic improvement (mostly normalization) of visual acuity and visual field, even in severe cases of compression neuropathy. Lagophthalmus and motility were markedly improved by the retroposition of the eyeball, addition squint or lid surgery was necessary in a minority of patients only. The technique enables the surgeon to control the extent of eye retro-position (maximum achieved: 11 mm). It proved important to consider surgical treatment as effective alternative before optic nerve atrophy develops, if grade IV to VI patients do not improve after conservative treatment.

References

[1] Buschmann W: Zur diagnostik und Therapie von Optikustomoren. fortschr. Ophthalmol. 79 (1982) 66 - 69

[2] Buschmann W: Glaukom bei endokrinen Exophthalmus. Klin. monatsbl. Augenheilk. 188 (1986) 138 - 140

[3] Buschmann W, Linnert D: Wandel der Indikationen und der Technik in der Chirurgie retrobulbärer Oritatumoren. Klin. Monatsbl. Augenheilk. 172 (1978) 1 - 12

[4] Buschmann W, Richter W: Ophthalmo-rhinochirurgische Entlastungsoperationen bei malignem endorkinen Exophthalmus. Klin. Monatsbl. Augenheil. 185 (1984) 1 - 8

[5] Buschmann W, Richter W, Kruse PH, Neumann O: Functional results in Graves' disease following ophthalmo-rhinosurgical orbital decompression. Orbit 5 (1986) 117 - 121

[6] Richter W CH, Kley W, Buschmann W: Ethmoidektomie und Orbitadekompression bei endokriner Ophthalmopathie. Laryng. rhinol. Otol. 63 (1984) 356 - 360

[7] Waller RR, Samples JR, Yeatts RP: Eyelid malpositions in graves' ophthalmopathy. In: gorman CA, Waller RR, Dyer JA (eds.): The Eye and Orbit in Thyroid Disease. Raven Press, New York, 1984, pp. 263 - 300

Further literature is given in the above quoted publications [4, 6]

Extended pterional decompression of the orbit: An alternative treatment in endocrine orbitopathy

J. M. Gilsbach, G. Kommerell, W. Seeger

Introduction

In endocrine orbitopathy, the neuropathy of the optic nerve is probably caused by pressure exerted by the ocular muscles. Accordingly, surgical enlargement of the orbit is followed usually by rapid improvement of visual acuity. Most ophthalmic and ENT surgeons enlarge the orbit by removing the medial and lower walls of the orbit [2, 4, 5, 6, 8, 9, 10]. However, although this enlarged ethmoidectomy provides sufficient room, it is often complicated by strabismus and occasionally by occlusion of the frontal sinus. In a case of a secondary visual deterioration after previous ethmoidectomy we enlarged the orbit additionally by removing the sphenoid wing. The visual acuity of the patient recovered rapidly thereafter. This case prompted us to explore the possibilities of pterional decompression [7, 13] for therapy resistant endocrine orbitopathy further.

Surgical technique

Surgery is performed under general anaesthesia. The head is fixated in a Mayfield-clamp. The skin is incised along the hairline starting from the preauricular region. There, the frontal branch of the facial nerve must be preserved. The skin flap is turned anteriorally until the region of the zygomatic process of the frontal bone and the frontal process of the zygoma are visible. The fascia of the temporal muscle is cut off the anterior part of the superior temporal line and zygoma, so that the muscle can be pulled posteriorly away from the temporal fossa. With high frequency drills (diamond) the larger wing of the sphenoid is removed until the frontal and temporal dura can be identified. With a microscope the lateral half of the lesser wing of the sphenoid is removed. In doing so, the upper bony border of the superior orbital fissure and the lateral half of the orbital fissure and the lateral half of the orbital roof are also removed. The lower and lateral borders of the superior orbital fissure are successively removed until the level of the floor of the orbit is reached (Figs. 1, 2). After removal of the lateral parts of the bony orbital roof the periorbity (periosteum of the orbit) is incised so that the orbital contents can expand into the created periorbital room (periosteum of the orbit) is incised so that the orbital contents can expand into the created periorbital room.

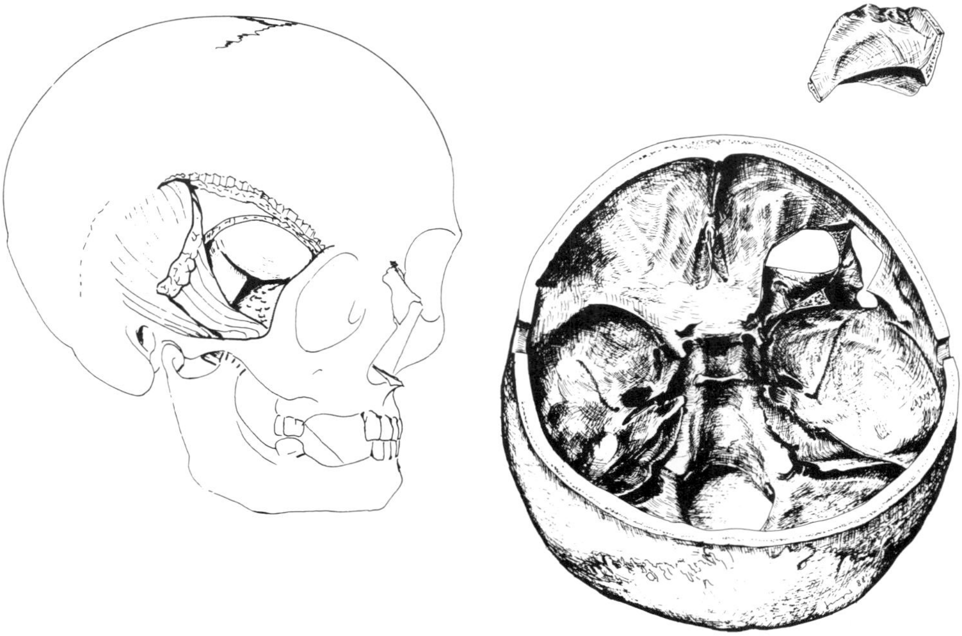

Fig. 1: Extended resection of bone in pterional orbital decompression for endocrine orbitopathy

Patients

Our series comprised seven orbits in six patients (Fig. 3). In six orbits, optic neuropathy prompted surgical intervention. The criteria for compression of the optic nerve were: reduction of visual acuity, defective colour vision, defective visual fields and an afferent pupillary defect. One orbit was decompressed because of an ulcer of the cornea caused by incomplete lid closure. In four of the seven orbits ethmoidectomies had been performed previously (open squares in Fig. 3). Additional decompression by pterional approach was performed because of recurrent deterioration of visual acuity. In three orbits pterional decompression was preferred as primary surgery after conservative measures like steroids and retrobulbar radiation had failed (filled squares in Fig. 3).

Results

In all cases, visual acuity improved. The relation between preoperative and postoperative visual acuities is depicted in Fig. 3. In 6 orbits we found a reduction of the exophthalmus of 3 mm, in one orbit of 4 mm. These values are comparable to those found after extended ethmoidectomy. In one patient, a strabismus that was caused by a previous ethmoidectomy improved. No new cases of strabismus were seen. No other complications occurred.

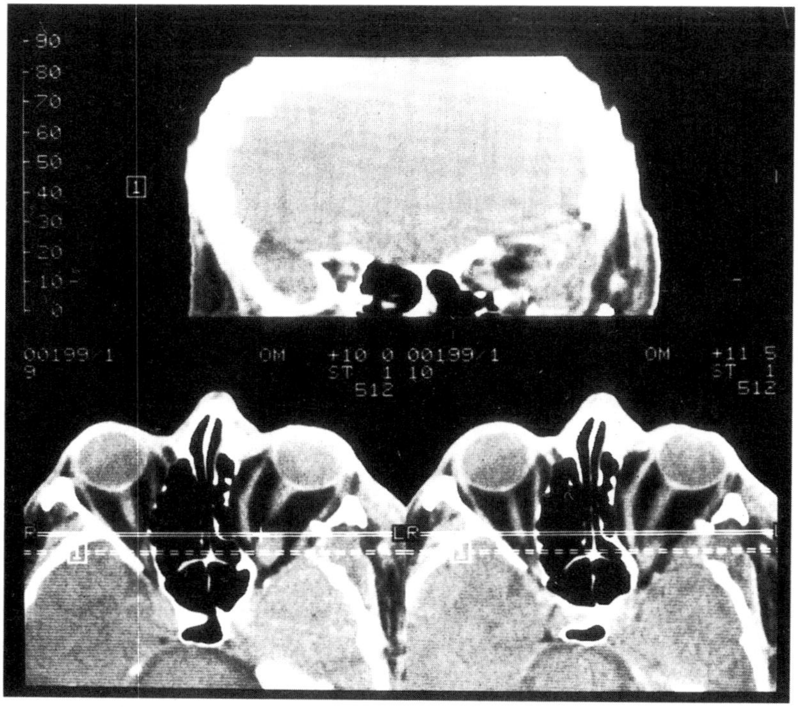

Fig. 2: CT scan after pterional decompression of the orbit after a previous ethmoidectomy and failed to improve visual acuity. The lateral orbital wall including the adjacent parts of the roof and apex have been removed

Discussion

The pterional approach for decompression of the orbit in endocrine orbitopathy is not a new one [1, 3, 7, 11, 13, 14]. Despite its effectiveness, this type of orbital decompression has never become very popular. After familiarizing ourselves with the pterional approach in tumours of the middle and anterior cerebral fossa, we decided to employ this technique in cases of recurrent deterioration of visual acuity due to endocrine orbitopathy.

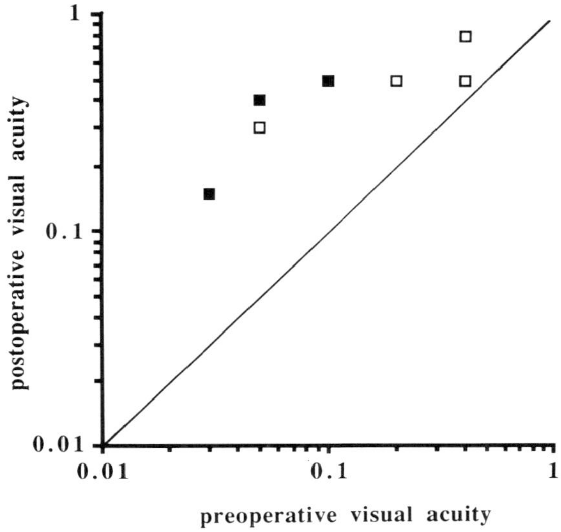

Fig. 3: Improvement of visual acuity after pterional decompression. Open squares correspond to patients with previous ethmoidectomies

Pterional decompression features the decompression of the apex of the orbit including the superior orbital fissure. This means decompressing the narrowest part of the orbit. Venous outflow may also be improved by the procedure, decreasing the volume load further.

Preservation of normal ocular motility is an important advantage of the pterional approach, as compared to ethmoidectomy. In none of the 7 operations the motility of the eye deteriorated. In contrast, the extended ethmoidectomy is often followed by convergent strabismus because the medial rectus muscle prolapses through a relatively small aperture into the ethmoid and, hence, cannot function properly [12]. In CT-scans, made after ethmoidectomy, the incarcerated medial rectus can be seen to curve strongly. After pterional decompression, however, the prolapse covers a larger surface area, interfering less with the functional anatomy of the orbital contents.

An additional advantage of the pterional approach as compared to ethmoidectomy may be that future increases of volume can be compensated, because the bony limit of the orbit is replaced by elastic frontal and temporal dura. Theoretically, removal of the bony walls of the orbit could result in pulsating exophthalmus. In none of our cases, however, this sign was present.

Interference with the drainage of the frontal sinus occurs occasionally after extended ethmoidectomy, necessitating secondary surgical reconstruction of the communication between the frontal sinus and the nose.

The risk of producing a CSF fistula is low in both procedures. Should the dura inadvertently be torn during a pterional approach, the danger of meningitis is less imminent, because no communication with contaminated areas like the nose results.

Scars are not visible if the skin incision is placed behind the hairline, in contrast to those in the ethmoidal approach. Experience with the pterional approach in cases of frontobasal tumors and aneurysm shows that palsies of the frontal branch of the facial nerve, a rare occurrence, almost always recover within half a year.

References

[1] Algverne P, Almquist S, Backlund EO: Pterional orbital decompression in progressive ophthalmopathy of Graves disease; 1./short term effects. Acta opthalmol 51 (1973) 467 - 74

[2] Anderson RL, Linber JV: Transorbital approach to decompression in Graves' disease. Arch Ophthalmol 99 (1981) 120 - 124

[3] Backlund E-O,: Pterional approach for orbital decompression. Acta ophtal (Kbh) 46 (1968) 535 - 540

[4] Buschmann W, Richter W: Ophtalmorhinochirurgische Entlastungsoperation bei malignem endokrinem Exophtalmus. Klin Mbl Augenheilk 185 (1984) 1 - 8

[5] Busse H, Stoll W, Promesberger H, Müller R-P: Operative Behandlung des malignen endokrinen Exophthalmus. Klin Mbl Augenheilk 182 (1983) 322 - 324

[6] Calcaterra TC, Thompson JW: Antral-ethmoidal decompression of the orbit in Graves' disease: Ten years experience. The Laryngoscope 90 (1980) 1841 - 1949

[7] Hamby WB,: Pterional approach to the orbits for decompression or tumor removal. J Neurosurg 21 (1964) 15 - 18

[8] Kennerdell JS, Maroon JC: An orbital decompression for severe dysthyroid exophthalmus. Ophthalmology 89 (1982) 467 - 472

[9] Kommerell G, Münker G: Operative Erweiterung der Augenhöhle zur Behandlung schwerer endokriner Orbitopathien. Z prakt Augenheilkd 6 (1985) 246 - 252

[10] Linberg JV, Anderson RL: Transorbital dedcompression. Arch Ophthalmol 99 (1981) 113 - 119

[11] Mac Carty CS, Kenefick TP, McConahey CS, Kearns TP: Ophthalmopathy of Graves disease treated by removal of roof, lateral walls and lateral sphenoid ridge. Mayo Clin Proc 45 (1970) 488 - 493

[12] Shorr N, Neuhaus RW, Baylis HI: Ocular motility problems after orbital decompression for dysthyroid ophthalmopathy. Ophtalmology 89 (1982) 323 - 326

[13] Welti H, Offret G: Indications et technique de la trépantion décompressive de l'orbite dans le traitement des exophtalmie maligne basedowienne. Lyon Chir 38 (1948) 542 - 555

[14] Welti H,: Resultats éloignés de dix tréphinations decompressives de l'orbite pour exophthalmie maligne. Rev Neurol 83 (1950) 389 - 393

Results of surgical orbital decompression in Graves' disease

F.X. Brunner, W. Kley, P. Plinkert

Introduction

From 1982 to 1987 more than 100 surgical orbital decompressions were performed in cooperation with rhino- and ophthalmosurgeons in the University of Würzburg. The surgical procedure was the technique developed by BUSCHMANN and RICHTER (1, 4).

Surgical technique

After a so-called Kilian-incision the anterior bony wall of the ethmoid cells is exposed. The ethmoid cells and the infundibulum of the frontal sinus are opened. The processus trochlearis is exposed and dissected free. Preserving the attachment of a small piece of bone to the tendon of the muscle allows its correct refixation without problems. The periostium of the lamina papyracea is elevated. The ethmoid arteries are cauterized. Afterwards the cell system of the ethmoid in an anterior posterior direction and the bone of the lamina papyracea can be removed. The bone of the orbital floor in a lateral direction is removed to the border of the canalis infraorbitalis. A surgical cavity surrounding the ethmoid cells, parts of the frontal sinus and parts of the maxillary sinus is created. After multiple incision of the orbital periostium the orbital fat is able to extend and occupy the space of the newly created surgical cavity. The medial or nasal wall of the ethmoid cells is preserved and strengthened with lyodura. The aeration of the maxillary sinus is maintained by creating a nasal antral window below the inferior turbinate, the aeration of the frontal sinus is secured in cases of surgical decompression of only one side by resection of the septum of the frontal sinus. In cases of surgical decompression of both sides, the aeration of the frontal sinus is made possible by resecting the bone of the lamina perpendicularis anterior to the alfactory area, according the procedure of MAYER (2, 3).

Postoperative controls

Normally the natural exits of the maxillary sinuses and frontal sinuses are resected, granulation tissue and scars in the area of the new ostium can then cause complaints. After-care of these patients by the ENT-surgeon are therefore necessary. In this investigation the results of these controls of 34 patients who underwent surgical orbital decompression from April 1984 to July 1987 are compared and discussed.

Results

In figure 1 the age structure of the population is illustrated and shows, that the patients reached mostly the age of 50 or 60 years before coming to surgery. In 9 patients the operation was done unilaterally, in 25 bilaterally. The male-female relationship was 1:2. The average age of the males was about 57 years, the average age of the females 48 years.

In a period of 3 weeks after the operation, 12 patients (= 35%) had no complaints (Tab. I). The remaining 65 % complained of diffuse headache of inconstant durancy.

Table I: Postoperative complaints n = 34

up to three weeks	Yes 22/65 %	No 12/35 %	Lasting more than six months	Yes 10/29 %	No 19/56 %	not classified 5/15 %
headache	11/32 %			6/18 %		
sensibility disorder V_1	8/24 %			4/12 %		
paraesthesia V_1	5/15 %			2/6 %		
neuralgiform pain V_1	2/6 %			1/3 %		
eyelid swelling	5/15 %			4/12 %		
healing disturbances	3/18 %			1/3 %		
tear duct disturbances	1/3 %					
retrobulbar heamatoma	1/3 %					
relapse of exophthalmos	1/3 %					

25 % of the patients had sensory disturbances in the region of the n.supraorbitalis. Paraesthesias in this area and eyelid swelling occured in 5 patients, neuralgiform complaints in 2 patients. The pain was permanent and of varying intensity in the region of the n.supraorbitalis, in one case also in the area of the n.infraorbitalis, in one case also in the area of the n.infraorbitalis. 3 patients had wound healing disturbances. A temporary disturbance of lacrimal drainage and a relapse of exophthalmus resulted in at least one case.

Only 10 patients had complaints lasting more than 6 months. Headache was the main complain. 4 patients reported of swollen eyelids while 2 of them complained about it only 20 minutes in the morning after waking up. In one case the wire used for refixation of the trochlea caused inflammation and abscess. After removing the wire no more disturbances occured.

By performing the ethmoidectomy the nasofrontal ducts and the ostiums of the maxillary sinuses are resected. Therefore the aftercare of the newly created openings has to be carried out, because an occlusion of the nasal antral window or the newly created openings of the frontal sinus is possible. Complications with the possibility of mucoceles formulation can result.

Testing the patency of the nasal antral window with a probe under local anaesthesia is not difficult. The nasal antral windows in cases of unilateral surgical procedure allowed probing in 89 % (Tab. II) and in cases of bilaterally surgical procedure in 80 %. It is more difficult to probe the new openings of the frontal sinuses. Also, the frontal sinuses can be tested with endoscopic techniques. In 72 % of the cases of bilaterally surgical procedure these openings were free and could be seen clearly. In 12 % of the cases they could not be seen endoscopically but they were probe-patent. In the remaining 4 patients no frontal sinuses were developed.

Table II: Postoperative control of maxillary and frontal sinuses

	unilaterally OP (n = 9)	bilaterally OP (n = 25)
nasal antral window easily to probe	Yes 89 % No 1/11 %	Yes 40/40 % No 10/20 %

Endoscopic control of the new opening of the frontal sinus (bilaterally OP n = 25)

Nasal frontal window free and visible	18/72 %	Nasal frontal window not visible but to probe	3/12 %	Aplasia of frontal sinuses	4/16 %

X-ray examinations of the paranasal sinuses (Tab. III) should be done 6 weeks after the operation, and repeated after one year if there are no complaints. The x-ray pictures of the 34 patients showed that even in nearly all cases, where the nasal antral windows could not be proved, a satisfactory aeration of the maxillary sinuses was still present. Only in one case the maxillary sinus was radiologically opacificated and not to be reached with the probe. In this case a second operation to open the nasal antral window was necessary.

32 (94 %) of the patients were satisfied with the results of the operation. The visible reduction of the exophthalmos and the improvement of visual function after the operation were considered as the most important results of the surgical treatment.

Discussions

Follow-up ENT examinations are necessary to avoid complications. In one case of 34 patients the nasal antral window became closed by scar tissue and had to be opened in a second operation. X-ray examinations of the paranasal sinuses should be performed 6 weeks after the operation and 1 year after surgery. Further controls should be performed every year.

Table III

X-ray controls

		unilateral OP (n = 9)	bilateral OP (n = 25)
maxillary sinus	normal	8/89 %	48/98 %
	opacification	1/11 %	1/2 %
frontal sinus	normal	6/67 %	42/100 %
	opacification	1/11 %	
	aplasia	2/22 %	4/16 %
sphenoidal sinus	normal	23/100 %	

In the opinion of the 34 patients the most important points of a successfully performed surgical orbital decompression are a visible reduction of the exophthalmos and the improvement of visual function. In nearly every case both could be achieved. Postoperative disturbances, such as sensibility disorders, paresthesia and eyelid swelling were estimated not to be so important. These disorders are disadvantages of the Kilian-incision, by which it can not be avoided to cut some branches of the supraorbital nerve. The advantage of this incision is a very good survey. The rhinosurgeon is able to create as much space as needed to push back the eyeball after the incisions of the orbital periostium are done.

The new openings of the paranasal sinuses can be created so that by longterm follow-up no complications could be found.

Summary

Surgical orbital decompression is necessary in severe cases of Grave's disease. According to the technique of BUSCHMANN and RICHTER, via an external approach, the ethmoid cells are removed. The functional results of the operation in 34 patients treated from 4/87 to 6/87 are discussed. Functional problems of nose and paranasal sinuses did not arise in any case.

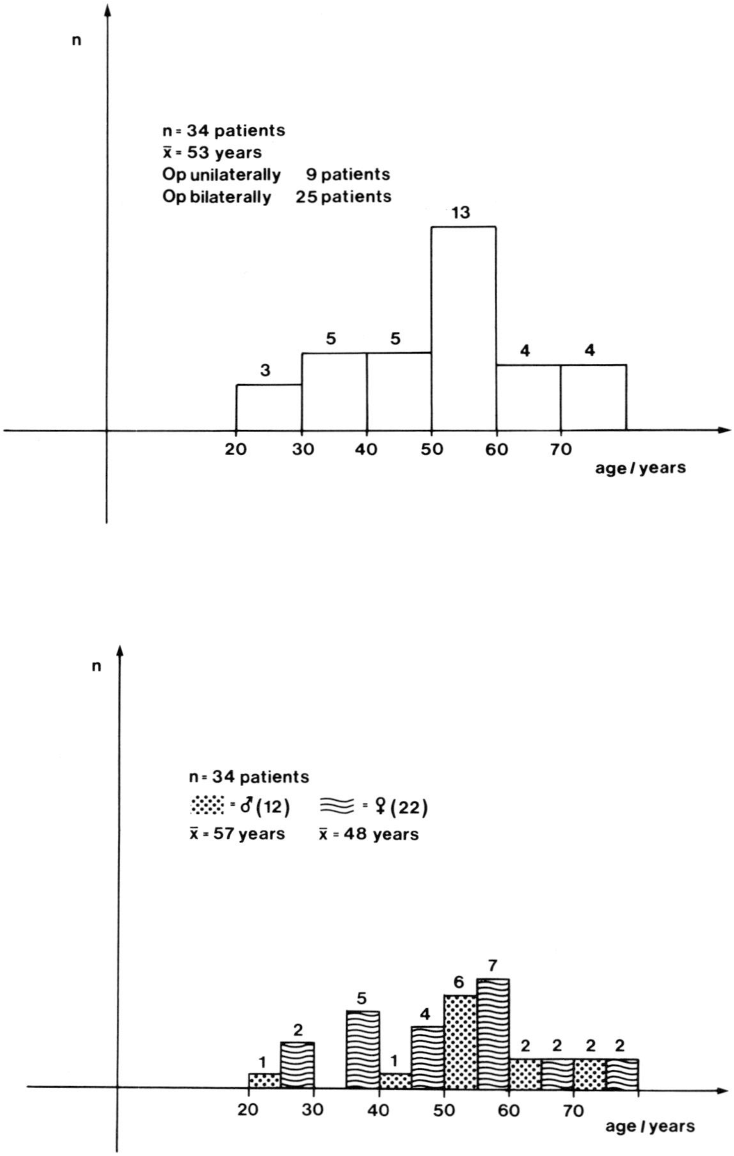

Fig. 1: Surgical orbital decompression - age of patients

References

[1] Buschmann W, Richter W, Kruse PH, Neumann O: Functional results in Graves' disease following ophthalmorhinosurgical orbital decompression. Orbit 5 (1986) 117

[2] Krenner A: Die Indikation zur Median- und Kontralateraldrainage der Stirnhöhle und deren Durchführung. Arch Ohr Nas Kehlkopfheilk 157 (1950) 28

[3] Mayer O: Über die Herstellung einer breiten Verbindung mit der Nase bei der wegen chronische Entzündung vorgenommenen radikalen Stirnhöhlenoperation. Arch Ohr Nas Kehlkopf 148 (1940) 282

[4] Richter W, Kley W, Buschmann W: Ethmoidektomie und Orbitadekompression bei endokriner Orbitopathie. Laryng Rinol Otol 63 (1984) 356

Long-term study of endocrine ophthalmopathy (A retrospective observation of 297 patients)

G. Kahaly, H. Böckmann, U. Cordes, J. Beyer

Summary

The objective of the study was long-term observation of endocrine orbitopathy with regard to clinical and clinical chemical parameters and possibilities of therapy. The progress observation of 297 patients, (44 ± 14 years, 248 female, 48 men; 5 : 1) was made between 1975 and 1986 with inclusion of data from the history and clinical data as well as the results of imaging techniques (CT and sonography of the orbit). In addition, the patients whose last investigation was made more than one year previously were interviewed with regard to the further disease course on the basis of a questionnaire.

Two hundred and fifty-three patients were hyperthyroid, 36 euthyroid and eight had latent to manifest hypothyroidism. The staging was: I 13, II 54, II 113, IV 95, V 5, VI 8. The HLA typing in 89 patients showed the following results: DR3 42 %, A3 33 %, B8 31 %, DR4 28 %, DR5 27 %. In 104/210 patients (50 %), there were raised microsomal antibodies. In 27/205 (18 %), there were raised thyroglobulin antibodies. 158/250 patients (63 %) received immunosuppressants: corticosteroids in 100 % (1 x in 75 %, 2 x in 30 %, 3 x in 10 %, 4 x in 3 %), cyclosporin A (Cy A) in 28 cases, ciamexon in 26 cases. The retrobulbar irradiation was performed in 23 cases, and total thyroidectomy in 17 cases. Significant differences were observed in combined Cy A + prednisone therapy (Hertel values: 21.8 ± 0.7 as compared to 18.8 ± 0.7; p less than 0.001) and in total thyroidectomy (Hertel values: 21.23 ± 3.9 as compared to 18.4 ± 3.7; p less than 0.05)

None of the therapies applied constitutes an optimal treatment with regard to the long-term course. Because of the suspected autoimmunogenesis, nonsteroid immunosuppressants are being used to an increasing extent. Combined immunosuppressant treatment is superior to steroid monotherapy with regard to the rate of recurrences, but has a higher rate of side effects.

Introduction

Endocrine ophthalmopathy (EO) is an autoimmune disease of which the pathogenesis is still obscure (3, 13, 19, 25). Different suspected pathomechanisms have led to different approaches to therapy (14 a), without providing the desired definitive result. Retrospective observations in small patient populations have already been published (8, 10, 11, 24). In the three of these studies mentioned, comparative data with regard to the existing possibilities of therapy are lacking. The lack of objectively appraisable parameters in the fourth study does not allow a precise evaluation of the course. In our patients, the long-term observation was to be evaluated on the basis of these objectively appraisable parameters (Hertel values, vision, intraocular pressure, computer tomogram, ultrasonography). The question as to the possibilities of therapy, changes in treatment schedules and their results received special consideration.

A. Patients

The patient records of 297 patients with endocrine ophthalmopathy (248 female, 49 male; ratio f : m = 5 : 1, age 16 - 78 years, mean value ± standard deviation = 44 ± 14 years). These comprised 242 patients who had been investigated (and treated in most cases) in the period from 1975 to 1986 in the Department of Internal Medicine, Endocrinology and Metabolism, Mainz University Medical School, and 55 patients who presented between 1983 and 1986 at the endocrinological practice of Prof. Cordes. A single investigation was carried out in 47 out of 297 patients, so that their data could only be included in part in the analysis (for detailed presentation of the patient data, see Tab. I).

B. Methods

The records of all patients in whom an endocrine ophthalmopathy had been diagnosed on the basis of the history, clinical values and clinical laboratory investigations (in some cases by imaging techniques: computer tomogram, sonography of the orbit) were analysed. The following parameters which were evaluated in the analysis of the patient records with regard to long-term course.

I. (1) Age of the patients at the beginning of therapy

(2) Age of the patients at the beginning of the disease, when this could be determined from the history

(3) Time relation between the occurrence of endocrine ophthalmopathy and hyperthyroidism (if present at all)

(4) Duration of therapy and control period

II.(1) The individual stage of endocrine ophthalmopathy at the beginning of therapy and in the course, in accordance with the classification of the Thyroid Section of the German Society of Endocrinology (17). Stage III = protrusio bulbo sive bulborum was established from a protrusion = 17 mm or in the case of unilaterality with a difference = 3 mm between the two eyes in the measurement according to Hertel. Only the Hertel values which were bases on identical basic values in the progress measurement were analysed.

II.(2) Additional detection of the subjective symptoms (e.g. light sensitivity, tear flow, feeling of retrobulbar pressure, blurred vision)

III.(1) Clinical laboratory values of the thyroid hormones before therapy and the course. T3, T4 and TSH were measured radioimmunologically (18). Normal values: T3 80 - 200 ng/dl, T4 4.5 - 10.5 μg/dl, basal TSH value 0 - 7 IU/ml, TSH after TRH stimulation 2.5 - 25 IU/ml but at least 2.5 IU/ml.

(2) Detection of microsomal and thyroglobulin antibodies before and after therapy was carried out by means of an ELISA method (23)

(3) Results of HLA typing

IV.(4) Type of therapy applied, if possible previous therapy attempts

VI.(1) Ophthalmological consultative investigation with special consideration of vision and intraocular pressure in the course of therapy

VII.(1) Computer tomographic investigations of the orbit

The patients whose last checkup was dated more than one year previously were interviewed with a questionnaire. Symptoms of endocrine ophthalmopathy still present were to be explored and the question as to whether a fresh therapy was necessary in the meantime (owing to a recurrence) was to be clarified.

For appraisal of the course with consideration of the therapy, the patients were subdivided into five groups (see Tab. II).

C. Statistics

In general, the data are specified as mean value and standard deviation. The comparison of Hertel values, vision and intraocular pressure before and after therapy was carried out by means of the Wilcoxon test for pair differences in dependent random samples. A value = 0.05 was considered to be significant.

Results

1) Results of therapy

In 250 out of 297 patients, the course and therapy of endocrine ophthalmopathy were appraised retrospectively. In 37 %, a specific therapy in terms of systemic immunosuppression or retrobulbar irradiation was not necessary (in five patients, there had already been a prior steroid treatment). Local protective measures ensured alleviation of symptoms (dark glasses, eye ointment, artificial tears). When hyperthyroidism was present, this was treated with thyrostatics (as a rule, metimazole, or with radioiodine therapy or strumectomy).

Table I

Clinical data 1

	N	m	f	age onset of therapy	average duration of symptoms at time of onset	average duration of control period
group 1	92	12	82	41,5±13,0 (16-77)	1,2±2,9 (-3,6-14,9)	2,2±2,3 (0,0-11.9
group 2	84	13	71	42,6±13,5 (17-18)	1,3±5,3 -0,1-44,5)	2,3±2,4 (0,1-8,9)
group 3	37	6	31	50,9±12,7 (22-76)	1,5±3,1 (-0,2-17,7)	1,7±1,4 (0,0-7,2)
group 4	27	5	22	48,4±12,0 (22-69)	3,8±9,1 (0,1-34,2)	4,2±3,2 (0,4-11,3)
group 5	10	3	7	47,6±13,9 (19-65)	3,1±5,8 (0,2-20,2)	2,8±3,7 (0,3-22.5)
group 6	47	8	39	45,4±14,7 (20-72)	4,3±8,0 (0,1-32,4)	

84/250 patients received glucocorticoids in the form of split course therapies. This was carried out once in 57 patients (mean dose 50 mg). Absence of therapeutic results and recurrences led to a double (mean dose 50 mg) steroid administration in 18 patients, and to a triple (mean dose 67 mg) steroid administration in six patients, and finally a quadruple steroid administration in one patient. In this group, such a therapy had already been carried out previously in 16 cases, and there had been prior retrobulbar irradiation in two patients. Three further retrobulbar irradiations after the therapy at the University Hospital were revealed by questionnaire.

Table II

Subdivision of the patients into therapeutic groups

Group 1:	Patients without specific therapy of endocrine ophthalmopathy; in hyperthyroidism, thyrostatic therapy
Group 2:	Patients with steroid therapy
Group 3:	Patients who received nonsteroid immunosuppressants in combination with steroids
Group 4:	Patients with retrobulbar irradiation or total thyroidectomy or a combination of both
Group 5:	Patients with multiple combination therapy: steroids, nonsteroid immunosuppressants, total thyroidectomy, retrobular irradation
(Group 6:	Patients investigated once)

Beside application of prednisone or prednisolone, group 3 was characterized by its having received nonsteroidal immunosuppressants (cyclosporin and ciamexon). Group 3 comprised two irradiated patients and 11 patients with prior prednisone treatment. Sixteen of these 37 patients received glucocorticoids several times. Total thyroidectomy and retrobulbar irradiation were each carried out in 11 patients, and a combination of the two treatments was given in five patients. This measure was combined with immunosuppressive steroid application. As in group 3, earlier attempts had also been made in this direction (30 %). In addition, there was a prior irradiation in 19 % of the patients.

Finally, group 5 contains the therapy-resistant cases, of whom the number amounted to 4 % of the total. Besides multiple administration of steroids in all patients, azathioprine (n = 1), cyclophosphamide (n = 1), cyclosporin (n = 7), ciamexon (n = 7), total thyroidectomy (n = 3) and retrobulbar irradiation (n = 7) were applied.

The fact that one could refer to stepping up of therapeutic measures in groups 1 - 5 is also reflected in the distribution of the individual stages before therapy. Accordingly, group 3 - 5 contained almost exclusively patients from stage III and even after therapy a displacement from the higher stages mostly stops at this "boundary". Stages V and VI were attained in 4 %. An improvement could be attained in this stages, apart from two measures: one case involved a discontinuation of therapy by the patient, and in the other case there was already an incomplete optic nerve atrophy (a decompression operation was recommended here). Table III shows a decline of the Hertel values in the longterm course. 73 % of the patients who had answered the questionnaire reported a subjective improvement of protrusion, 24 % stationary protrusion and only one patient reported an increase of the exophthalmos.

Table III

Clinical data 3

HERTEL VALUES

	Right eye before	Right eye after	Left eye before	Left eye after
group 1	19,0±3,1	18,7±2,0	18,8±2,9	18,3±2,3
	(p>0,05)		(p>0,05)	
group 2	19,9±3,0	17,8±2,5	19,9±3,0	18,0±2,5
	(p>0,05)		(p>0,05)	
group 3	21,8±0,7	18,8±0,7	21,9±0,67	18,9±0,4
	(p<0,001)		(p<0,001)	
group 4	21,2±3,9	18,4±3,7	20,8±3,8	18,7±3,8
	(p<0,05)		(p<0,05)	
group 5	23,3±3,7	21,0±2,2	24,1±4,5	21,0±2,2
	(no statistic evaluation possible)			

The appraisal of vision and intraocular pressure (see Tab. IV, V) had also to be carried out almost exclusively by means of mean value ± SD, but the low percentage presence of stage VI with loss of vision corresponds to the fact that no major alterations in vision before and after therapy were present in the majority of cases in the mild stages (below III). As shown by the results in group 3, marked successes in terms of a lowering of pressure were doubtless to be registered in consistent, comparative measurement. Figure 1 shows a synoptic presentation of the staging before and after therapy.

2) Clinical chemical values

In 91 % of patients suffering from endocrine ophthalmopathy, this was accompanied by hyperthyroidism substantiated in the history or by clinical chemical values. The ophthalmological symptoms preceded the hyperthyroidism in 10 % of the cases, the two diseases were manifested at roughly the same time in 52 %, and the hyperthyroidism followed the E.O. in 38 % (this in turn most frequently in the first six months after beginning of the thyroid hyperfunction (Fig. 2). The average T3 value was 280 ± 180 ng/dl in the hypothyroidism's group. T4 exceeded the upper range of normal only to a small extent (11.2 ± 6.9 μg/dl) owing on the one hand to isolated T3 hyperthyroidism and on the other hand to thyrostatic therapy which has already been commenced.

Twenty patients displayed a euthyroid metabolic situation during the entire control period which was also substantiated in the history. In 15 TRH stimulation tests available at the beginning of therapy, five did not show any rise of TSH after TRH administration. In addition, the microsomal thyroid antibodies were also raised in one third of the cases in this group, and TAK only in one out of 16 determination.

Hyperthyroidism as a manifestation of a past thyroiditis was present in three patients, MAK was positive in all three patients, and TAK in one. Apart from in group 1, which showed raised titers for MAK in more than 50 % and raised titers for TAK in more than 15 %, these markedly decreased in the remaining groups (MAK: 22 % - 36 %, TAK: 10 % - 12 %). The HLA typing (see Fig. 3) was carried out in about one third of the patients. the raised occurrence of HLA B8 and DR3 which has already been described many times was shown, but HLA A3 was also very prominently represented (33 %). It was interesting in this connection to investigate the occurrence of other autoimmune diseases within the patients: a type I .diabetes mellitus was found in six patients, an atrophic gastritis in three patients, a chronic polyarthritis in two patients, an idiopathic Addison's disease and a myasthenia gravis were found in one patient each.

3) Imaging techniques (computer tomogram and ultrasound)

In 69 out of 92 patients, involvement of the extraocular muscles could be demonstrated at the beginning of therapy. The medial rectus muscle and the inferior rectus muscle predominated, and the lateral rectus muscle was affected most rarely. There was a marked atrophy of individual eye muscles under combined Cy A/prednisone therapy in half of the patients. Since this study otherwise only enables qualitative statements, its appraisal validity with regard to the effects of therapy on the straight eye muscles is very limited. Nevertheless, 89 % of patients investigated by computer tomography in the period from 12 to 24 months after the beginning of therapy showed thickened eye muscles, and this went up to 95 % more than 24 months after the beginning of therapy which is probably based on a negative selection. Parallel results were found in sonography.

Discussion

In this paper, the course of endocrine orbitopathy was evaluated over a maximum of 22.5 years. The question was examined as to whether a conclusion can be drawn with regard to therapy recommendations or schedules on the basis of the results in the different kinds of treatment, also bearing in mind that several forms of therapy were applied at the same time in a proportion of the patients.

Table IV

Clinical data 4

VISUAL ACUITY

	Right eye before	Right eye after	Left eye before	Left eye after
group 1	0,86±0,26	0,67±0,32	0,77±0,28	0,77±0,32
	(no statistic evaluation possible)			
group 2	0,83±0,27	0,85±0,21	0,80±0,31	0,92±0,09
	(p>0,05)		(p>0,05)	
group 3	0,59±0,05	0,89±0,03	0,56±0,03	0,87±0,03
	(p<0,001)		(p<0,001)	
group 4	0,47±0,34	0,69±0,28	0,57±0,37	0,75±0,24
	(p<0,05)		(p<0,05)	
group 5	0,77±0,29	0,80±0,17	0,62±0,36	0,66±0,30
	(no statistic evaluation possible)			

Compared to GORMAN (8) the results of this retrospective study showed a lower proportion of male patients with similar age distribution. However, the patient population at the Mayo Clinic exclusively involved patients in whom decompression was foreseen. Severe ophthalmopathy, which necessitates such a surgical operation, occurs four times more frequently amongst men (on the basis of the lower incidence of hyperthyroidism in men) than in women (3, 6, 7) and thus explains the shift in the sex ration. The number of patients who have never been hyperthyroid is higher in this investigation, probably due to the fact that the observation was only made up to the time of operation and the hyperthyroidism possibly following the E.O. was no longer registered. The duration of the presence of the ophthalmological symptoms average 12 months in the euthroid patients in this group. Both his and our own results with regard to the time relation between the onset of E.O. and the hyperthyroidism show that the ophthalmological manifestations precede the thyroid hyperfunction by months to years in about 10 % - 15 % of the cases. Complete agreement also prevails with regard to GORMAN's assertion that about 80 % of the patients developed the ophthalmological symptoms in a period of 18 months before and after diagnosis of the hyperthyroidism. Compared to this, the data of SCHIFFERDECKER (24) are based on similar values. However, the exact chronological breakdown before the onset of hyperthroidism is lacking here. In addition, the published number of just under 5 % ophthalmological manifestations before the beginning of hyperthyroidism appears to be relatively low.

The fact that about 50 % of the patients checked by SCHIFFERDECKER did not require any specific therapy, whereas this number was very much lower in our investigations might be due a negative selection within the observation groups (as also at GORMAN). Patients with slight orbitopathy merely receive local measures or are treated with corticosteroids at outside hospitals, as proved by the numberous pretreatments of our patients. Severe stages of disease are then handed over to experienced therapist. In addition, 80 % of the untreated patients of SCHIFFERDECKER did not undergo any improvement. As already demonstrated at an early stage by HALES and RUNDLE (9), a persistence or indeed a deterioration of the E.O predominated compared to improvement, even if there is no specific therapy. A stage III or IV as a residual stage of an ophthalmopathy which is inactive in the meantime must frequently be accepted, but should not be the objective of therapy.

However, there is agreement that mild stages (less than stage III) do not require any immunosuppressants, and on the other hand severe conditions should be treated at an early stage. With regard to the partial remissions described in the literature (1, 12, 26), our study shows on the one hand that a spontaneous decline of the protrusion or the diplopia (possibly an improvement of vision) hardly occurs, and that on the other hand mild stages, e.g. upper eyelid retraction may regress under conservative treatment.

Corticosteroids are the standard treatment of E.O. (14 a). However, their known side effects restrict their chronic application. Earlier papers (5, 14, 21) and results of this study revealed of this study revealed a lasting improvement in a few patients. They were often imployed several times in succession and afterwards required other therapeutic measures because of the high rate of relapses. The new immunosuppressant or immunomodulator products of the new generation (cyclosporin A, ciamexon) have a very much more specific action on the immune system (14 a) and possess less general side effects, and these are mostly reversible when the dose is reduced. In this respect they are superior to the drugs such as methotrexate, azothioprine and cyclophospahmide employed earlier and allow a combined treatment at an early stage with glucocorticoids in florid ophthalmopathy. The retrospective evaluation of the objective parameters such as Hertel values, vision, intraocular pressure, stages of E.O. indicate a significant effect of the combined immunosuppressant therapy (Cy A plus prednisone) (14 a, 14, 15) which is confirmed by other authors (28, 19). Because of the not inappreciable side effects of the products specified, these substances should be regarded as complementary to steroid therapy and should not be administered on their own.

Table V

Clinical data 5

INTRAOCULAR PRESSURE

	Right eye before	Right eye after	Left eye before	Left eye after
group 1	16±3 (12-26)	16±1 (15-18)	16±3 (13-26)	16±1 (15-18)
	(no statistic evaluation possible)			
group 2	13±8 (15-25)	17±2 (14-20)	18±4 (12-26)	17±1 (15-19)
	(no statistic evaluation possible)			
group 3	17±4 (11-25)	15±2 (11-19)	17±4 (12-32)	14±1 (12-16)
	($p<0,05$)		($p<0,05$)	
group 4	16±3 (12-24)	17±3 (12-19)	16±3 (12-22)	17±1 (15-18)
	(no statistic evaluation possible)			
group 5	18±4 (12-25)	16±1 (14-18)	17±4 (13-25)	17±2 (15-22)
	(no statistic evaluation possible)			

Retrobulbar irradiation combination with glucocorticoids, even if it is superior to steroid therapy alone (2) has proved effective with regard to bringing a progressive process to a standstill (10, 11), but leaves diplopia and exophthalmos largely unaffected (24, 27). Many of our patients had already been irradiated before the period of observation, but then showed fresh signs of activity and progression.

On the basis of the notion that a thyroid antigen plays a role in the pathogenesis of E.O., total thyroidectomy was propagated (4, 5, 16, 20). This study confirmed that the operation in combination with steroids in the course led to a significant decline of the hertel values, to an improvement of vision, and in many of our patients to a stabilization of E.O. over long periods of time. However, it was unfortunately associated with residual states in the form of eye muscle pareses. It remains reserved for the severe forms.

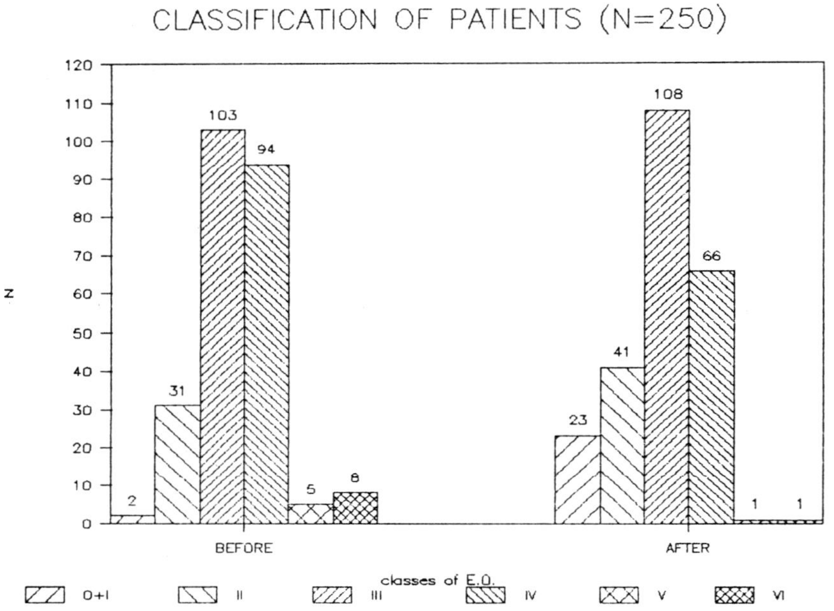

Fig. 1:

Orbit decompression has the aim of restoring or preserving a threatened visual capacity, safeguarding the function of the outer ocular muscles, eyelid closure and not least has the objective of favourably influencing the cosmetic result (22). As shown by GORMAN's large patient population, the operation is performed very much more frequently in America than in Europe, and several possibilities of access to the orbit gave rise to divergent results (13). During the period of the study, such an operation was not necessary in any of the patients. However, orbit decompressions have been performed in two cases in the last year with satisfactory results and may indicate an increase of surgical therapy of E.O. in Europe, too.

The results show the limitations of a retrospective observation. In a controlled prospective study, the problem to be analysed, the objectives and the progress parameters were laid down at the beginning, so that the analysis was to be complete in principle and well-founded. In comparison, there are limitations of this study in relation to the different subjective answers of the patients which are difficult for the investigator to evaluate, and which in some cases do not correlate with subjective findings, e.g. in the computer tomogram. A change of doctor within the observation period led to alterations in the basic values in the Hertel measurements, so that the number of reference values was restricted in the course and made it difficult to verify the results of therapy by statistical means. In complete documentation led to the same difficulties. A concept of the therapy at the beginning could not always be laid down in view of the recurrent and divergent course of the disease, so that often several forms of treatment were employed until the results were stabilized.

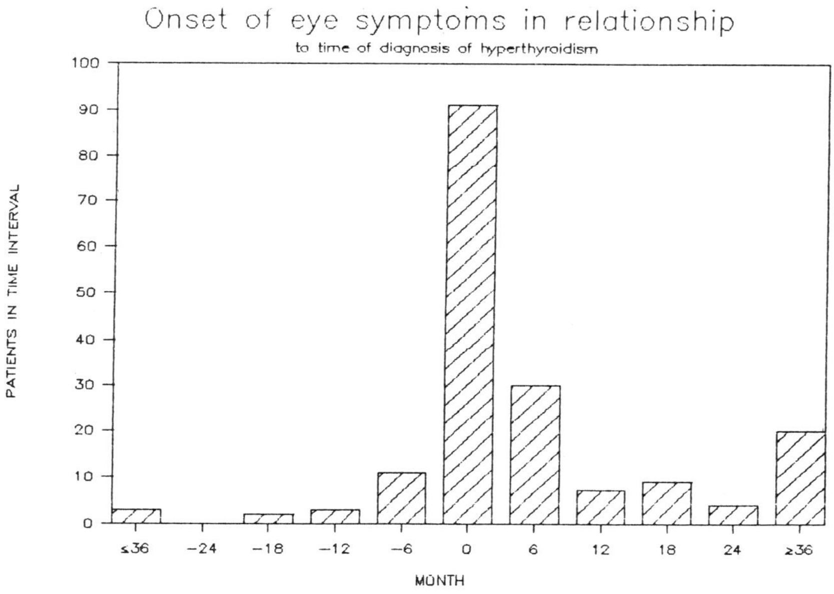

Fig.2

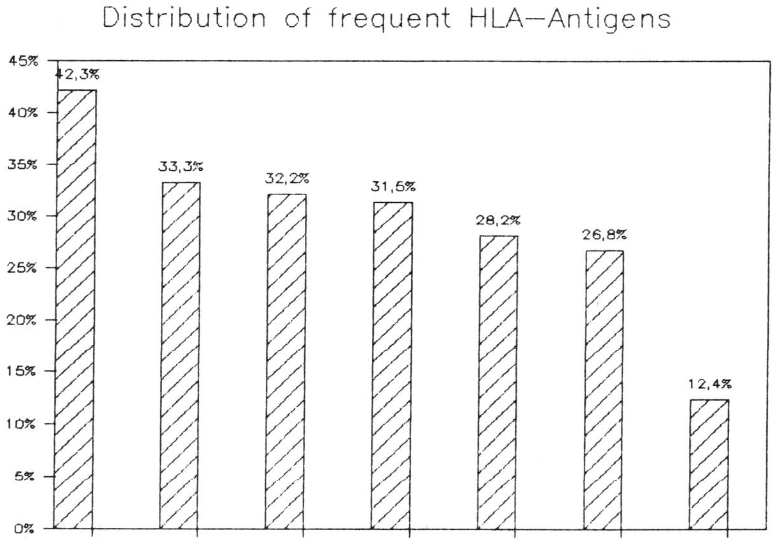

Fig. 3

Finally, it could be emphasized that none of the therapies applied constitute an optimal treatment with regard to the long-term course. Because of the suspected autoimmune genesis of endocrine ophthalmopathy, we consider systematically administered corticosteroids and nonsteroid immunosuppressants as the primary, causal form of treatment. Compared to this, orbit peak irradiation and the entirely successful decompression technique are local (if anything, palliative) in nature. An initial specific antiinflammatory and immunosuppressant treatment thus appears to us to be indicated in florid orbitopathies from stage IIb/c, without wishing to underestimate the side effects of immunosuppressants.

References

[1] Aranow H, Day RM: Management of thyrotoxicosis in patients with opthalmopathy: Antithyroid regimen determined primarily by ocular manifestations. J. Endocrinol. 25 (1965) 1

[2] Bartalena L, Marcocci C, Chiovato L, Laddaga M, Lepri G, Andreani D, Cavallagi G, Baschieri L, Pinchera A: Orbital cobalt irradiation combined with systemic cortocsteroids for Graves' ophthalmopathy: comparison with systemic coticosteroids alone. J Clin Endocrinol Metab 56 (1983) 1139 - 1144

[3] Beyer J, Kahaly G: Pathogenetische Vortstellungen und Klinik der endokrinen Ophthalmopathie in: Beyer J, Kahaly G (Hrsg.): Fortschritte in Diagnostik und Therapie der endokrinen Ophthalmopatie pmi Verlag GmbH, Frankfurt/Main, 1987

[4] Beyer J, Brandstetter K, Dieser I, Czackert J, Cordes U, Atzpodien W, Rochels R, Nover A: Therpaie der schweren endokrinen Orbitopathie. In: Scriba PC, Rudorff KH, Weinheimer B (Hrsg.): Schilddrüse 1981. Gedrg Thieme Verlag Stuttgart, New York 1982

[5] Beyer J, Brandstetter K, Dieser I, Czackert J, Cordes U, Atzpodien W, Rochels R, Rothmund M, Kümmerle F: Die totale Thyreoidektomie im Behandlungsplan der endokrinen Orbitopathie-Gesichertes und nicht Gesichertes einer ablativen Maßnahme. In: Röher HD, Wahl RA (Hrsg.): Chirurgische Endokrinologie, Georg Thieme Verlag Stuttgart, New York 1983

[6] Dobyns BM: The influence of thyroidectomy on the prominence of the eyes in the guinea pig and in man. Surg Gynecol Obstet 80 (1946) 526

[7] Dobyns BM. Present concepts of the pathologic physiology of exophthalmos. J Clin Endocrinol 10 (1959) 1202

[8] Gorman CA: Temporal relationship between onset of Graves' ophthalmopathy and diagnosis of thyrotoxicosis. Mayo Clin Proc 58 (1983) 515 - 519

[9] Hales JB, Rundle FF: Ocular changes in Graves' disease. Q J Med 29 (1960) 113

[10] Horst W, Glanzmann CH: Diagnostik und Therapie der endokrinen Ophthalmopathie. Therapiewoche 32 (1982) 4848 - 485

[11] Horster FA, Wildmeister W: Endokrine Orbitopathie: Therpaieerfolge bei 148 Patienten unter Berücksichtigung neuer pathogenetischer Aspekte. Dtsch med Wschr 108 (1983) 413 - 415

[12] Hüfner M, Hess HG, Grußendorf M, Ziegler R: Der Langzeitverluaf der endokrinen Orbitopathie unter thryriostatischer Therapie: eine retrospektive Studie. In: Scriba PC, Rudorff KH, Weinheimer B (Hrsg.): Schilddrüse 1981. Georg Thieme Verlag Stuttgart, New York (19829

[13] Jacobson DA, Gorman CA: Endocrine ophthalmpathy: current ideas concerning etiology, pathogenesis, and treatment. Endocr Rev 5 (1984) 200 - 220

[14] Kahaly G, Beyer J: Derzeitiger Stand der medikamentösen Therapie der endokrinen Ophthalmopathie in: Beyer J, Kahaly G: Fortschritte in Diagnostik und Therapie der enokrinen Ophthalmpathie. pmi Verlag GmbH, Frankfurt/Main

[15] Kahaly G,Schrezenmeir J, Krause U, Schweikert B, Meuer S, Müller W, Dennebaum R, Beyer J: Ciclosporin and prednisone versus prednisone in treatment of Graves' ophthalmopathy: A controlled, randomized and prospective study. Eur J Clin Invest 16 (1986) 415

[16] Kahaly G, Schrezenmeir J, Schweikert B, Müller W, Krause U, Beyer J: Remission-maintaining effect of cyclosporin in endocrine ophthalmpathy. Transplantat Proc, XVIII, No 4 (1986) 844

[17] Kirmse L, Lahrtz HG, Schemmel K, Waschulik G: Totale Thyreoidektomie bei progredienter endokriner Orbitopathie. Dtsch med Wschr 100 (1975) 535 - 537

[18] Klein E, Kracht J, Krüskemper HL, Reinwein D, Scriba PC: Klassifikation der Schilddrüsenkrankheiten. Internist 15 (1974) 181 - 183

[19] Krause U: vollautomatischer radioimmunoassay. Ein Jahr Erfahrung mit dem ARIA II. NuCompact 13 (1982) 6

[20] Kriss JP, Konishi J, Herman M: Studies on the pathogenesis of Graves' ophthalmopathy (with some related observations regarding therapy). rec Progr Horm Res 31 (1975) 533 - 566

[21] Müller W, Schemmel K, Uthgenannt H, Weissbecker L: Die Behandlung des malignen Exophthalmus durch totale Thyreoidektomie. Dtsch med Wschr 92 (1967) 2103 - 2106

[22] Oberdisse K: Die endokrine Ophthalmopathie (endokrine Orbitopathie), die endokrine Dermatopathie und die Akropachie. In: Oberdisse K, Klein E, reinwein D: Die Krankheiten der Schilddrüse, Georg Thieme Verlag Stuttgart (1980) 370

[23] Richter WC, Kley W, Buschmann W: Ethmoidektomie und Orbitade-kommpression bei endokriner Ophthalmpathie. Laryng Rhinol Otol 63 (1984) 356 - 360

[24] Roman SH, Korn F, Davies TF: Enzyme-linked immunosorbent microassay and hemagglutination compared for detection of thyroglubulin and throid microsomal autoantibodies. clin Chem 30 (1984) 246

[25] Schifferdecker E, Schulz F, Rosak C, Hennning-Althoff P: Verlauf der endokrinen Ophthalmopathie und Effektivität der etablierten therapeutischen Maßnahmen. Med Klin 81 (1986) 779 - 783

[26] Schleusener H: Die Pathogenese der Hyperthreose und der "endokrinen" Orbitopathie. SM 4, heft 1 81981) 37 - 44

[27] Solem JH, Seegard E, Ytteborg J: The course of endocrine ophthalmopathy during antithyroid therapy in a prospective study. Acta Med Scand 205 (1979) 111

[28] Uhlenbrock D, Fischer HJ, Rohwerder R: Strahlentherapie der endokrinen Ophthalmopathie - Auswertung von 56 fällen Strahlentherapie 160 (1984) 485 - 491

[29] Utech C, Wulle KG, Biegler EU, Pfannenstiel P, Panitz N, Kiefer H: Treatment of severe Graves' ophthalmpathy with ciclosporin A. Acta endocrinol 110 (1985) 493 - 498

[30] Weetman AP, Ludgate M, Mills PV, McGregor AM, Beck L, Lazarus JH: Cyclosporin improves Graves' ophthalmopathy. Lancet II (1983) 486

V

CAROTID CAVERNOUS FISTULA - DISTURBANCES OF CIRCULATION

Carotid Cavernous Fistula: Anatomical Clinical correlations and Clinical Signs

R. Renella, S. Hussein, H. Dietz

Carotid cavernous fistulas (CCF) are typically due to an abnormal communication between the internal carotid artery and the cavernous sinus, following laceration of the arterial wall.

The incidence of CCF in head injuries is very low. SEDZIMIR (37) encountered three cases in 1100 admissions for cranio-facial trauma. HAUSER (19) was able to find only 25 CCF in 6792 patients with head injuries (0.4 %). FRIEDMANN (12) reported an incidence of 0.4 % in all observed cranio-cerebral trauma and of 2.2 % in severe head injuries.

In most cases the etiology is traumatic. The typical pattern of cranio-cerebral injury includes basal skull fracture at the level of the anterior or middle cranial fossa, with a fracture line through the sphenoid bone. In some posttraumatic cases, however, objective lesions can be very mild or absent. Latrogenic CCF following a Fogarty catheter thrombarterectomy or a postganglionic procedure for trigeminal neuralgia are also reported (1,19, 23, 44).

In 25 - 30 % of patients CCF occurs as a spontaneous arteriovenous shunt and women are affected more often. These fistulae most frequently resulted from a rupture of intracavernous carotid aneurysms or from the development of spontaneous dural fistulae in the cavernous area. Spontaneous shunts occasionally develop during pregnancy or postpartum, especially in multipara. Various other conditions were proposed to explain their occurrence. arteriosclerosis, inflammatory lesions in autoimmune diseases, mycotic aneurysms, arteritis luetica as well as autosomal dominant disorders of connective tissue and rare vascular diseases (6, 13, 16, 34, 35). The classic findings in CCF include pulsating exophthalmos, conjunctival congestion and intracranial bruit in association with headache, diplopia and visual disturbances. More commonly the clinical signs are unilateral at the site of lesion. However, they can develop contralaterally or bilaterally. Knowledge of the anatomy of the arterial contributions and of the drainage patterns is the key to an understanding of clinical features of cavernous sinus shunts. This study deals with the clinical aspects of CCF as a consequence of the anatomical situation.

Clinical material and methods

This series includes 24 cases of CCF who were treated at the neurosurgical Department of the Hannover Medical School from 1973 to 1985.

They represent 1,5 % of the total 1583 head injuries operated in our department during this period.

Of the 24 patients, 22 had moderate to severe head injury caused in almost all cases by a road accident. There were 16 men and 8 women (age range: 23 to 68 years, mean: 39.2). In 2 women the CCF occured spontaneously without any demonstrable trauma. There was a marked prevalence of young male patients in the second and third decades, while most of the older patients were female. clinical data concerning the 24 patients are listed in tab. I.

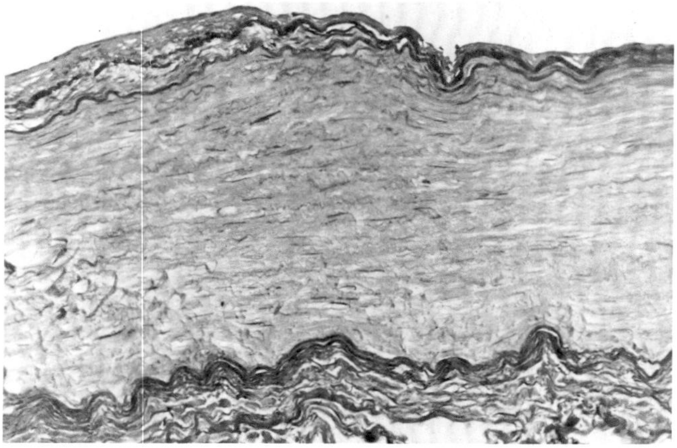

a)

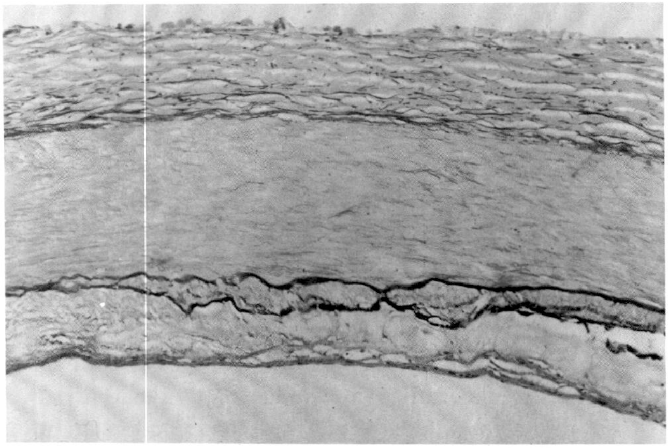

b)

Fig. 1a): Internal carotid artery, extracranial portion. Typical elastic artery with well developed adventitial and media layers and thin internal elastic lamina.

b) Internal carotid artery, intracavernous segment. Typical muscular artery with few elastic fibers and thin media layer.

The fistula was located on the right side in 11 cases and on the left side in 10, while bilateral fistulae were demonstrated in three cases. 16 patients had unilateral ocular symptoms, on the ipsilateral side, four had an unilateral fistula with bilateral symptomas and one showed contralateral exophthalmos by unilateral shunt.

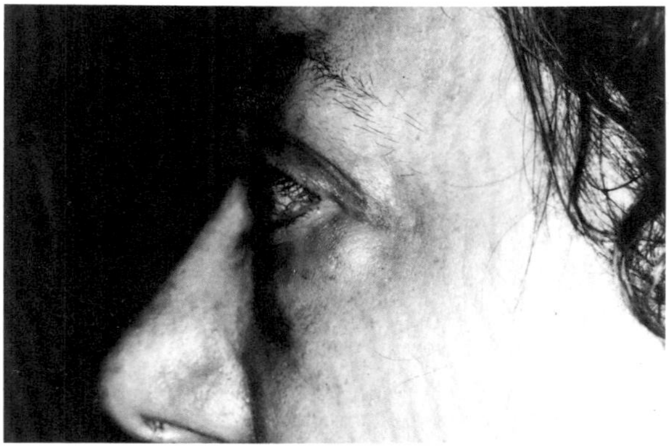

a)

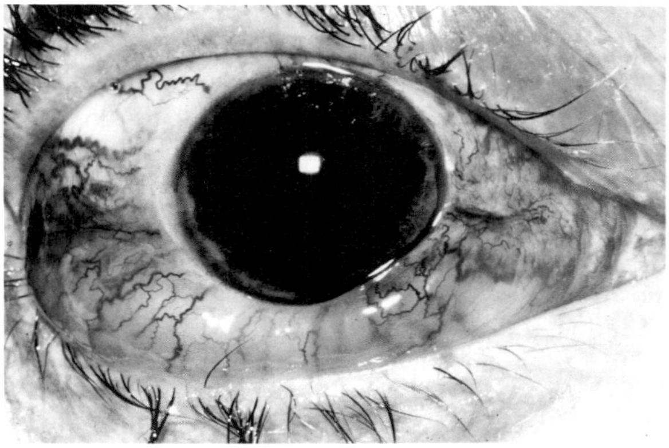

b)

Fig. 2: Ocular changes in carotid-cavernous fistula. Exophthalmos and congestion of the periorbital region (a), thickened tortuous arterialized conjunctival veins and mydriasis by amaurosis (b).

To assess anatomical clinical correlation 20 cavernous sinuses were dissected in routine autopsy material using microsurgical techniques. The peculiar feature of CCF were demonstrated in a patient presenting bilateral CCF, who died following head trauma a few hours after admission.

Results and discussions

1. Anatomical consideration

The cavernous sinus develops very early in embryonal life (7 mm embryo) as an ampullar dilatation of the venous system on the medial side of the Gasserian ganglion, draining in the superior cardial vein. Up to the stage of the 20 mm embryo it assumes the entire cerebral venous drainage. Parallel to the further development of the main sinusoidal channels, the primitive cavernous sinus differentiates in a plexus-like structure around the internal carotid artery and the cranial nerves III, IV, V and VI (50 mm embryo).

Prior to the development of the internal jugular vein, the pterygoid region is drained by the cavernous sinus through embryonal basal emissary veins, this observation explains the important anastomotic network between the pterygoid plexus and the cavernous sinus that persists in some adults. The pattern of the cavernous sinus as a trabeculated blood lake was critically reviewed by TAPTAS (41) and BONNET (5) on the basis of embryological evidences. The definitive dura mater results from the fusion of the primitive dural layer with the periosteum. The inhibition of this process by interposed neural or vascular structures results in a local dural fold (repli duremerien) outlining a cavity. This space is filled with a venous plexus around the neurovascular elements. Indeed the definitive structure of the cavernous sinus depends mainly on the involution of the venous plexus superor-lateral to the carotid wall, as observed by GOLASSOL (15) in a 4 month-old foetus. This view is supported by the microscopic study of MICHAILOV (25) on 165 anatomic casts and by the reports of OLIVER and PAPAMILTIADES (29) and COPPINI (8).

The shape of cavernous plexus results from the evolving changes of the adjacent structures. In the 40 mm embryo the development of the pituitary gland determined a lateral shift of the internal carotid artery and associated venous plexus with a related adjustment of the lateral sphemoid bone. The development of the temporal lobes and of the middle cerebral fossa in the 140 mm embryo outlines the definitive shape of the sinus. Racial factors also influence configuration of the sinus and the arrangement of its contents. A long and flat cavernous cavity is a typical finding in dolicocephalic subjects. On contrary, brachicephalies reveal a deep and short sinus. The syphon knee is more pronounced in the latter (25).

The adult cavernous plexus is a paired pyramidal space between the basal dural layer and the periosteum of the sphemoid bone and its adjacent part of the ala major. The periosteum covers the superior and lateral sides of the sphenoid bone and the dorsum of their ala major. The dura mater is separated from the periosteum at the inferior recess of the pituitary fossa, rises obliquely to its superor-lateral border and reaches finally the diasphragma sellae (32). The venous plexus formes three main compartments with respect to the intracavernous carotid wall: the antero-inferior, below its first knee, the medial between the pituitary gland and the carotid wall and the posterior, between the dorsal carotid and sinus roof (18). According to RABISHONG (32) the main connections of the plexus are with the orbit (superior and inferior ophthalmic vein), the dura mater (middle meningeal vein), the transverse sinus (superior petrosal sinus), the jugular bulb (inferior petrosal sinus), the pterygoidal plexus (basal emissary veins), the cerebral hemispheres (middle and inferior cerebral vein) and the facial veins (ophthalmic veins).

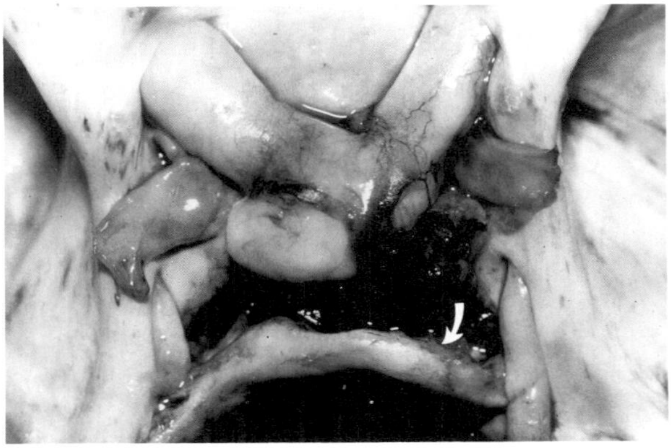

a)

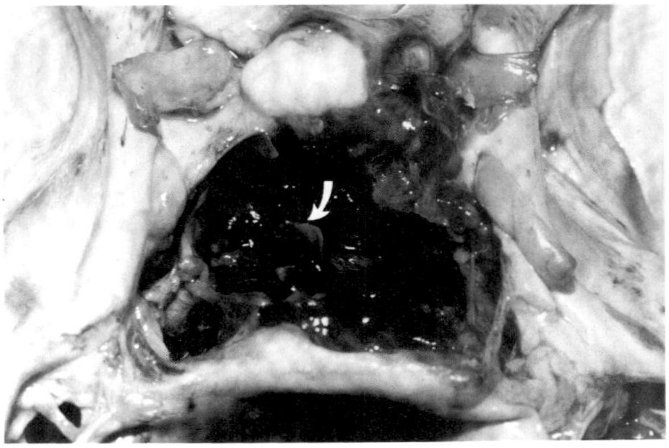

b)

Figs. 3: Pathological findings in carotid-cavernous fistula. a) Cross fracture of the cranial basis with avulsion of the dorsum sellae (arrow). b) The sphenoidal sinus is filled with hematoma and free bone fragments (arrow). The sphenoidal sinus communicate bilaterally with the cavernous cavity.

The intercavernous sinuses run in the dura mater of the sellar floor as anastomotic channels. The anterior intracavernous sinus is the largest and lies anterio-superiorly beneath the sellar tubercle. The inferior connection is localised below the pituitary gland, sometimes as a delicate plexus. The posterior intracavernous sinus is variable in structure and lies beneath the posterior clinoids (21).

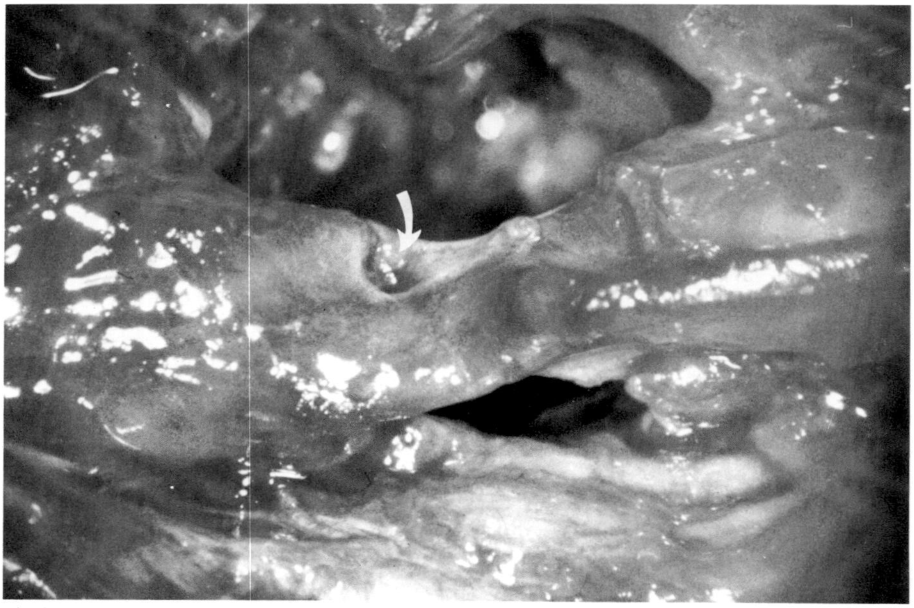

Fig. 3c: Pathological findings in carotid-cavernous fistula. The wall of the internal carotid artery is lacerated at the level of the horizontal segment (arrow).

The presence of valve-like formations in the walls of the intracavernous and petrosal sinuses suggest the possibility of a venous blood flow regulation (25, 26).

The intracavernous carotid artery lies between the foramen lacerum and the medial side of the anterior clinoid process. Few data concerning the histological structure of the intracavernous artery are reported in the literature (7, 25). Our study on 5 specimens agrees with the observations of MICHAILOV (25). The intracranial course of the internal carotid artery was accompanied by progredient loss of elastic fibers in the arterial wall and thinness of the media layer, starting in its intrapetrous portion. The intracavernous segment and its branches showed the typical features of a muscular artery (fig. 1).

Table I: Clinical features of carotid-cavernous fistulae

	MARTIN and MABON 1943 (22) n = 224	present series n = 24
bruit	191	24
exophthalmos (pulsating)	178	13
exophthalmos (non pulsating)	-	10
dilated epibulbar veins	-	24
chemosis	159	15
visual disturbance	66	11
amaurosis	-	3
diplopia	76	14
headache	71	4

Before it perforates the sinus roof, the carotid artery ascends toward the posterior clinoid process and then turns forwards in a horizontal segment. In the present study the largest intracavernous branch, the meningohypophyseal tract and the inferior artery of the cavernous sinus were present in all and in 18/20 of the specimens respectively. Less frequently we encountered capsular (5/20) and dorsal meningeal arteries (2/20).

According to RENN and RHOTON 8359 the ophthalmic artery arises within the sinus in 8 % of the cases, more frequently on the right side. proximal to the branching of the ophthalmic artery the intracavernous carotid show a typical narrowing of its lumen. In 6 % of the cases the ophthalmic artery entered the intracranial end of the optic canal, in 2 % it reached its floor through a formaen in the bone. In our material we were able to demonstrate intracavernous origin of the ophthalmic artery in 2 cases. In all but three specimens its extrasinusal segment was very short (1 - 2 mm) and strongly adherent to the basal dura. this anatomical arrangement emphasized the hazard of ophthalmic occlusion in trapping procedures.

The intracavernous carotid branches showed an important anastomotic network specially with the opposite side and the basal dural afferent. apart from these normal anastomoses, persistent embryonal vessels are seldom describes.

Embryonic carotid-basilar anastomoses include the Aa. trigemina, optica and hypoglossa primitiva. These can be involved exceptionally in a vascular pathology of the cavernous area (11, 14, 30).

The entry and the intracavernous course of the oculomotor, trochlear, abducent and of the first divison of the trigeminal nerve are described in detail by several authors (2, 18, 24, 31, 42).

Our findings in 20 specimens confirm the statements of PATOUILLARD (32) and UMANSKY (42). The lateral wall of the cavernous area was found to be formed by a superficial dural layer and by deep layer including the sheaths of the nerves III, IV, $V_{1,2}$ as well as a delicate membrane with constant perforations.

2. *Clinical features*

Clinical signs of CCF include intracranial bruit, exophthalmos, pulsations of the eyeball, enlargement of the orbital veins, visual impairment and extraocular palsy. The pulssynchronised bruit is the more constant manifestation in CCF. In most cases it is demonstrated by auscultation of the ipsilateral temporal or orbital regions and may irradiate contralaterally. Intensity and frequence of noise can fluctuate, depending on arterial pressure, rest and emotional factors. In two cases of the present series the bruit was perceived only after digital compression over the eyeball. The maneuver is through out to reverse the drainage pattern of small fistulae from the orbital region into the petrosal sinuses (37). The usefulness of carotid compression test in the appraisal of the hemodynamic situation of CCF is questionable. In our experience abolition of bruit throught the carotid compression indicates at best the dominance of the ipsilateral carotid flow in filling the fistula. An ineffective compression, however, is almost invariabily indicative of an arteriovenous shunt with mixed afferentes. Compression test also proved to be of little value in differentiating bilateral from pseudobilateral fistulae.

Enlargement, tortuosity and cork-screw-like dilated reddish vessels on the surface of the eyeball were encountered in all the cases (fig. 2). Lid edema and chemosis were most frequently observed in patients with immediate onset of symptomatology. Unilateral or bilateral exophthalmos was present in all patients but one. According to HAMBY (17) pulsation may not be visible at all, however, it is usually palpable as a thrill over the bulbus of the angular vein. In our series we observed pulsations in half of the CCF. In severe proptosis (more than 5 mm) the venous congestion results in displacement and fixation of the ocular bulb (4 cases of the present series). In this instance the eyeball is displaced mostly down and outwards, related to the location of the major orbital vein.

Impairment of visual acuity is quite frequent in the course of CCF and represents its most dramatic complication. Amaurosis was reported in 25 % of the cases until 1925 (22). Sudden visual loss in CCF is related to stretching of the optic nerve in severe head injury or to alterations in its blood flow (40, 43). The latter mechanism is supposed to be responsible for the decrease of visual acuity during the course of CCF, as observed in 11 patients of the present series. According to SANDERS and HOYT (36), CCF induces a reduction of the retinal arteriovenous gradient and perfusion pressure, an increase in retinal venous pressure as well as a rise in intraocular pressure resulting in pronounced vascular insufficiency. By effective compensatory changes visual acuity can be preserved for along time. Additional imbalance in retinal microcirculation, however, produces a brisk visual impairment.

Impaired ocular movements were observed in 14 of our 24 patients. The extraocular muscle involvement may be a direct outcome of the head injury, a consequence of the venous orbital congestion of a stretching effect of severe proptosis (40).

Although hyposmia is often associated with basal skull fractures, this symptom is rarely reported in the literature. In the series of TÖNNIS, however, hyposmia was noticed in 9 of 44 cases (12). the incidence of the trigeminal involvement is difficult to appreciate. FRIEDMANN (12) did not find any sensory disturbance in his 44 patients. In our literature study we were able to find only a single case with palsy of the trigeminal motor branch (27). Deafness and facial palsy can occur from a cross fracture of the petrous bone.

3. Anatomical clinical correlations

PARKINSON (21) described two types of CCF: direct rupture of the intracavernous carotid artery (type I) and avulsion or distal rupture of their intracavernous branches, especially the meningohypophyseal trunk (type II). The occurrence of type II fistulae is supported by the frequency of CCF localized at the first posterior knee of the syphon, i.e. the typical point of origin of this branch. Microanatomic evidences suggest that type II fistulae can occur without significant head trauma. Intracavernous vessels namely showed a short free initial segment followed by a long intradurally fixed portion. Brisk traction of the basal dura by acceleration trauma is supposed to sever the small branch at their origin or at the junction of the two segments (3).

The cranial nerves IIIrd, IVth and V_1 are widely protected against a direct trauma. On the contrary the abducent nerve show very intimate relation to the intracavernous carotid and can be harmed directly. A typical case of CCF is demonstrated in fig. 3a - d. The development of clinical symptoms depends on the diameter, and the location of the arteriovenous shunt as well as on the structure of the venous drainage (39).

The diameter of the fistula influences the shunt volume and therefore the cerebral blood flow (CBF) distal to the rupture point. HEYCK (18) reported an impressive rise of CBF in three patients with large fistulas (232.7 - 400.5 ml/100 g/min) and demonstrated that CBF was reduced at levels nearly to normal following carotid ligature. NORNES (28) measured shunt volumes from 95 to 975 ml/100 g/min. This mechanism may be responsible for ischemic complications in CCF. However, there is no correlation between the shunt volume and the ocular symptoms. When considering the pathophysiology of CCF, another important factor is the location of the shunt. If there is a low flow fistula sited on the junction of the horizontal and the posterior ascending intracavernous carotid, the posterior compartment of the cavernous sinus may be sufficient for its drainage. A patient of our series with a fistula on the posterior carotid segment presented only a subjective bruit.

In our experience the clinical presentation of CCF is mostly a consequence of the anatomy of the venous pathways of the cavernous area. BICKERSTAFF (14) divided CCF in unilateral, bilateral, contralateral, with exophthalmos at the side opposite the toe carotid rupture, and alternating fistula, as a consequence of an ipsilateral occlusion of the ophthalmic veins, diverting the blood to the contralateral orbit.

Based on our observations and on the literature we divided CCF in six distinct types (tab. II).

Table II: Anatomical clinical correlations

type	ipsilateral ophthalmic veins	contralateral ophthalmic veins	intracavernous connections	ipsilateral to fistula	contralateral to fistula
I	patent	patent or hypoplastic	hypoplastic	+	∅
II	patent	patent	patent	+	+
III	thrombosed or hypoplastic	patent	patent	∅	+
IV	unilaterally thrombosed or hypoplastic		patent or hypoplastic	unilateral	
V	bilateral patent		patent or hypoplastic	bilateral	
VI	thrombosed or hypoplastic	patent or hypoplastic	hypoplastic	none	

I: conventional unilateral CCF, II: pseudobilateral CCF, III: paradoxical CCF, IV: pseudounilateral CCF, V: bilateral CCF, VI: silent CCF

1. Conventional unilateral CCF results from the drainage of the shunt volume into the ophthalmic veins in presence of inconsistent intracavernous connections. In this instance one can expect the familiar clinical features of an intracavernous shunt (19 of 24 cases).
2. Pseudobilateral CCF occurs when the arterial blood can also be diverted into the contralateral sinus cavity through patent intacavernous sinuses. Ocular symptoms therefore develop bilaterally and or usually symmetrical depending upon the degree of patency and on the relative importance of these connections (5 of 24 cases).
3. If there is an occlusion of the ipsilateral ophthalmic veins and patent intracavernous channels, ocular symptoms are observed on the side opposite to the fistula (paradoxical CCF: 1 of 24 cases). This unusual presentation may occur in course of a conventional CCF, following thrombosis of the superior ophthalmic vein (alternating CCF).

4. Pseudounilateral CCF are bilateral fistulae with unilateral ocular symptoms. Hypoplasia, primary or secondary thrombosis of the ophthalmic veins as well as an abnormal orbital drainage are responsible for this unusual clinical presentation.
5. When both superior ophthalmic veins are patent, bilateral intracavernous carotid rupture causes bilateral ocular symptoms (2 of 24 cases).
6. Silent CCF are observed by thrombosis or hypoplasia of the ipsilateral ophthalmic vein and negligible intracavernous connections (1 of 24 cases).

References

[1] Barker WF, Stern WE, Krayenbühl H, Senning A: Carotid endarterectomy complicated by carotied cavernous sinus fistula. Ann. Surg. 167 (1986) 568 - 572

[2] Beford MA: The cavernous sinus. Br. J. Ophthalm. 50 (1966) 41 - 46

[3] Besson G et al.: Fistule carotido-caverneuse par arrachement our ruptur du tronc meningo-hypophysaire ou de l'une de ses branches. Neurochirurgie (Paris) 22, 5 (1976) 477 - 491

[4] Bickerstaff ER: Mechanisms of presentation of carotido-cavernous fistulae. Br. J. Ophthalm 54 (1970) 186 - 190

[5] Bonnet R: La loge caverneuse et les syndromes de la loge caverneuse. Arch Ophthalm 15 (1955) 357 - 372

[6] Chavany JA: Anéurysme arterioveineux de siège carotido-caverneux d'origine traumatique sur un terrain syphylitique. Presse Med. XLVI (1983) 859 - 860

[7] Cherubino M: Structure of internal carotid artery in the intrapetrous and intracavernous portions. Arch. de Vecchi per Anat. Pat. and Med. Clin. 9 (1947) 533 - 552

[8] Coppini L, et al.: Alcuni dati sul seno cavernoso. Boll. soc. ital. Sper. 53 (1977) 2122 - 2129

[9] Dandy WE, Follis RH: On the pathology of carotid cavernous aneurysms. Am. J. Ophthalm. 24 (1941) 365 - 385

[10] Eggers F, et al.: Latrogenic carotid cavernous fistula following fogarty catheter thromboendarterectoma. J. Neurosurg. 51, 4 (1979) 543 - 545

[11] Enomoto T, et al.: Carotid cavernous fistula caused by rupture of a primitive trigeminal artery aneurysm. J. Neurosurg. 46, 3 (1977) 373 - 376

[12] Friedmann G, et al.: Karotis-Sinus cavernosus Aneurysmen. fortschr. neurol. Psychiatr. 38 (1970) 57 - 79

[13] François P.: Maladie d'Ehlers-Danlos avec anéurysme artérioveineux intracrânein. Bull. Soc. Ophthalm. Fr. 5 (1955) 392

[14] Gerlach J, et al.: Traumatic carotid cavernous fistula combined with persisting primitve hypoglassal artery. J. Neurosurg. 20 (1963) 885 - 887

[15] Gerlach J, et al.: Traumatic carotid cavernous fistula combined with persisting primitve hypoglassal artery. J. neurosurg. 20 (1963) 885 - 887

[16] Golassol B: Les veins du sinus caverneux du foetus humain de 4 mois. Cr ASS Anat. 149 (1970) 1009 - 1015

[16] Graf JC: Spontaneous carotid cavernous fistula, Ehler-Danlos syndrome and related conditions. Arch. Neurol. (Chicago) 13 (1979) 662 - 672

[17] Hamby WB: carotid cavernous fistula. Thomas, Springfield, 1966

[18] Harris FS, Rhoton AL: Antomy of the cavernous sinus. a microsurgical study. J. neurosurg. 45, 2 (1976) 169 - 180

[19] Hauser K: Das arteriovenöse Aneurysma der Arteria carotis interna im Sinus cavernosus. Ein therapeutisches Problem. Inaugural dissertation, Zürich, 1966

[20] Heyck H: Beitrag zur Hämodynamik der cerebralen arteriovenösen Aneurysmen und Fisteln des Sinus cavernosus. Deutsche Zeitschr. Nervenheilk. 177 (1958) 327 - 347

[21] Kaplan HA, Browder J: Intracavernous connections of the cavernous sinuses. The superior and inferior circular sinuses. J. Neurosurg. 45, 2 (1976) 166 - 168

[22] Martin JD, Mabon RF: Pulsating exophthalmos. Review of all reported cases. JAMA 121 (1943) 330 - 334

[23] Matajeme A, Keifer JW: Carotid cavernous sinus fistula as a complication of carotid endarterectomy. Radiology 108 (1973) 83 - 84

[24] McGrath P: The cavernous sinus. An anatomical survey. Aust. NZ J. Surg. 47 (1977) 601 - 613

[25] Michailov SS: Macro and microscopic investigations of the structure of the cavernous sinus. anat. Az. 115 (1964) 233 - 255

[26] Michailov SS: Reflexes influencies from the cavernous sinus on the cerebral arterial blood flow. Fiziol. Zh. SSSR Secenov. 52 (1966) 883 - 887

[27] Nieden D: Arch. f. Augenheilk., Ergänzungsheft 1881 641

[28] Nornes H: Hemodynamic aspects in the management of carotid-cavernous fistula. J. Neurosurg. 37 (1972) 687 - 694

[29] Oliver F, Papamiltiades M: The cavernous sinus. Cr. Ass. anat. 38 (1951) 769

[30] Ostheim-Dzerowycs W: Traumatic carotid cavernous sinus fistula in a case of persistent branchial arch artery. wien. med. Wochenschr. 120 (1970) 875 - 876

[31] Parkinson D: A surgical approach to the cavernous portion of the carotid artery. anatomical studies and case report. J. Neurosurg. 23 (1965) 474 - 476

[32] Patouillard P, Vanneuville G: Les parois du sinus caverneux. Neurochirugurgie (Paris) 18 (1972) 551 - 559

[33] Rabishong P: Haemodymic approach to the fuctional significance of the cavernous sinus. neurochirurgie (Paris) 18 (1972) 613 - 622

[34] Rad von M: Spontaneous carotid cavernous fistula in a case of hereditary heamorrhagic teleangiectasia. J. neurol. 209, 3 (1975) 237 - 242

[35] Renn WH, Rhoton AL: Microsurgical anatomy of the sellar region. J. Neurolsurg. 43 (1975) 288 - 298

[36] Sanders MD, Hoyt WF: Hypoxic sequeelae of carotid cavernous fistulae. Brit. J. Ophthalm. 53 (1969) 82 - 97

[37] Sattler CH: Pulsierender Exophthalmus. Handbuch der gesmaten Augenheilkunde. Vol. 9 (2nd Ed.) Springer, Berlin, 1920

[38] Sedzimir CB: Treatment of carotido cavernous fistula by muscle embolisation and Jaeger's maneuver. J. neurosurg. 27 (1967) 309 - 314

[39] Stern WE, Brown WJ, et al.: The critical challenge of carotid cavernous fistula: the critical role of intracranial circulatory dynamics. J. Neurosurg. 27 (1967) 298 - 308

[40] Sugar HS, Mayer ST: Pulsating exophthalmos. Arch. Ophthalm. 23 (1940) 1288 - 1321

[41] Taptas JN: Les aneurysmes arterioveineux carotido-caverneux (étude pathogénique). Neurochirurgie (Paris) 8 (1962) 385 - 394

[42] Umansky F, Nathan H: The lateral wall of the cavernous sinus. With special reference to the nerves related to it. J. neurosurg. 56 (1982) 228 - 234

[43] Weinstein JM, et al.: Optic nerve flow and its regulation. Invest. Ophthalm. Vis. Sci. 23, 5 (1982) 640 - 645

[44] Wepsic JC: Carotid cavernous fistula due to extradural subtemporal retrogasserian rhizotoma. J. Neurosurg. 37 (1972) 498 - 500

[45] Zimmermann R, et al.: Carotid cavernous fistula associated with intracrainal fibromuscular dysplasia. Radiology 122 Suppl. 2 (1977) 725 - 726

Ophthalmological problems in patients with spontaneous AV-Fistulas affecting the orbit

R. Guthoff, J.S. Jürgens

Abstract

An ophthalmological follow up is presented on 24 patients with spontaneous AV-fistulas of a period from 6 months to 8 years. Leading symptoms have been unilateral episcleral venous congestion with mild proptosis and raised intraocular pressure. the age at the time of diagnosis ranged from 51 - 89 years. A spontaneous closure occurred in 80 % of the patient within 12 weeks in 3 patients with recurrent symptoms after several months. Ocular findings due to severe venous congestion included papilledema, exudative retinal detachment and central retinal vein thrombosis. diagnostic and therapeutic possibilities are discussed with special emphasis on contact B-scan ultrasound.

Two types of carotid cavernous fistulas have to be distinguished. Fistulas of traumatic origin formes a well known clinical entity (SATTLER, 1920, SUGAR et al., 1940). In patients without any trauma in history, clinical signs are much more subtile so that diagnosis often is delayed. Unilateral injection of conjunctival and episcleral vessels which does not respond to local treatment is often the only symptoms. These spontaneous fistulas originate in shunts between small branches of either the external or internal crotid artery and the cavernous sinus (CASTAIGNE et al., 1966). The anatomical basis for these symptoms has been worked out using selective angiographic techniques (NEWTON et al., 1970, PETERS et al., 1979) in ophthalmological literature they are known as "red-eye-shunt-syndrome" (PHELBS et al., 1982).

Material and Methods

We report on our clinical findings and follow up of 24 of these patients, we have seen since 1977 in our department. Routine examination included complete ophthalmological test including b-scan ultrasonography. CT-examination was performed in 15, carotid angiography in 7, orbital venography in 4 patients.

Results

Ophthalmological signs during the first examination are summarized in table I. The main symptom was a red eye. In 16 of 24 patients there was a proptosis of more than 4 mm. In 12 patients diplopia occurred at least in some directions of gaze (tabl. I).

Table I: Presenting symptoms of patients with spontaneous carotid cavernous fistula

Red eye	24
Proptosis of more than 2 mm 16	16
Orbital pain ± headache	4
Noise in the head	3
Diplopia due to:	12
Restricted eye movements (unspecific)	8
Abduction weakness	4

(n = 20, age: 51 - 89 years, w. 17, m. 7)

Patients were referred with a wide range of differential diagnosis (see table II), only in 3 patients the correct diagnosis was suspected prior to admission.

At the initial ophthalmological examination 3 signs are constantly present:

1: Episcleral venous dilatation
2: Retinal venous congestion sometimes even with hemorrhages and
3: a clearly visible superior ophthalmic vein on B scan ultrasound which starts pulsating on orbital compression.

Intraocular pressure ranged from 12 - 50 mm Hg. Tonography was performed in 5 patients and showed a normal to slightly elevated outflow facility. CT-scans made the diagnosis most likely in 6 patients in whom the superior ophthalmic vein was unilaterally enlarged. In 4 out of 6 an arterialization of the vein by sequential CT-scan after venous injection of contrast medium was suspected. On conventional carotid angiograms AV-shunts were found in all patients, but the exact localization could not be identified.

Follow-up

During the follow-up (table III) in 4 patients out of 24 the fistula closed within 3 months. In 4 patients between 6 and 18 months after the diagnosis. In 2 patients the ophthalmic vein seems to be thrombosed with or without an involvement of the cavernous sinus. Ocular complications were seen rather frequently of which a thrombosis of central retinal vein was the most serious one.

Discussion

The diagnosis of a spontaneous carotid cavernous fistula can be made on clinical grounds. Most constant findings are unilateral dilated episcleral veins and mild to moderate unilateral increase of intraocular pressure. the diagnosis can be proven by demonstrating a pulsating ophthalmic vein on B-scan ultrasound (GUTHOFF et al., 1983). Vessels with an internal diameter of about 1,0 mm are well outlined using this technique (Fig. 1). Carotid angiography seems to be not necessary unless surgical treatment is considered. The course of the disease in our patients was unpredictable and we were unable to find a correlation between the caliber of the dilated vein, the extent of the protrusion and the incidence of spontaneous fistula closure. No lasting ophthalmoplegia as reported by LEONHARD et al. (1984) in traumatic cases was present.

Table II: Suspected diagnosis on referral in patients with spontaneous carotid cavernous fistula (n = 24)

Orbital myositis	5
Orbital tumor	3
Orbital pseudotumor	4
Conjunctivitis	3
Thrombosis of central retinal vein	12
Angle closure glaucoma	1
Grave's disease	3
AV-fistula	3

Table III: Follow-up of patients with spontaneous carotid cavernous fistula

Spontaneous closure within 3 months	14
closure after 6 - 18 months	4
Still patent	1
Presumed thrombosis of ophthalmic vein ± cavernous sinus	2
No follow-up	3

Ocular complication

Central retinal vein thrombosis	5
neovascular glaucoma	2
Secondary open angle glaucoma	3

(5 months to 7 years; n = 24)

There is no standard conservative treatment available. Intermittend digital occlusion of the external carotid artery is advocated by some authors. To deal with the glaucoma ensuing from the raised episcleral venous pressure the intraocular pressure must be higher for the circulation of the aqueous humor to continue (NORDMANN et al., 1961). The effect of antiglaucoma therapy will therefore be limited. In none of our patients a filtering procedure was performed partly because of the quick spontaneous occlusion of the fistula, partly because the expected complications such as spontaneous choroidal effusion as reported by BELLOWS et al. (1979). Some authors advocate to lower the systemic blood pressure or the evaluate blood viscosity to promote thrombosis of the fistula (VIRNO, 1982, VINUELA et al., 1984). Ocular complications such as central retinal vein thrombosis occurred to a higher percentage in our cases than reported in literature (PHELBES et al., 1982). Whenever the eye has reached the stage of painful complete glaucoma which may well happen to some of our patients in the future, the surgeon should be careful consider the orbital circulation before planning an enucleation as PURCELL (1979) reported a nearly fatal bleeding during enucleation in a case of unsuspected carotid cavernous fistula.

References

[1] Bellows AR, Chylack LT, Epstein Jr DLIT, Hutchinson BT: Choroidal effusion during glaucoma surgery in patients with prominent episceral vessels. Arch. Ophthal. 97 (1979)493

[2] Castaigne P, Laplane D, Djindijian R: Communication artério-veineuse spontaée entre la carotide externe et le sinus caverneux. Rev. Neurol. 114 (1966) 5

[3] Guthoff R, Hamnn KU, Kühne D: diagnostische und therapeutische Möglichkeiten orbitaler Gefäßveränderungen unter besonderer Berücksichtigung der Sinus cavernosus-Fistel. fortschr. Ophthal. 79 (1983) 388 - 390

[4] Newton TH, Hoyt W: Dural arteriovenous shunts in the region of the cavernous sinus. Neuroradiology 1 (1970) 71 - 81

[5] Nordmann J, Lobstein A, Gerhard JP, Levy J: A propos de 14 cas de glaucome par hypertension veineuse d'origine extraoculaire. Ophthalmologica 142 (suppl.) (1961) 501

[6] Peeters FLM, Kröger R: Dural and direct cavernous sinus fistulas. Amer. J. Radiol. 132 (1979) 599 - 606

[7] Phelbs CD, Thompson HS, Ossoinig KC: The diagnois and prognosis of atypical carotid cavernous fistula (red eye shunt-syndrome). Amer. J. Ophthal. 93 (1982) 423 - 436

[8] Sattler W: In: Graefe-Saemisch: Handbuch der gesamten Augenheilkunde, 2nd edn., chapter 9, 1920

[9] Vinuela F, Fox AJ, Debrun GM, Peerless SJ, Drake CG: Spontaneous carotid-cavernous fistulas: Clinial, radiological and therapeutic considerations. J. neurosurg. 60 (1984) 976 - 984

[10] Virno M, Malagola R, Motolese & Giraldi JP: Bluthyperosmolarität durch Azetazolamid und Augeninnendrucksenkung. In: Medikamentöse Glaukomtherapie. G.K. Krieglstein and W. Leydhecken, eds. J.F. Bergmann-Verlag, Munich, 1982

Dopplersonographic Findings in Retinal Stroke and Chronic Ocular Ischemia - Their Pathogenetic Implications

M. Schlenker, C. Weilles, A. Mertens, S. Wolf, E.B. Ringelstein

Abstract

The results of extracranial Doppler sonography in 62 consecutive patients referred because of chronic ocular ischemia or of retinal strokes of different degrees of severity are reported.

Of the 3 patients with chronic ocular ischemia, two had a homolateral occlusion of the internal carotid, one a pseudoocclusion. In all of these patients there was a severe disturbance of cerebral blood flow homolaterally, as could be shown by a severe decrease of the vasomotor reactivity to CO_2.

On the other hand, in the 59 cases of retinal strokes of different degrees of severity (transient monocular blindness, individual artery of central artery occlusions) a hemodynamically relevant stenosis of the homolateral internal carotid could be demonstrated in only about 1/3 of all patients. This, once more, indicates that most cases of retinal stroke are supposedly of embolic, rather than hemodynamic, origin.

Introduction

Both retinal strokes and chronic ocular ischemia are often associated with carotid vascular disease. Retinal strokes of different degrees of severity (transient monocular blindness, occlusion of an individual retinal artery or of the central retinal artery) are thought to be mainly of embolic origin by most authors, after the pioneering work of FISHER (2), who demonstrated embolic material in the retinal arteries directly during transient monocular blindness by fundoscopy. In a previous study, we could demonstrate a hemodynamically relevant homolateral carotid stenosis in only 1/3 of patients with retinal stroke (10). In another 1/3 we found lowgrade stenoses, often exulcerated and therefore potentially thrombogenic.

In 1963 HEDGES (4) and KEARNS and HOLLENHORST (6) calles attention to the fact that venous stasis-retinopathy is associated with homolateral internal carotid artery occlusion. The full picture of chronic ocular ischemia or ischemic oculopathy includes additional changes in the anterior segment of the eye, the most important being due to neovascularization. These are episcleral vascular congestion, rubeosis iridis and neovascular glaucoma (5, 8).

With all of these findings in mind, the dopplersonographic examination of the carotids in all patients with acute or chronic ischemic retinal disease has become standard procedure in our hospital. We report on the dopplersonographic findings in

62 consecutive patients referred by our Department of Ophthalmology. Three of the had chronic ocular ischemia, the others had retinal strokes.

Methods

All patients were examined by continuous wave Doppler sonography using the standard procedure described by the Freiburg School (9).

Results

Among the 62 patients, three individuals suffered from monocular chronic ischemic ophthalmopathy (chronic group), whereas 59 individuals had experienced acute, stroke-like monocular symptoms (acute group). The clinical and angiological findings in the chronic group are summarized in Table 1. In brief, all of them had complete ipsilateral ICA occlusion or quasi-occlusion (11), often combined with additional occlusive disease of the external carotid or contralateral internal carotid arteries. During CO_2-induced vasomotor reactivity measurement, all of these patients demonstrated a severe low-flow state of the ipsilateral cerebral hemisphere, with VMR values of less than 20 % (normal range: 86 $\pm$ 16 according to Ringelstein et al., 1988). The typical ophthalmoscopic aspect of an eye with ischemic ophthalmopathy (= chronic ocular ischemia or ischemic oculopathy) is demonstrated in Fig. 1. Figure 2 displays the CO_2-reactivity of patient N. 1 on both sides. On the side with the patent carotid artery, the CO_2-response was normal. (VMR = 83.7 %), but was severely curtailed on the occluded side (VMR = 9.8 %).

Table I: Dopplersonographic findings in three patients with ischemic oculopathy

	Pat. 1 male, 67 yrs.	Pat. 2 male, 55 yrs.	Pat. 3 fem., 47 yrs.
homolateral	IC-occlusion	IC-occlusion EC - 80% stenosis	IC-pseudo-occlusion EC-subtotal occlusion
contralateral	∅	∅	IC - 70% stenosis EC- 80% stenosis

IC: internal carotid artery
EC: external carotid artery

The findings in 59 patients with acute retinal strokes are summarized in Table II. A typical fundoscopic finding of acute embolic retinal stroke is shown in figure 3, displaying branch occlusion of a retinal artery. Fundoscopy was normal in every patient with transient monocular blindness (= amaurosis fugax).

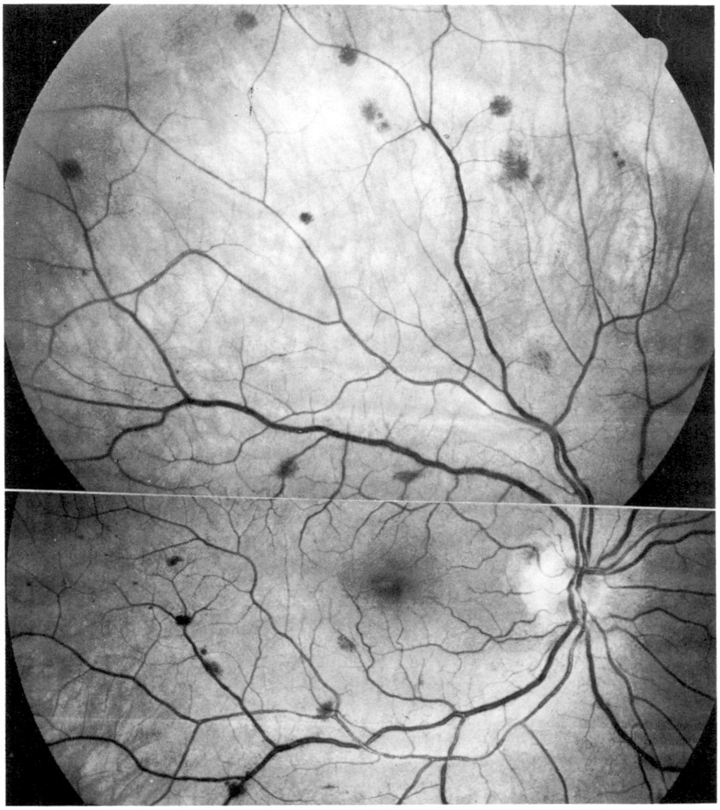

Fig. 1: Fundoscopic appearance of chronic ischemic oculopathy (case No. 1). The typical signs of venous-stasis retinopathy are visible. The caliber of the veins is enlarged and the veins are congested. Multiple preretinal hemorrhages are also visible (dark spots). Ischemia has not yet lead to neovascularization.

Even if a hemodynamically relevant stenosis or occlusion of the ipsilateral internal carotid artery was found in these patients, CO_2-test always revealed VMR values greater than 40 % and was even completely normal in a few ICA occlusions with obviously excellent intracranial collateralization.

Discussions

If all three different groups of retinal strokes are taken together, Doppler sonography revealed a hemodynamically relevant lesion of the homolateral internal carotid in only about 1/3 of all patients. This is the same percentage as in a previous study (10). In this previous study an angiographic examination of the 19 patients described was performed as well as a Doppler sonographic examination. Angiography revealed potentially thrombogenic lesions (low-grade stenoses and/or ulcerations) in another 1/3 of all patients.

Table II: Dopplersonographic findings in the homolateral internal carotid in retinal strokes

		trans. monocular blindness	individual artery occlusion	central artery occlusion
hemodynamically relevant	IC-occlusion	4	3	3
	IC-pseudo -occlusion	2	0	0
	IC-sten. 90 %	2	0	1
		---------	---------	---------
		n = 8	n = 3	n = 4
hemodynamically not relevant	IC-sten. 60 - 90%	2	1	2
	IC-sten. - 60%	1	1	1
	IC normal	14	7	15
		---------	---------	---------
		n = 17	n = 9	n = 18
% hemodyn.		32 %	25 %	18 %

These findings, once more, indicate that hemodynamic factors do not play a major role in the pathogenesis of retinal strokes. The incidence of hemodynamically relevant lesions was about as high in those patients with certain embolic origin of their retinal stroke, that is those with individual artery occlusion, as in the others. In our opinion, this indicates that even in those patients with hemodynamically relevant lesions embolization from this lesion rather than the hemodynamic effect itself plays a major role in the pathogenesis of retinal strokes.

Our study was not concerned with the direct demonstration of thrombogenic sources by B-scan, electrocardiography and echocardiography or by the new method of radioactive platelet-labelling. All these methods have to be used singly or in combination in these patients, according to the individual clinical situation.

a

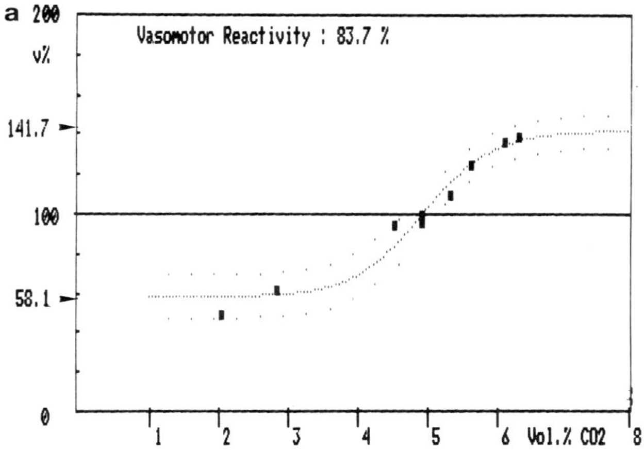

Fig. 2a: Vasomotor reactivity (VMR) of the middle cerebral artery territory in patient No. 2 with ipsilateral ischemic oculopathy. On the non-occluded side, the relative velocity changes (V %) within the middle cerebral artery (MCA) form a sigmoid curve depending on the end-tidal CO_2 Vol % values. The distance between the asymptotes is 83.7 % and reflects a normal VMR

Not surprisingly, all our patients with chronic ocular ischemia had a homolateral occlusion or pseudoocclusion of the internal carotid. In a completion of previously published data CARTER (1) showed that 90 % of 30 patients with venous stasis retinopathy or ischemic oculopathy had a homolateral occlusion of the common carotid or the internal carotid, 24 % a bilateral. In our three patients bilateral occlusion did not occur. In all patients, however, insufficient collateralization from the other side could be proven by the test of vasomotor reactivity to CO_2-stimulation using transcranial Doppler sonography. the method and the results for patients with chronic ocular ischemia are described elsewhere (3). The finding of a severe decrease of vasomotor reactivity in the homolateral cerebral hemisphere in all patients with chronic ocular ischemia indicates that in those patients there is always a severe, hemodynamic, disturbance of cerebral blood flow in the cerebral hemisphere which is on the side of the affected eye. These patients, therefore, have a very high risk of cerebral stroke. In 1979 KEARNS et al. (7) suggested extracranial-intracranial bypass surgery for patients with venour stasis retinopathy or ischemic oculopathy. To our knowledge, there is still no controlled study solving the question, whether IC/EC-bypass surgery can indeed safe the afflicted eye in patients with venous stasis retinopathy or ischemic oculopathy. In those few cases, where the ipsilateral internal carotid is not completely occluded but only tightly stenotic, endarterectomy should be performed. If there is occlusion of the homolateral internal carotid with, at the same time, high-grade stenosis contralaterally, endarterectomy on the other side should be considered.

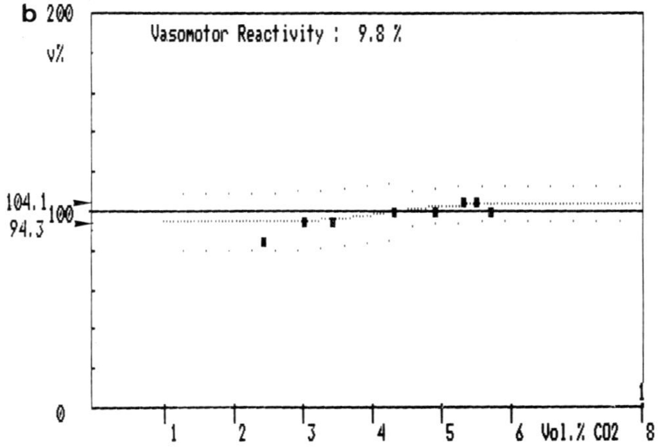

Fig. 2b: On the side with chronic oculopathy, hemispheric VMR is nearly exhausted and is only 9.8 %. This indicates a very severe disturbance of the hemispheric blood supply and insufficiency of collateral pathways

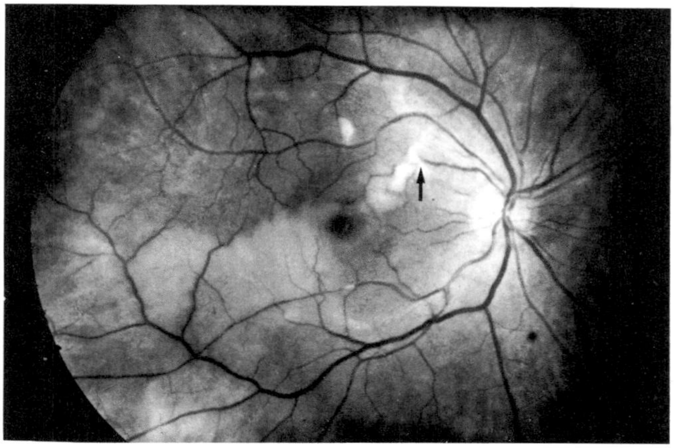

Fig. 3: Fundoscopic findings in a patient with sudden amaurosis fugax and subsequent visual field defect on the same eye. Arrow indicates embolic occlusion of a major branch of the superior temporal retinal artery with surrounding infarcted retinal tissue (light area). This patient had a medium-grade ipsilateral ICA stenosis

References

[1] Carter JE: Chronic ocular ischemia and carotid vascular disease. Stroke 16, Nr. 4 (1985) 721 - 728

[2] Fisher CM: Observations of the fundus oculi in transient monocular blindness. Neurology 9 (1959) 333 - 347

[3] Grosse W, Ringelstein EB: CO_2-Reaktivität bei Verschlußprozessen der A. carotis interna. In: Widder B (ed): Transkranielle Dopplersonographie bei zerebrovaskulären Erkrankungen. Springer Verlag, Berlin-Heidelberg-New York, 1987

[4] Heges TR: Opthalmoscopic findings in internal carotid artery occlusion. Am J Opthalmol 55 (1963) 1007 - 1012

[5] Hoefnagels KL: Rubeosis of the iris associated with occlusion of the carotid artery. Opthalmologica 148 (1964) 196 - 200

[6] Kearns TP, Hollenhorst RW: Venous-stasis retinopathy of occlusive disease of the carotid artery. Mayo Clin Proc 38 (1963) 304 - 312

[7] Kearns TP, Siekert RG, Sundt jr TM: The ocular aspects of bypass surgery of the carotid artery. Mayo Clin Proc 54 (1979) 3 - 11

[8] Knox DL: Ischemic ocular inflammation. Am J Ophthalmol 60 (1965) 995 - 1002

[9] Reutern von GM, Bündingen HJ, Hennerici M, Freund HG: Diagnose und Differenzierung von Stenosen und Verschlüssen der Arteria carotis mit der Doppler-Sonographie. Arch Psychiat Nervenkr 222 (1976) 191

[10] Ringelstein EB, Körber N, Zeumer H, Hunold W: Arterielle retinale Durchblutungsstörungen: Eine dringende Indikation zur dopplersonographischen Untersuchung der Carotis-Strombahn. Klin Mbl Augenheilkunde 182 (1983) 133- 140

Quantitative video-fluorescenceangiography: Retinal circulation in internal carotid occlusion

S. Wolf, B. Bertram, J. Rebstock, CH. Teping, M. Reim, M. Schlenker, E. Ringelstein

Summary

In 20 patients with internal carotid artery occlusion video-fluorescenceangiograms were performed. In all patients we found significantly prolonged retinal blood flow parameters compared to healthy volunteers. In these patients the mean arm retina time (ART) was 45 %, the mean arterio-venous passagetime (AVP) 189 % longer compared with healthy volunteers. The mean dye bolus velocity (MDV) was reduced to 33 % of the values of healthy volunteers.

In 55 % of our patients we found pulsative arterial filling. This indicates that the diastolic blood pressure in the central retinal artery may be lower than the intraocular pressure. In addition the markely prolonged retinal blood flow parameters in these patients showed a severely reduced ocular blood flow. since in 5 out of 11 patients with pulsative filling of the retinal artery an obstruction of the contralateral internal carotid artery was also found, it may be concluded that pulsative filling points to reduced collateral supply of the affected side.

Further investigations of the retinal blood flow are needed to demonstrate the correlation between ocular blood flow parameters and the development of the ophthalmological symptoms of ischemic ophthalmopathy in patients with internal carotid artery occlusions.

Introduction

The poor correlation between the angiographic and ultrasonic findings of the internal carotid artery on one side and the associated ophthalmological and neurological symptoms on the other side has stimulated the interest in the research of internal carotid artery occlusion (1, 8, 12, 15). Previous results have shown that the number of patients with internal carotid artery occlusion suffering also from chronic ischemic ophthalmopathy was less impressive than expected (4, 5).

The evaluation of ocular blood flow by means of video-fluorescenceangiography in patients with internal carotid artery obstructions makes it possible to obtain a new understanding of the pathophysiology of chronic ischemic ophthalmopathy (13, 17). For neurologists data about retinal circulation are of interest as well because of histopathological correlations between retinal and cerebral microcirculation (10, 11, 14). The major emphasis in this investigation was based on video-fluorescenceangiography (6, 9, 16) for the measurement of retinal blood flow parameters.

Methods

The ophthalmological examination emphasized assessment of visual acuity, visual fields, intraocular pressure, anterior segment findings on slit lamp examination and gonioscopy, ophthalmoscopy and video-fluorescenceangiography.

Video-fluorescenceangiograms were performed by means of a Zeiss funduscamera FK 50 with adapted videosystem. For the evaluation of the video angiograms a picture analysis system (HP9826, as control unit for the analyser, Microvideomat 3, C. Zeiss) was used. By means of the picture analysis system dye dilution curves were registered as intensity curves over the time axis from the recordings (16). From the dye dilution curves provided by the analyser the following parameters (6, 16) were taken:

a) The time required for the dye to appear in the retinal arteriols: arm - retina time (ART)
b) The time required for the dye to pass the areas of microcirculation between a retina arteriole and corresponding venule: arterio-venous passage time (AVP)
c) The mean dye bolus velocity (MDV) in retinal arteriols. it is calculated from the time difference (dt) of the appearance of the dye between two areas of measurement on the same arteriole, separated by a known distance (s). ($MDV = dt/2^{*}s$)

Patients

In 20 patients with internal carotid arterial occlusion aged 15 to 79 years (mean 59 ± 14 years) the ophthalmologic examinations were performed. 11 patients (55 %) were suffering from systemic hypertension, 1 (5 %) from diabetes mellitus. The average systolic blood pressure was 133 ± 16 mmHg, the diastolic value was 84 ± 11 mmHg. 14 of these patients were treated neurologically because of transient ischemic attacks, amaurosis fugax or lacunar strokes. The occlusion of the internal carotid artery was confirmed by Doppler ultrasound examination and by cerebral angiography.

Results

The ophthalmologic examination demonstrated normal findings in visual acuity, visual fields, intraocular pressure, anterior segment findings and morphology of the fundus. Video-fluorescenceangiograms showed disturbances of retinal circulation. The retinal blood flow parameters in these patients with internal carotid artery occlusion and in healthy volunteers are summarized in Table I.

In all patients we found significantly prolonged retinal blood flow parameters compared to healthy volunteers. In these patients the mean arm retina time (ART) was 4 %, the mean arterio-venous passagetime (AVP) 189 % longer compared with healthy volunteers. The mean dye bolus velocity (MDV) was reduced to 33 % of the values of healthy volunteers. In 11 patients pulsative changes of dye velocity could be observed. Especially in these patients the man dye bolus velocity was markedly reduced in these patients and arterio-venous passagetime was increased up to very high values. The data of these patients are demonstrated in Table II. The retinal blood flow parameters were significantly worse in the patients with pulsative arterial filling than in the other group. Even the group with normal arterial filling showed markly reduced mean dye bolus velocity and significantly increased arterio-venous passagetime (AVP) in relation to the normal values. In 5 (45 %) of 11 patients with pulsative arterial filling hemodynamically significant stenoses (> 90 %) of the contralateral internal carotid artery were observed. In the other normal filling group in 3 (33 %) patients the contralateral internal carotid artery was affected by hemodynamically significant stenosis. Clinical data in both groups were similar.

Table I: Age, arm retina time (ART), arterio-venous passagetime (AVP) an mean dye bolus velocity (MDV) in patients with internal carotid artery occlusion and in healthy volunteers

Diagnosis	N	Age (years)	ART (s)	AVP (s)	MDV (mm/s)
Healthy volunteers	55	32 ± 13	11 ± 3	1,34 ± 0,4	6,0 ± 2,3
Internal carotid occlusion	20	59 ± 14	16 ± 5	3,87 ± 2,1	1,9 ± 2,9
P-value		<0,01	<0,05	<0,001	<0,001

Discussion

Our patients with internal carotid artery occlusion showed no morphologic signs of ischemic ophthalmopathy. It is reported (18), that the ophthalmologic findings in these patients depend on the severity of reduction of retinal blood flow. We found in our patients a wide variation of retinal blood flow parameters. This could be due to the degree of collateralisation and the prior status of the cerebral, orbital and retinal vasculature (2, 3, 5, 7). Other factors might have been involved as well.

In 55 % of our patients we found pulsative arterial filling. This indicates that the diastolic blood pressure in the central retinal artery may be lower than the intraocular pressure. In addition the markely prolonged retinal blood flow parameters in these patients showed a severely reduced ocular blood flow. The decreased mean dye bolus velocity and the prolonged arterio-venous passage time in these patients presumably were due to a reduced ocular perfusion pressure. Since in 5 out of 11 patients with pulsative filling of the retinal artery an obstruction of the contralateral internal carotid artery was also found, it may be concluded that pulsative filling points to reduced collateral supply of the affected side. the other group with normal arterial filling showed a less severe reduction in the ocular blood flow.

Table II: Age, arm-retina time (ART), arterio-venous passagetime (AVP) and mean dye bolus velocity (MDV) in patients with non pulsative and pulsative arterial filling

Diagnosis	N	Age (years)	ART (s)	AVP (s)	MDV mm/s)
non pulsative arterial filling	9	64 ± 11	14,9 ± 4,0	2,3 ± 0,3	3,3 ± 2,1
pulsative occlusion	11	55 ± 15	17,4 ± 5,6	5,2 ± 2,0	0,8 ± 0,7
P-value		n.s	<0,05	<0,001	<0,001

Further investigations of the retinal blood flow are needed to demonstrate the correlation between ocular blood flow parameters and the development of the ophthalmological symptoms of ischemic ophthalmopathy in patients with internal carotid artery occlusions.

References

[1] Copetto JR, Wand M, Bear L, Sciarra R: Neovascular glaucoma and carotid artery obstructive disease. Am J Ophthalmol 99 (1985) 567 - 570

[2] Deweese JA, May AG, Lipchick EO, Rob CG: Anatomic and haemodynamic correlations in carotid artery stenosis. Stroke 1 (1970) 149 - 157

[3] Gaul JJ, Marks SJ, Weinberger J: Visual disturbance and carotid artery disease. Stroke 17 (1986) 393 - 398

[4] Hedges TR: Ophthalmoscopic findings in internal carotid artery occlusion. Bull John Hopkins Hosp 111 (1962) 89 - 97

[5] Hollenhorst RW: Ocular manifestations of insufficiency or thrombosis of the internal carotid artery. Am J Ophthalmol 47 (1957) 753

[6] Jung F, Kiesewetter H, Körber N, Wolf S, Reim M, Müller G: Quantification of characteristic blood-flow parameters in the vessels of the retina with a picture analysis system for video-fluorescence angiograms: initial findings. Graefe's Arch Clin Exp Ophthalmol 211 (1983) 133 - 136

[7] Kearns TP: Ophthalmology and the carotid artery. Am J Ophthalmol 88 (1979) 714 - 722

[8] Kobayashi S, Hollenhorst RW, Sundt TM: Retinal arterial pressure before and after surgery for carotid artery stenosis. Stroke 2,5 (1971) 569 - 575

[9] Körber N, Gesch M, Kiesewetter H, Reim M: Fluoreszenzangiography der Retina - Neue technische Aspekte. Graef's Arch Clin Exp Ophthalmol 213 (1980) 65 - 70

[10] Lodato G, Brancato G: Glaucome neovasculaire secondaire à une occlusion veineuse de branche et à une deficit de la circulation carotido-encephalique: correlations pathogeniques. J Fr Ophthalmol 7 (1984) 615 - 621

[11] Lund OE: Der Augenhintergrund bei allgemeiner und cerebraler Arteriosklerose. Fortschr Med 81 511 - 518

[12] Ringelstein EB, Körber N, Zeumer H, Hunold W: Die Diagnose der Carotisthrombose durch den Augenarzt (Hager 1962) - Aktualisierung dieses Auftrages durch die Doppler-Sonographie. Fortschr Ophthalmol 80 (1983) 66 - 69

[13] Raitta CH, Eisalo A, Folgholm R, Takki K: The ocular pulse wave in health and in occlusive disease of the cervical arteries. Graefe's Arch Clin Exp Ophthalmol 187 (1973) 265 - 272

[14] Sakries NJC, Shilling JG, Burnand KG, Browse NL, Russel RW: Assessment by fluoresceinangiographie of surgical treatment of occlusive carotid artery disease. Stroke 18 (1987) 585 - 590

[15] Steuhl KP, Rohrbach JM, Diener HCH: Augenveränderungen bei Stenosen der Arteria carotis interna- histologsiche und klinische Befunde. Klin MBL Augenheilk 189 (1986) 302 - 307

[16] Wolf S, Jung F, Körber N, Kiesewetter H, Reim M: Measurement of retinal blood flow parameters by means of image analysis system for video - fluorescence angiography. XXV Acta int Congress Ophthal Roma, Kugler Publications 1987 in press

[17] Wolf S, Körber N, Reim M, Ringelstein EB: Ocular blood supply in internal carotid obstructions. In: Benezra D, Ryan SJ, Glaser BM, Murphy RP (eds): Ocular circulation and neovascularisation. martinus Nijhoff/Dr W. Junk Publishers, Dortrecht-Boston-Lancaster 1987

[18] Young LH, Appen RE: Ischemic oculopathy: A manifestation of carotid artery disease. Arch Neurol 38 (1981) 358 - 361

Amaurosis fugax: Sonographic findings and follow-up

A. Valentin, R. Karnik, H.P Ammerer, J. Slany, H. Brenner

Summary

Within 52 months 83 (= 1,25 %) of 6650 patients examined for carotid artery disease suffered from amaurosis fugax.

Continous-wave sonography identified hemodynamically significant lesions of the carotid artery in 40 patients. these patients had a higher incidence of risk factors and vascular disease than those with inconspicuous doppler sonographic findings. Cerebral angiography was performed in 26 patients, of these 22 had abnormal arteriograms. 4 - 56 (median 20) months after the first examination, follow-up of 48 patients was available. of these, 5 patients have died, 9 patients underwent surgery and 1 case each had suffered a stroke or a recurrence of amaurosis fugax. Duplex sonographic examination was performed in 37 patients. all operated patients showed normal ultrasonic findings in the surgically treated area. Complete normal findings of the carotid artery system on both sides were found in 9 out of 37 patients. Amaurosis fugax seems to be a rare but important indicator for extracranial carotid artery disease. Duplex sonographic examination should be performed in all these patients to rule-out hemodynamically non-significant and exulcerated lesions.

Introduction

Amaurosis fugax is a result of temporary retinal ischemia, and like transient neurologic deficits, a warning sign of an impending stroke. Imbolization of cholesterol, fibrin, or platelet aggregates from the carotid artery, or impaired blood flow distal to a hemodynamically significant lesion is usually thought to cause transient monocular visual loss (8). Following the suggestions by HEDGES (4) and HARRISON (3) we defined amaurosis fugax as a painless fleeting attack of partial to total blindness lasting from seconds to minutes with no evidence of ocular disease. The aim of our retrospective study was to report doppler ultrasonic and angiographic findings of patients refered to us with the diagnosis amaurosis fugax. Clinical follow up and Duplex sonographic findings of these patients complete the report.

Patients and Methods

From January '83 to April'87, Doppler sonographic examinations of the carotid arteries were performed in 6650 patients at our department. In '83 (1,25 %) of these patients, amaurosis fugax was the cause for referal. There were 48 men and 35 women with an average age of 62,8 and a range from 19 to 92 years. Periorbital Doppler was performed in all patients, and direct insonation of the carotid arteries by continous-wave Doppler sonography in 60 of the patients. In 26 subjects the supraaortic vessels were examined by angiography. In the first retrospective part (period I) of the study we analysed data and findings of all patients with the primary diagnosis of amaurosis fugax. In the second part (period II) patients were investigated again clinically, and by Duplex sonography (Disonics scanner CV 400 with a 10-MHz imaging transducer and a 3,0-MHz Doppler transducer) of the carotid arteries (2)m 4 - 56 months after the first examination. Analysis of these findings was restricted to patients with symptoms in accordance with the above mentioned definition.

Results

Period I

Continous-wave Doppler sonography identified hemodynamically significant lesions of the carotid arteries in 40 patients (group I). 43 patients with normal findings formed group II. Table I shows the patients characteristics of both groups. 3 patients in group I and 7 in group II were younger than 50 years. Visual symptoms appeared several times in 13 patients of group I, but only once in all patients of group II. Non-simultaneous transient ischemic attacks occured in 9 patients of group I and 3 of group II. Risk factors and associated vascular disorders are listed in Table II. There was a higher incidence of ischemic heart disease, peripheral vascular disease, cerebral vascular disease (history of stroke or carotid endarterectomy), smoking and hyperlipidemia in group I.

Table I: Patients characteristics

	group I n = 40	group II n = 43
Sex (m/w)	29/11	19/24
Age	46,3	61,3
Repeated visual symptoms	13	0
TIA	9	3
History of stroke	2	2

26 patients were studied by cerebral angiography. Stenosis exceeding 50 % of the lumen was found in the extracranial internal carotid artery (ICA) in 11 patients and in the common carotid artery (CCA) in 1 patients. Stenosis of the carotid siphon was

seen in 1 patient. Complete occlusion of the ICA was present in 5 patients and of the CCA in 1 patients. There was 1 case each of kinking of the ICA, fibromuscular dysplasia, and extatic origin of the CCa. 4 symptomatic patients had both, normal Doppler sonographic findings and normal arteriograms.

Table II: Risk factors and associated vascular disorders

	group I n = 40	group II n = 43
Smoker	12	6
Hypertension	14	14
Diabetes	8	7
Hyperlipidemia	5	2
Oral contraceptives	2	1
Ischemic heart disease	6	4
Peripheral vascular disease	6	2
Cerebral vascular disease	4	2

Period II

4 - 56 (median 20) months after the first examination, information about 56 patients was available. 27 patients were lost to follow-up. In 8 patients the given definition of amaurosis fugax was not verifieable, therefore the follow-up involved 48 patients (25 of group I and 23 of group II). Group I (N = 25): 1 patient had died, 8 patients underwent carotid endarterectomy and in 1 patient EC-IC bypass was performed. No patient of this group had further neurological symptoms. In 22 out of these 25 patients, Duplex sonography of the carotid arteries was performed. Abnormal findings were recorded in 17 patients (77 %). Group II (n = 23): 4 patients had died, 17 patients had no further neurological symptoms, 1 patient had suffered a stroke. In 15 out of these 23 patients Duplex sonography was performed, abnormal findings were seen in 11 patients (73 %).

Table III shows the findings of the non surgically treated subjects. There is no significant difference in the incidence of stenosis or occlusion between the symptomatic and asymptomatic sides except in the case of exulcerated plaques. 6 patients had normal findings on both sides. Duplex findings of the surgically treated patients are listed in Table IV. In all patients with carotid endarterectomy the IVA was judged normal. 3 of these patients had a thrombendarterectomy on both sides.

Table III: Dublex findings: non-surgically treated patients (N = 28)

	CCA s/a	ICA s/a	ECA s/a
exulc. plaques	1/0	4/0	0/0
stenosis 0 - 25 %	3/2	8/7	1/1
26 - 50 %	0/2	1/3	0/1
51 - 80 %	0/0	1/2	0/1
81 - 99 %	0/0	1/0	1/0
occlusion	1/0	2/2	0/0

Discussion

Amaurosis fugax seems to be a rare event. SÖRENSEN (7) reported in an unselected material an incidence of 1 patient per 5000 per year in an ophthalmic practice. SANDOK (6) found in a group of 1080 patients studied by carotid angiography, 43 who experienced amaurosis fugax. Due to different patient groups data are not comparable, but the trend seem to be substantiated by our results, where an incidence of 1,25 % was found in patients referred for vascular investigation. Reported results of arteriography in patients with amaurosis fugax differ markedly (1, 3, 6), due to various selection principles and different definitions of amaurosis fugax (4). In our study the high number of positive arteriograms could be explained by Doppler sonographic screening.

Only a part of our patients was available for follow-up, therefore we avoid to give data about mortality and morbidity. POOLE and ROSS RUSSEL (5) reported in a study of 110 patients 4 times higher incidence of stroke and 1,4 times greater mortality than in the general population, 6 years after amaurosis fugax. Ischemic heart disease was the most frequent cause of death. These findings suggest amaurosis fugax to be a marker of more generalised arteriosclerotic disease.

Table IV: Dublex findings: patients with carotid endarterectomy (= 8) and EC-IC bypass (n = 1)+

	CCA s/a	ICA s/a	ECA s/a
exulc. plaques	1/0	0/0	0/0
stenosis			
0 - 25 %	1/2	0/1	0/0
26 - 50 %	3/0	0/2	1/0
51 - 80 %	1/1	0/1	0/0
81 - 99 %	0/0	0/0	0/0
occlusion	0/0	1+/0	0/1

s/a = symptomatic/asymptomatic side

In period II of our study only 6 out of 28 non-operated patients showed normal duplex sonographic findings of the carotid arteries. It could not be answered retrospectively, wether there is any causal connection to the primary symptoms. Duplex sonography is a new method useful for detecting hemodynamically non-significant lesions and exulcerated plaques, which may be missed by Doppler examination. Therefore, in all patients presenting amaurosis fugax with normal Doppler sonographic findings, a Duplex sonography should be performed.

References

[1] Adams Jr HP, Putman SF, Corbett JJ, Sires BP, Thompson HS: Amaurosis fugax: The results of Arteriography in 59 patients. Stroke 14 (1983) 742 - 744

[2] Garth KE, Carroll BA, Sommer FG, Oppenheimer DA: duplex ultrasound scanning of the carotid arteries with velocity spectrum analysis. Radiology 147 (1983) 823 - 827

[3] Harrison MJG, Marshall J: Arteriographic comparison of amaurosis fugax and hemispheric transient ischaemic attacks. Stroke 16 (1985) 795 - 797

[4] Hedges THR: The terminology of transient visual loss due to vascular insufficiency. Stroke 15 (1984) 907 - 908

[5] Poole CJM, Ross Russel RW: Mortality and stroke after amaurosis fugax. J Neurol, Neurosurg, Psych. 48 (1985) 902 - 905

[6] Sandok BA, Trautmann JC, Ramirez-Lassepass M, Sundt Jr TM, Houser OW: Clinical angiographic correlations in amaurosis fugax. Amer J Ophthal 78 (1974) 137 - 142

[7] Sörensen PN: Amaurosis fugax, a unselected material. Acta ophthal. 61 (1983) 583 - 588

[8] Wilson LA, Ross Russel RW: Amaurosis fugax and carotid artery disease: Indications for angiography. brit Med J 2 (1977) 435 - 437

Hemodymanic in central vein occlusion

Ch. Teping, M. Reim, B. Bertram, S. Wolf

Summary

44 patients were examined by video-fluorescenceangiography. With the onset of the first symptoms a significant decrease of retinal blood flow was determined by prolonged arterio-venous passage time (AVP) and diminution of mean dye bolus velocity (MDV). A correlation between the extend of the impeded retinal perfusion in the acute phase and the severity of the clinical appearance could not be found. In 35 of 44 patients a favourable clinical course was observed. An initially markedly reduced retinal perfusion improved under inpatient care (iso- or hypervolemic hemodilution, fibrinolysis, panretinal lasercoagulation) and remained stationary during the further course of time. A complete normalisation of the arterio-venous passage time (AVP) and of the mean dye bolus velocity (MDV) could not be found in any of these patients. We suppose that even several months after the onset of clinical symptoms some disturbance of retinal perfusion persisted. We encountered 16 % of patients with retinal stasis syndrom who progressed to develop a hemorrhagic central venous thrombosis. In our opinion the videoangiographic follow up of patients with retinal stasis syndrom is of essential importance for early detection of further reduced retinal perfusion. Thus it may be possible to prevent the transition of these cases into a hemorrhagic central retinal vein occlusion by early treatment.

Introduction

Central retinal vein obstruction consists of two different entities: 1. venous stasis retinopathy; 2. hemorrhagic retinopathy [2, 13]. The retinal stasis syndrom shows thickening and tortuosity of veins and postcapillar venoles; usually there are only few hemorrhages observable, most numerously occuring in the more peripheral retina [12, 13]. In some cases the retina shows considerable hemorrhages of the posterior pole. Papilloedema can be observed in some cases [2]. Hemorrhagic central retinal vein occlusion is typically associated with papilloedema and extensive hemorrhages. Retinal hemorrhages are found peripapillarly and associated with the retinal veins. Usually the macula region shows hemorrhages and marked edema [2, 13].

Hemorrhagic central retinal vein occlusion has a poor visual outcome [7, 8]. Obliterated vessels, mainly veins, and tissue death of large areas of retinal parenchyme can be observed in the later stages. Hemorrhagic secondary glaucoma is the most severe complication [2, 10]. However, in the venous stasis syndrom only cystoid macular oedema or progression to cystoid degeneration, macular cyst, hole or premacular gliosis is reported as a complication [2]. The change of retinal stasis syndrom to hemorrhagic central retinal vein occlusion seems to be more frequent than reported [11, 12].

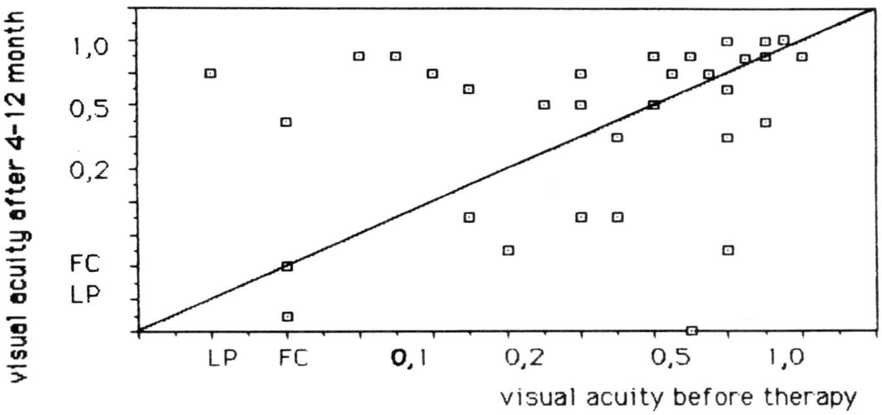

Fig. 1: Visual acuity in 32 patients with retinal stasis syndrom before (x-Axis) and 4 - 12 months (y-Axis) after therapy

The technique of video-fluorescenceangiography (3, 9, 15) enables a new understanding of the pathophysiology of impeded retinal circulation. In this paper we report on the retinal hemodynamics in the natural course of venous stasis syndrom.

Materials and Methods

44 patients with retinal stasis syndrom were examinated by video-fluorescenceangiography. The maximal time between first subjective symptoms and first clinical examination was 21 days, the mean time was 7,1 ± 7,7 days. 32 of these patients could be clinically observed for a period of at least 4 - 12 months. There were 18 males and 14 females aged from 28 to 80 years (mean: 59 ± 13 years). 15 (34 %) of these patients were suffering from systemic hypertension, 2 (5 %) from diabetes mellitus and 5 (11 %) from hyperlipoproteinaemia.

The ophthalmological examination emphasized assessment of visual acuity, visual fields, intraocular pressure, slit lamp examination, ophthalmoscopy and video-fluorescenceangiography. Video-fluorescenceangiograms were performed by means of a Zeiss funduscamera FK 50 with adapted videosystem. With an picture analysis system composed of a HP 9826 computer and the videoanalyser Microvideomat 3, C. Zeiss.

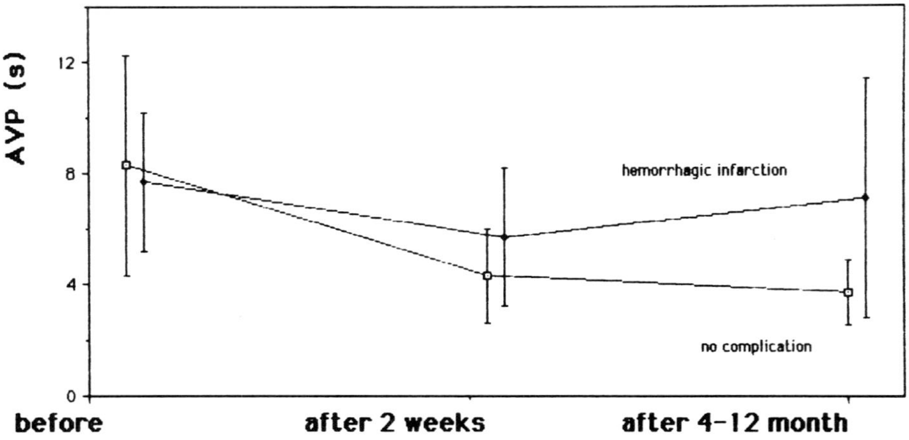

Fig. 2: Development of the arterio-venous passagetime of patients with hemorrhagic infarction (n = 7) and patients without hemorrhagic complication (n = 25)

Dye dilution curves were registered as intensity curves over the time axis from the recordings [15]. From the dye dilution curves the following parameters [3, 15] were taken:

a) The time required for the dye to pass the areas of microcirculation between a retinal arteriole and corresponding venole: arterio-venous passage time (AVP).
b) The mean dye bolus velocity (MDV) in retinal arteriols was calculated from the difference of time (dt) of the appearence of the dye between two areas of measurement on the same arteriole, separated by a known distance (s). (MDV = $dt/2^{*}s$)

In addition as hemorrheological parameters hematocrite (HCT), plasmaviscosity.v.plasmaviscosity; (PV) and fibrinogen(Fib) were quantified. In table I the examination methods are summarized.

Table I: Examination parameters, methods, symbol and reference values

parameter	methode (reference)	symbol	reference	values
hematokrit	impedance methode (4,6)	HCT	m: 39-52 % f: 34-50 %	
plasma-viscosity	capillary viscosimeter (4,5)	PV	1,14-1,34 mPas	plasma-
fibrinogen	Clauss (1)	FIB	2,0-4,0 g/1	
arterio-venous pas-sagetime	video-flourescence-angiography	AVP	0,5-2,1 s	(3,14,15)
mean dye bolus velocity	video-fluorescence-angiography	FBG	2,6-9,4 mm/s	(3,14,15)

Results

The development of visual acuity during the observation period is shown in figure 1.

In table II and III the hemorrheological parameters and retinal blood flow parameters are summarized. Normal hematocrit and fibrinogen values were found; plasmaviscosity was significantly increased. The arterio-venous passagetime (AVP) in our patients was about six times longer than the control values. The mean dye bolus velocity was significantly reduced. The initially significant increased plasmaviscosity was only marginaly reduced after 4 - 12 months. Retinal blood flow parameters were significantly improved during the first two weeks after the initial examination. After 4 - 12 months these parameters stabilized. It is remarkable that the retinal perfusion did not return within the normal range. There was no correlation between the functional reduction, perimetry and retinal perfusion parameters.

5 patients with retinal stasis syndrom developed a hemorrhagic central retinal vein occlusion. In 2 cases a hemorrhagic secondary glaucoma occured in spite of hemodilution therapy or panretinal lasercoagulation. 2 further patients showed beginning hemorrhagic infarction, however, further progression could be prevented

by immediate panretinal laser coagulation or fibrinolysis. These 7 patients did not differ in their initial clinical parameters from the other patients. In figure 2 the development of the arterio-venous passage time (AVP) of the 7 patients with the hemorrhagic infarction is compared with the values of the remaining 25 patients. During the first 2 weeks a similar AVP was found in both groups. However thereafter a significant prolongation of the AVP ($P < 0{,}05$) was observed in the complicated cases.

Table II: Hematocrite (HCT), plasmaviscosity (PV) and fibrinogen level (Fib) before therapy and after 4 - 12 months in 32 patients with retinal stasis syndrom

	normal values	before therapy	after 4 - 12 months
HCT(%)	m: 39-52 f: 34-50	m: 46 ± 3 f: 42 ± 4	m: 44 ± 4 f: 40 ± 3
PV(mPas)	1,14-1,34	1,38 ± 0,11	1,33 ± 0,10
Fib(g/l)	2,0-4,0	3,1 ± 0,9	3,2 ± 0,8

Discussion

Video-fluorescenceangiography conveys new information about the pathophysiology of central retinal vein obstruction. With the onset of the first symptoms a significant decrease of retinal blood flow was determined by prolonged arterio-venous passage time (AVP) and diminution of mean dye bolus velocity (MDV). A correlation between the extend of the impeded retinal perfusion in the acute phase and the severity of the clinical appearance could not be found. this is in aggreement with previous published data [12, 14]. In 35 of 44 patients a favourable clinical course was observed. 26 patients obtained a final visual acuity of 0.5 or better. An initially markedly reduced retinal perfusion improved under inpatient care (iso- or hypervolemic hemodilution, fibrinolysis, panretinal lasercoagulation) and remained stationary during the further course of time. A complete normalisation of the arterio-venous passage time (AVP) and of the mean dye bolus velocity (MDV) could not be found in any of these patients. We suppose that even several months after the onset of clinical symptoms some disturbance of retinal perfusion will persist.

6 of those 9 patients, who suffered a reduction of visual acuity of two or more lines during therapy, were found to have a hemorrhagic retinal infarction. The videoangiographic examination showed significant raise of arterio-venous passage time in these patients. The pathologic retinal perfusion results in chronic hypoxia of the inner retinal layers. This leads to a breakdown of the blood retinal barrier of small

and large retinal vessels and hemorrhagic infarction. In our study we encountered 16 % of patients with retinal stasis syndrom who progressed to develop a hemorrhagic central venous thrombosis.

*Table III: Age, arterio-venous passagetime (AVP) and mean dye bolus velocity (MDV) before therapy, after 2 weeks and after 4 - 12 months in 32 patients with retinal stasis syndrom (* P < 0,01 to the normal values; ** P < 0,01 to the initial values)*

	patients with retinal stasis syndrom n = 32			normal values n = 55(17)
	before therapy	after 2 weeks	after 4-12 month	
age (years)	59 ± 13*			32 ± 13
AVP(s)	8,2 ± 3,6*	4,6 ± 1,7**	4,6 ± 2,7**	1,3 ± 0,4
MDV(mm/s)	1,6 ± 0,8*	2,6 ± 0,9**	2,7 ± 0,9**	6,0 ± 1,7

	patients with retinal stasis syndrom n = 32			normal values n = 55(17)
	before therapy	after 2 weeks	after 4-12 month	
age (years)	59 ± 13*			32 ± 13
AVP(s)	8,2 ± 3,6*	4,6 ± 1,7**	4,6 ± 2,7**	1,3 ± 0,4
MDV(mm/s)	1,6 ± 0,8*	2,6 ± 0,9**	2,7 ± 0,9**	6,0 ± 1,7

In our opinion the videoangiographic follow up of patients with retinal stasis syndrom is of essential importance for early detection of further reduced retinal perfusion and by early treatment could prevent the transition into a hemorrhagic central retinal vein occlusion.

References

[1] Clauss A: Gerinnungsphysiologische Schnellmethode zur Bestimmung des Fibrinogens. Acta Hämat 17 (1957) 237

[2] Hayreh SS: Classification of central retinal vein occlusion. Am Ac of Ophthalmol 90 (1983) 458 - 474

[3] Jung F, Kiesewetter H, Körber N, Wolf S, Reim M, Müller G: Quantification of characteristic blood-flow parameters in the vessels of the retina with a picture analysis system for video-fluorescence angiograms: initial findings. Graefe's Arch Clin Exp Ophthalmol 211 (1983) 133 - 136

[4] Jung F, Kiesewetter H, Roggenkamp HG, Nüttgens HP, Ringelstein EB, Gerhards M, Kotitschke G, Wenzel E, Zeller H: Bestimmung der Referenzbereiche rheologischer Parameter: Studie an 653 zufällig ausgewählten Probanden im Kreis Aachen. Klin Wochenschr 64 (1986) 357 - 381

[5] Jung F, Roggenkamp HG, Schneider R, Kiesewetter H: Das Kapillarschlauch-Viskosimeter. Ein neues Meßgerät zur Quantifizierung der Blutplasmaviskosität. Biomed Techn 28 (1983) 248 - 252

[6] Kiesewetter H, Lazar H, Radtke H, Thielen W: Hämotokritbestimmung durch Impedanzmessung. Biomed Technik 27 (1982) 171 - 175

[7] Kohner EM: Central retinal vein occlusion: Natural history, associated medical conditions and treatment. Bull Soc belge Ophthal 201 (1982) 1 -13

[8] Kohner EM, Laatikainen L, Oughton J: The management of central retinal vein occlusion. Ophthalmology 90,5 (1983) 484 - 187

[9] Körber N, Gesch M, Kiesewetter H, Reim M, Schmid-Schönbein H: Fernsehfluoreszenzangiographie der Retina. Neue technische Aspekte. Albrecht v Graefes Arch klin exp Ophthal 213 (1980) 65 - 70

[10] Magargal LE, Brown GC, Augsburger JJ, Donoso LA: Efficacy of panretinal photocoagulation in preventing neovascular glaucoma following ischemic central retinal vein obstruction. Ophthalmology 89 (1982) 780 - 784

[11] Reim M, Kiesewetter H, Körber F, Jung F, Raemaekers B, Wolf S: Untersuchung der retinalen Blutzirkulation durch Videofluoreszenz-angiographie bei Verschlüssen der Zentralvene. Sitzungsbericht der 148. Versammlung des Vereins Rheinisch-Westfälischer Augenärzte (1986)

[12] Reim M, Kiesewetter H, Körber N, Jung F, Raemaekers B, Wolf S: Untersuchung der retinalen Blutzirkulation durch Video-Fluoreszenzangiographie bei Verschlüssen der Zentralvene. In: XXV. Acta int Congress Ophthal Roma, Kugler Publications 1987

[13] Reim M: Augenheilkunde Enke, Stuttgart 1985

[14] Wolf S, Bertram B, Kiesewetter H, Jung F, Reim M: Iso- and hypervolemic hemodilution in central retinal vein occlusion (CRVO). Clinical Hemorheology 7 (1987) 398

[15] Wolf S, Jung F, Körber N, Kiesewetter H, Reim M: Measurement of retinal blood flow parameters by means of image analysis system for video-fluorescence angiogrphy. In: XXV. Acta int Congress Ophthal Roma, Kugler Publications 1987

VI

TRAUMATIC LESIONS

Periorbital comminuted Fractures and their Relationship to the Facial Bones

E. Machtens, L. Heuser

Abstract

Periorbital comminuted fractures including maxilla and skull-base may not be viewed as an isolated problem. The principles of a stabilizing and occluding treatment require a solid osteosynthesis of the cranium. Qualified treatment planning starts with an extensive diagnostic approach to skullbase, orbital region and maxilla. The more accidental or arbitrary boundaries of the special lines may not restrict the patient's care. Rather on the contrary therapy should be optimized by integration of special knowledge. The fundamental principles are discussed by typical examples.

A

Specialities such as neurosurgery, otorhinolaryngology, ophthalmology and maxillofacial surgery have got a better understanding and increased knowledge of each other potentials requirements in diagnosis and therapy during the last years resulting in an improved treatment of facial and cranial injuries. Interdisciplinary clinical and scientific communication is essential for a successful therapy.

B

In the following the aspects of maxillofacial surgery concerning the stabilization of a torn-off maxilla in comminuted fractures of the skull-base and the periorbital bones are demonstrated. Muscular effects due to chewing, respiration, swallowing etc. cause permanent motility resulting in infection, liquorrhoe and remaining malfunctions.

Dislocation can be caused by the facial muscles, especially those who open the mouth (Fig. 1) but also by inappropiate compression in therapeutic wiring (Fig. 2). Therefore adequate fixation of the facial bones to the cranium is required (Fig. 3).

The maxilla is fixed to the lateral parts of the orbitas and/or to the middle of the frontal bone by craniofacial wires, internal wires, and maxillo-frontal wires. None of those techniques yields sufficient stability, which is the real problem in comminuted fractures of the skull-base and the medial and lateral parts of the frontal pilars.

C

There are two fundamental aspects in treatment:

- Periorbital and frontobasal traumata in combination with maxillary fractures require adequate, if necessary simultaneous operative approach by several special lines [2, 5]

- A stable resetting and reconstruction of the bony structures. In certain circumstances, such as life-threatening situations, a subsequent therapeutic approach by the different special lines has to be considered.

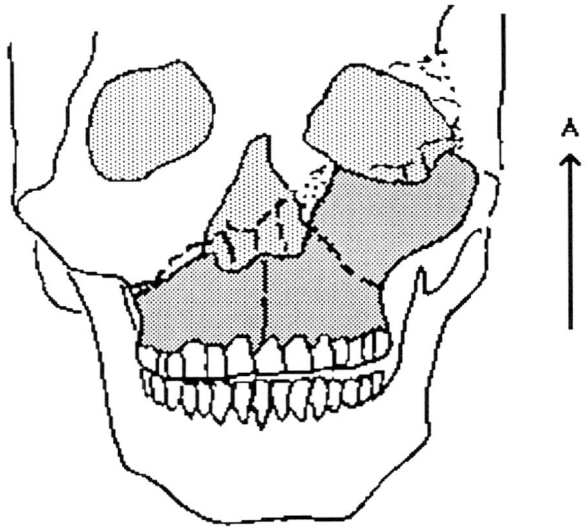

Fig. 1: Schematic drawing of a maxillozygomatic fracture with a compression induced dislocation

Diagnostic imaging starts with the plain film of the facial skull (Watersprojection) and is completed by high-resolution computed tomography [1, 3, 4].

In patients suffering from trauma of the neurocranium, the CT-examination should be extended to the facial skull when additional fractures of the facial bones are suspected. In cases presenting with maxillofacial trauma the CT-examination should always be extended to the skull-base.

D

During the past years a change has occurred in operative treatment. SCHWENZER [9] and others [7, 8] suggested wiring techniques for osteosynthesis of isolated impression fractures and comminuted fractures of the periorbital area. Despite their advantages these methods are insufficient when additional fractures of the maxilla are present.

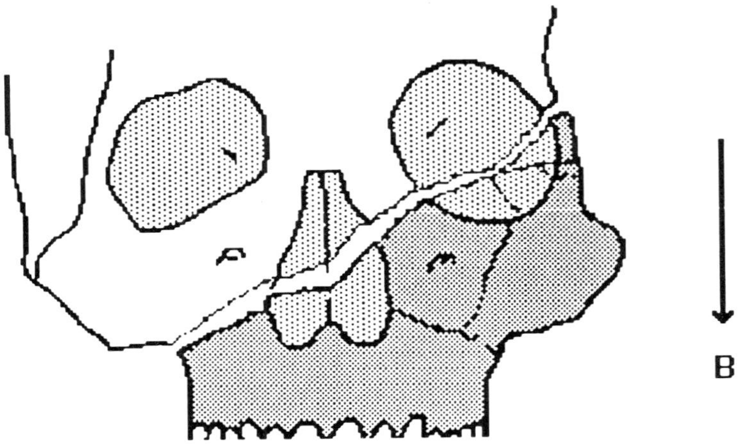

Fig. 2: Schematic drawing of a caudally dislocated maxillar and os zygoma fracture

The introduction of plate-osteosynthesis with and without compression therefore means a new dimension of operative therapy although this technique does not replace the wiring methods completely.

"State of the art" in treatment of combined frontobasal, periorbital and maxillar fractures is a most stable plate-osteosynthesis of all fragments combining also those of the upper face skull.

This is demonstrated in a case of a comminuted fracture of the lateral periorbital bones (Fig. 4).

The demonstrated treatment shows that sufficient suspension of the torn-off maxilla would not be achieved without stabilization of the multiple supraorbital and lateroorbital fragments.

Osteoclastic trepanation procedures of the frontal bone can not longer be accepted to fullfill the requirements stated above. On the other hand subtile reconstruction of the puzzle-like fragments takes plenty of time. In severe situations such as brain edema when primary osteosynthesis is not possible, the autologue bone material should be kept and stored for secondary implantation.

In cases presenting a leaking from the dura mater, the temporarily explanted fragments must be reimplanted after sealing.

Thus stable fixation of the dura mater is achieved, which is necessary for the prevention of haematomas.

The principles of restoration of the paranasal sinuses and their drainage are maintained, and there was no higher infection rate in all of our cases. Even in loss of the posterior wall of the sinus frontalis a stabilization of the frontal bone could be performed by plate osteosynthesis.

The secondary treatment is more lasting and safer done by plate-osteosynthesis which also yields better cosmetic and function results.

An example of secondary treatment of a dislocated periorbital comminuting fracture 3.5 weeks after an injury with severe contusion of the brain stem and epidural heamatoma is shown in Fig. 5.

Caudal displacement of the fragments can well be demonstrated in comparable projections. Complete reposition of the whole frontal and supraorbital region was achieved. Stable fixation was not possible by wiring osteosynthesis, as cicatricial connections would cause an elastic refraction. Safe reposition, therefore, required plate-osteosynthesis.

Plate-osteosynthesis with and without compression must be accepted as an improvement in definitive stable treatment of combined periorbital, frontobasal and maxillar fractures [5, 6].

Figures

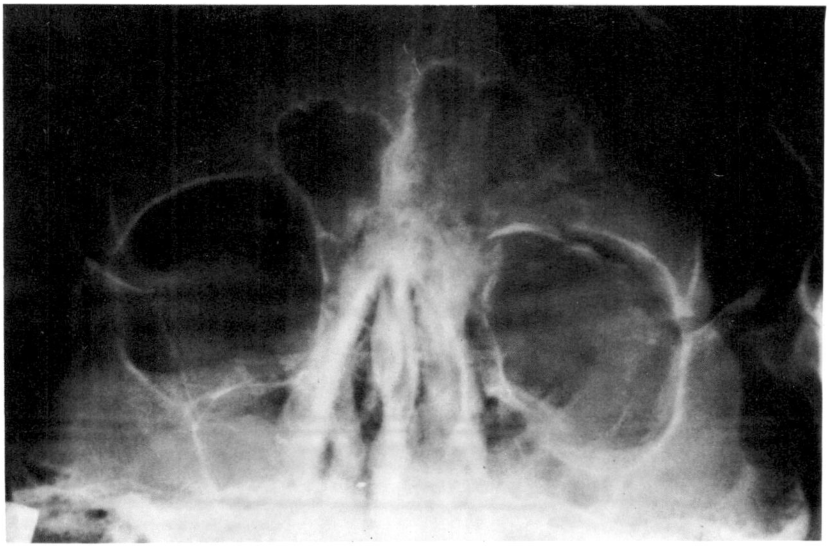

Fig. 3: Fractures of the frontal and zygomatic bones combined with a central fracture of the maxilla on the le Fort-II-level

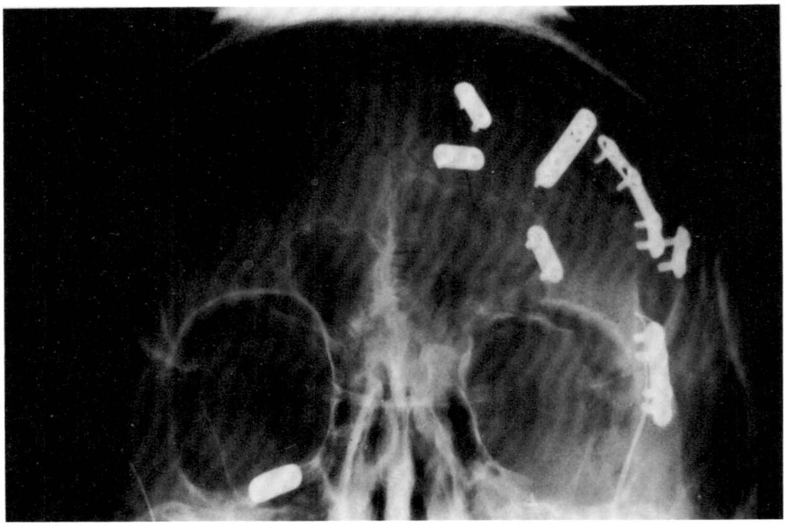

Fig. 4a: Stable osteosynthesis of the frontozygomatic region and craniofacial wiring. Close up Film in occipitonasal projection

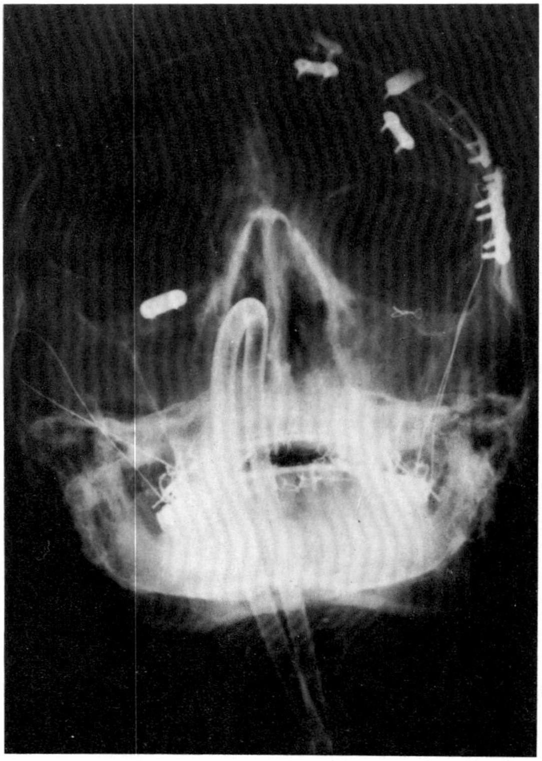

Fig. 4b: Plain film in Waters projection

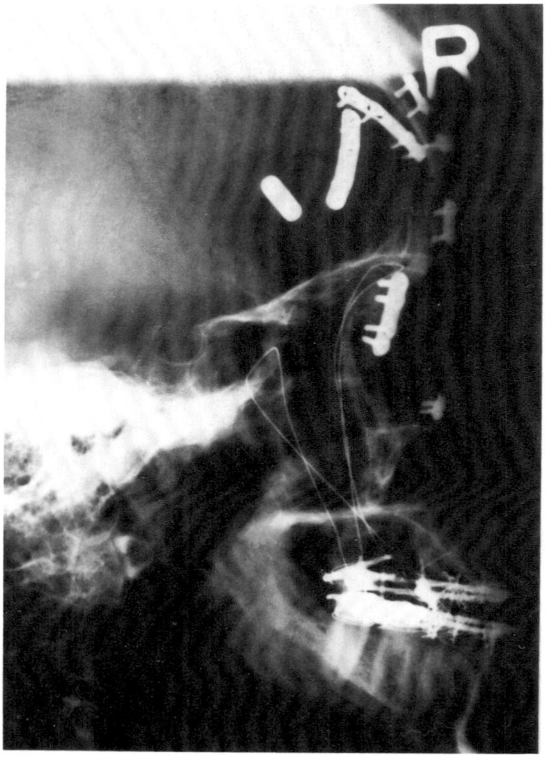

Fig. 4c: Lateral view

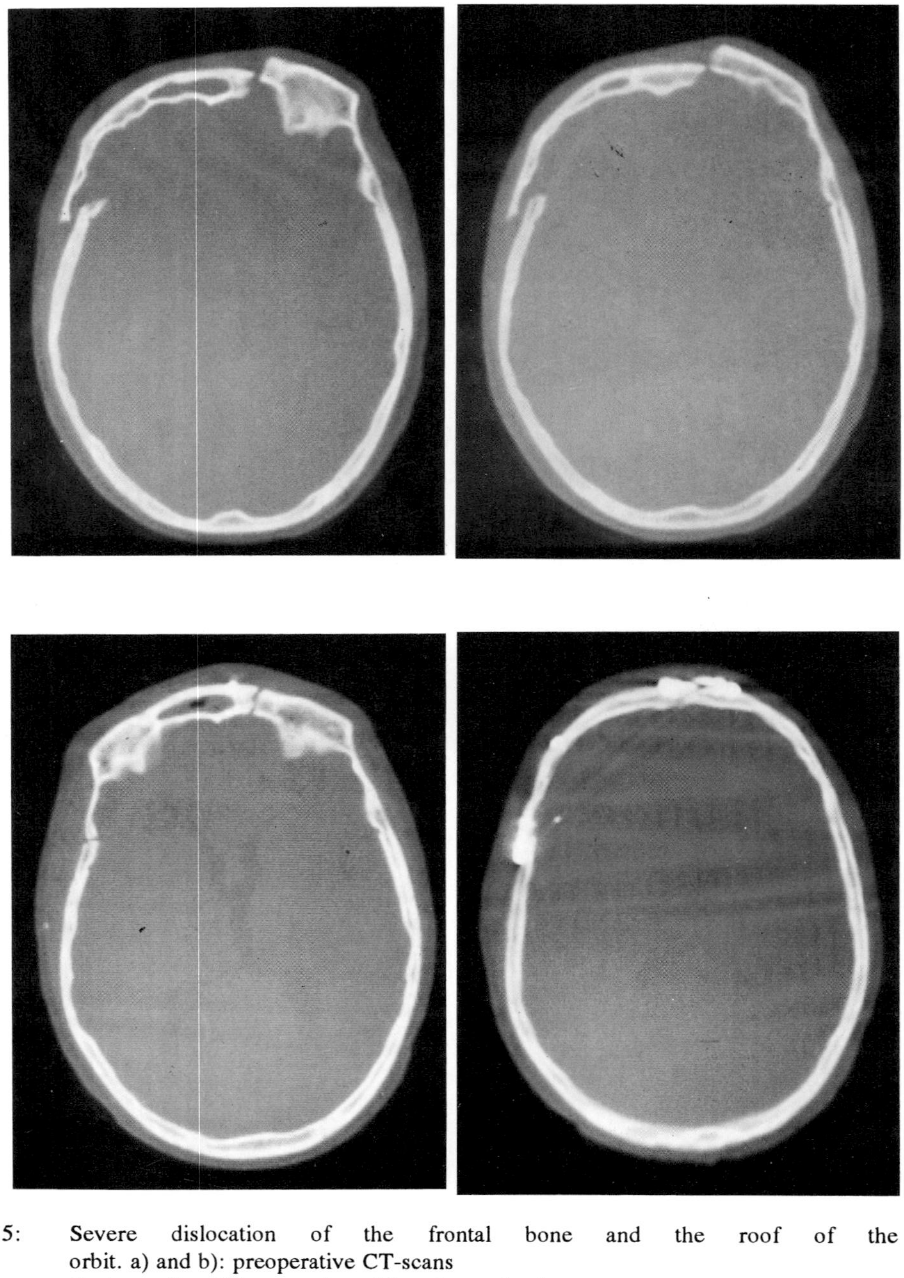

a,b)

c,d)

Fig. 5: Severe dislocation of the frontal bone and the roof of the orbit. a) and b): preoperative CT-scans
Postoperative CT-scans after plate osteosynthesis

References

[1] Brutish T, Mödder U: HNO Röntgenatlas - Pathologische Befunde - Springer 1986

[2] Deitmer T: Versorgung frontobasaler Schädelverletzungen. Welche Aufgaben hat der Rhinochirurg ? Klinikarzt 15 (1986) 543 - 548

[3] Johnson Jr H:CT of maxillofacial trauma. Radiologic Clinics of North America 22, Nr. 1 (1984) 131 - 144

[4] Koornneef L: The role of direct multiplanar high resolution CT in the assessment and management of orbital trauma. Radiologic Clinics of North America 25, Nr. 4 (1987) 753 - 766

[5] Machtens E: Diagnostik und Behandlungsablauf aus der Sicht des Mund-, Kiefer- und Gesichtschirurgen. In: Schwenzer N, Pfeifer G: Fortschritte der Kiefer- und Gesichtschirurgie, Band XXXII Thieme Verlag (1987) 221 - 223

[6] Machtens E: Chirurgische Versorgung von Mittelgesichtsfrakturen aus der Sicht des Kiefer- und Gesichtschirurgen. In: Majer EH und Zrunek M: Die Oto-Rhinolaryngologie in Kooperation mit Nachbardisziplinen. Verlag: Facultas, Universitätsverlag (1987) 11 - 17

[7] Rowe NL, Williams JL: Maxillofacial Injuries. Churchill-Livingstone, Edingburgh 1985

[8] Schwenzer N, Dieckmann J: Tierexperimentelle Untersuchungen zum Stabilitätsproblem bei der Drahtnaht im Gesichtsskelet. Stoma 24 (1971) 153

[9] Schwenzer N: Zur Osteosynthese bei Frakturen des Gesichtsskeletts. Thieme 1976

Primary and secondary reconstruction in the case of interdisciplinary surgical management of combined cranio-facial injuries

D. Schettler, K. Roosen, J. Heesen, Ch. Mohr

The number of serious traumatic lesions to the bony orbital margin and the mid-face region has shown a tendency to rise during the last two decades. According to the statistics of the Department of Maxillo-Facial Surgery of the University Clinic of Essen, the peak was reached in 1983 with 165 patients (Tab. I).

Since wearing a safety-belt in the car was made compulsory, the injuries by the simple cuts in the facial region have decreased considerably whereas the grave combined cranio-facial lesions have not changes as regards their number.

Amongst 810 patients with head injuries during the period from 1980 to 1984, there were 80 with cranio-facial trauma (Tab. II). Because of the concomitant trauma of the brain, other organs or the extremities, 65 of those patients were given primary conservative treatment. The occlusion in the region of the jaw first of all was stabilized by splints used for fractures of the jaw. To bridge the gaps when presented with extensive osseous defects, particulary polimerisates were used such as PMMA (Palacos^{R}).

Here necrosis of the skin has to be expected if the latter has been damaged badly and if the cutaneous circulation will be additionally impaired by implanting synthesis substances.

Therefore for many decades partical recovery was the chosen strategy (Fig. 1). By means of the later reconstruction with the help of synthetic material, polymerized by heat, very good results can also be obtained (Fig. 2).

During the last ten years various systems of the mini-plates have been developed with the help of which the burst fractures in the center of the face and in the region of the bony orbit can be extremely well stabilized. These operations, preferably performed at the secondary phase are like putting together a jig-saw-puzzle where by the tiny bone fragments are fixed in the required position like pearls on a string (Fig. 3).

Results of the healing process were surprisingly good and almost without complications. Not in a single case was there loss of bony fragments once they were stabilized, although next to the opened-up orbital cavity, the adjoining paranasal sinus as well as the maxillary sinus and the cells of the ethmoid were also exposed in the course of the trauma. Here we discovered a method to establish primary stable osteo-synthesis when dealing with severe cranial-facial lesions which include the center of the face, the area of the orbital as well as the cranium (Fig. 4).

It is extremely important for the neurosurgeon to realise that even minute bony fragment has to be preserved (Fig. 5). This osteo-synthesis with the help of mini-plates establishes a bony consilidation of the stabilized structure within the next two or three months. The mini-plate system used was of the "Study Group for Osteosynthesis" (A.O.) and that of Champy. The great advantage is to be found in the areas of the frontal bone and of the mid face where the dainty osseous structure between frontal sinus, orbita, nasal sinus, maxillary sinus and the cells of the ethmoid present best results when primary reconstruction is performed. The re-building of the pneumatized cavities and in particular of the frontal sinus is done completely preserving the mucous membranes, at the same time taking great care that every sinus has been provided with a wide and permanent opening. Amongst 842 patients from 1980 to 1986 not a single osteomyelitis or sequestration or meningitis occured, although numerous bony fragments were without their periosteum. This primary osteo-synthesis enables us to largely avoiding cranio-facial defects without having to fear that special complications might develop (Fig. 7 and 8). In general the implants will be removed 6 - 8 months later.

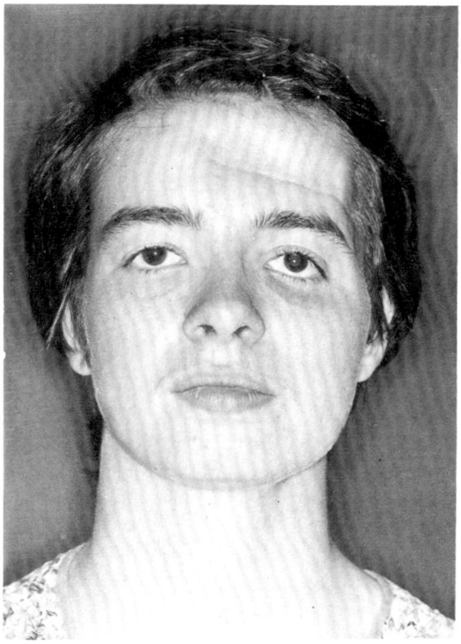

Fig. 1

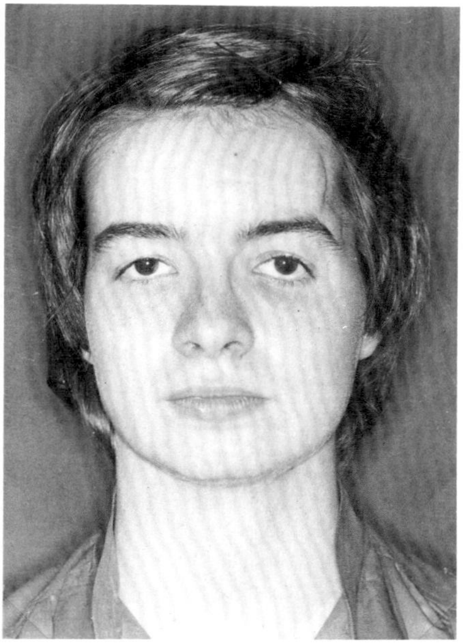

Fig. 2

Fig. 1, 2: Conditions after splinked fracture of the frontal bone and the partial recovery
Fig. 2: Reconstruction of the face by implantation of synthetic material

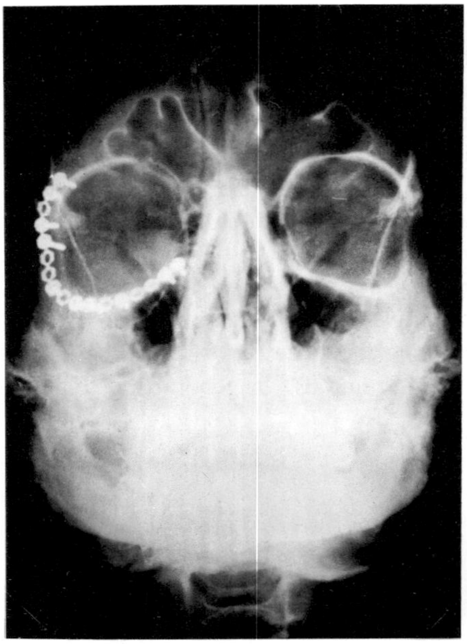

Fig. 3

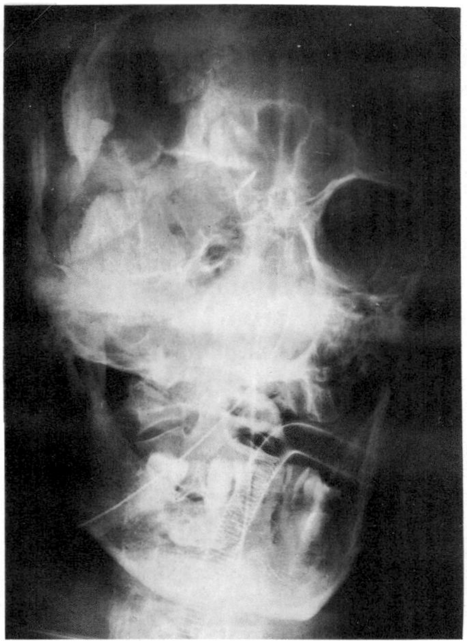

Fig. 4

Fig. 3: Fracture of right orbital ring and subsequent osteo-synthesis by mini-plates

Fig. 4: Most severe fractures on the right side of the skull, frontal bone, and orbit

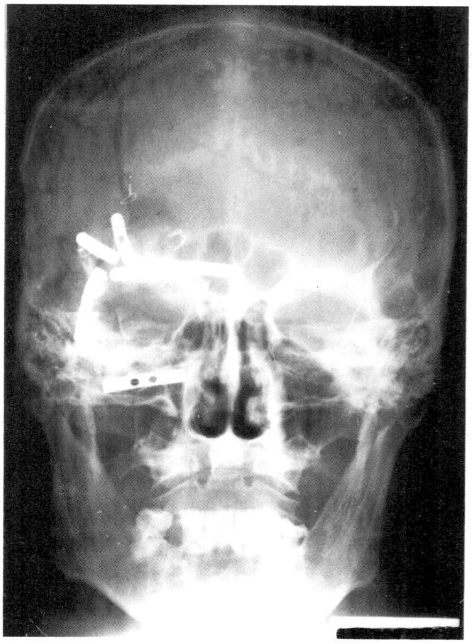

Fig. 5

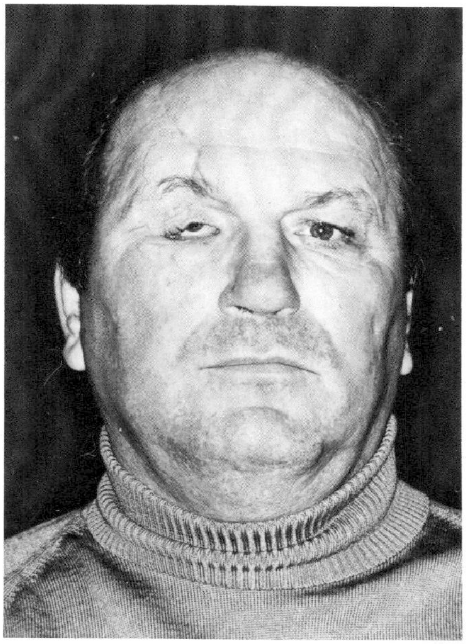

Fig. 6

Fig. 5: Solid osteo-synthesis by AO-mini-plates

Fig. 6: Condition after osseous healing of the extensive trauma

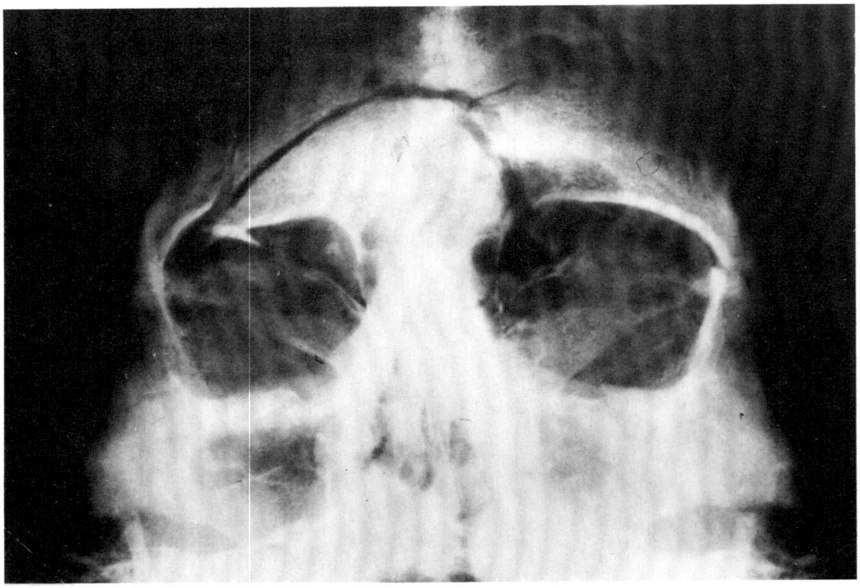

Fig. 7: Severe fracture of the frontal bone and mid-face

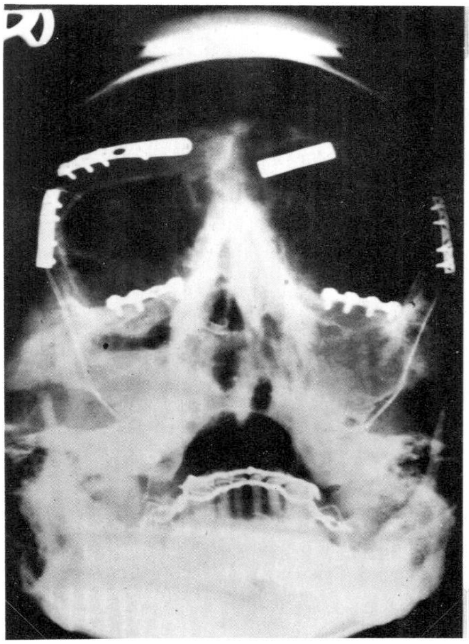

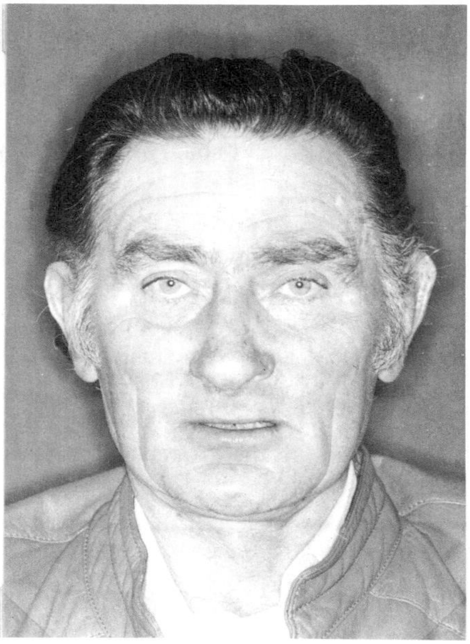

Fig. 8: Rearrangement and fixation by six-fold osteo-synthesis with the aid of mini-plates
Fig. 9: Sound healing of the bone without defects and without loss of bony substance within two months

Summarizing

It should be emphasized that the aim of an instant or early operation of cranio-facial lesions should be made the rule. As an absolute precondition a CGS (Glasgow Coma Score) of at least 12 is regarded, if possibly other concomitant injuries also permit this indication. As to the early secondary therapy, a period of three days is indicated as a maximum. Trauma of the bulbi oculi should be excluded in any case.

For the osteo-synthesis various system of mini-plates with or without compression are a matter of choice for the therapy. Essential with this procedure is to create a long-lasting opening (channel) in all the pneumatized sinus cavities leading to the nasopharyngeal space to prevent purulent infections within these closed-in areas.

The surgical strategy is based on three important factors:

1.) It is easier to carry out osteo-synthesis in the early primary or secondary phase than this is at a time when the fragments have become consolidated in displaced positions.
2.) There is only a minimal risk of infection or sequestration, so that all (even the minute) bony fragments can be re-implanted, even if they are no longer periosteally connected.

3.) The functional and aesthetic late results were far better after an early surgical intervention than in the case of the delayed reconstruction. It is very difficult and takes a long time to reconstruct either a dis-face or large areas of caved-in defects in the region of the frontal bone whereas the early attention produces good results.

Clinical and otolaryngological considerations of skull base injuries with special regard to bone plate fixation

F. X. Brunner

Abstract

Using all modern possibilities of surgical treatment of skull base fractures good results can be achieved. These results depend on the degree of primarily existing destructions of bone and soft tissue. bone and the midface. Very essential for a satisfactory medical treatment is a good cooperation between all specialists: The neuro-surgeon, the ophthalmosurgeon, the maxillofacial surgeon and otolaryngologist.

Introduction

Skull base fractures are often associated with multiple fractures of the nose, the anterior and posterior wall of the frontal sinus, the ethmoid bone and the midface.

Frontobasal fractures have to be considered as indirect open wounds, even in cases of no soft lesions of the face. 50 % of all midface fractures are combined with a rhinobasal fracture. Mucous membrane lacerations are always present. Therefore a risk of ascending infection to the endocranium is possible especially in cases of an existing dural injury. The extent of bone fractures and other traumatic complications are shown by computed tomography (Fig. 1). The evidence of liquor in the nasal secretion is easier since the possibility of biochemical identification of the liquor specified betatransferrin.

The conception of our surgical treatment worked out by BOENNINGHAUS [1] and KLEY [6] in 1967 to 1968 on principle is:

1. Closure of open fractures and indirectly open fractures is necessary, that means especially closure of the dura gaps and fractures of the frontal skull base in order to avoid endocranial complications.
2. Handling of soft-tissue lesions and facial bone fractures should take into account all aesthetical and functional aspects during primary treatment.

Operative techniques

Preexisting soft tissue wounds have to be considered in the surgical approach to the skull base. In cases of extended bone fractures without soft tissue wounds the coronal incision, opposite to the conventional eye brow incision, ensures a good survey [8]. From the coronal incision, the upper midface, the anterior and posterior wall of the frontal sinus, the orbital roof and the ethmoid cells can be reached and reconstructed easily without evident scars arising in the face. The orbital floor and the bony infraorbital region can be exposed from a subciliary incision.

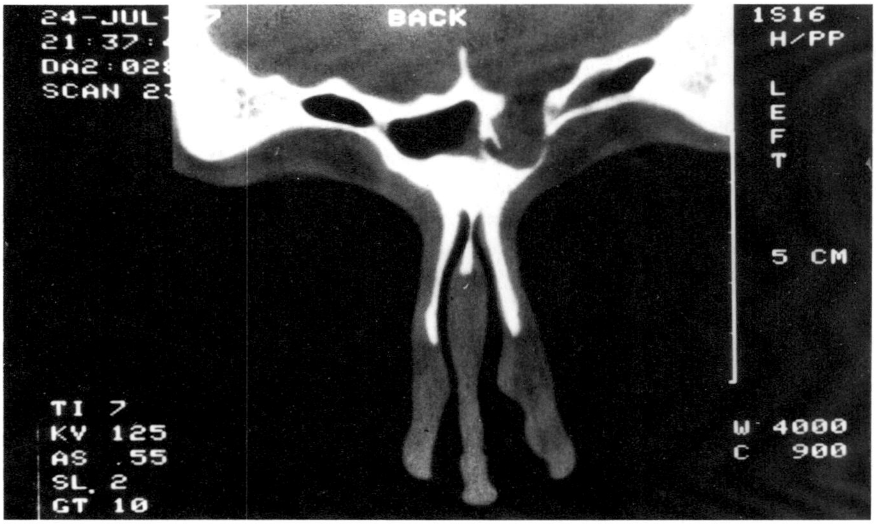

Fig. 1: Computed tomography, coronal view; with coronal sections fractures of the frontal skull base can be seen at best; in this case a fracture of the left posterior wall of the frontal sinus is illustrated

Frontal skull base defects can be, depending on their extent, covered with autologous fascia lata, with muscle periosteum of the frontal muscle, with fascia from the temporal muscle, with ceramic plates, with lyodura or with frontal or temporal muscle flaps. In the past the surgical approach to frontal skull base fractures has often been performed in an osteoclastic procedure. Frontal bone defects resulting for these patients were often unsatisfactory. Only in few cases a correction was possible with considerable effort. Even with wiring good results could not be achieved in all cases. With wiring bone fragments can be readapted, but a stable three-dimensional fixation, however, can not be achieved.

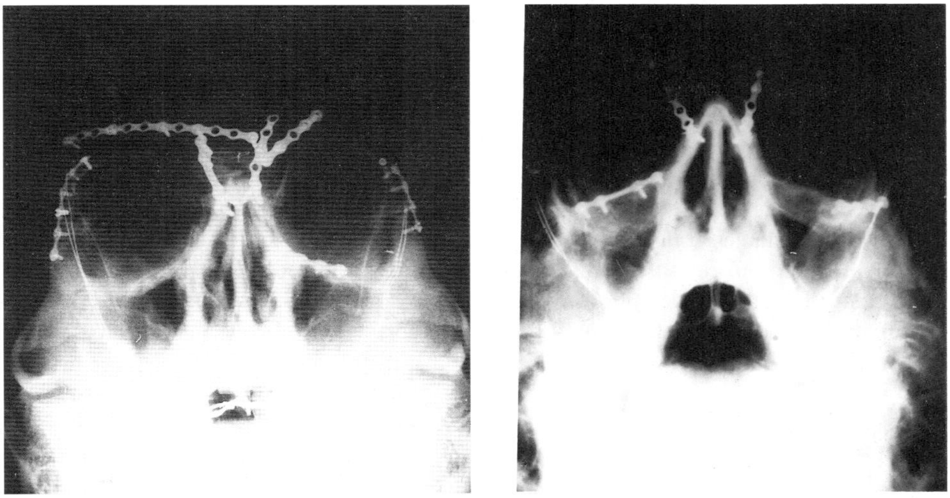

a) b)

Fig. 2a,b: Modified Water's x-ray views showing bone plate osteosynthesis to repair multiple glabellar fractures, fractures of the anterior wall of the frontal sinus, the supraorbital rim and Le Fort III fractures. a) Multiple fractures of the anterior wall of the frontal sinus, the supraorbital rim and Le Fort III fractures. The anterior wall of the frontal sinus has been reconstructed and fixed to the adjacent frontal bone; boneplate osteosynthesis involves the osseous base of the nose, the whole supraorbital rim of one side and the lateral midface, while the maxilla is suspended with wires

b) Fractures of the nose, the anterior wall of the frontal sinus, Le Fort II and III fractures. The nasal bone fragments and the fragments of the anterior wall of the frontal sinus were fixed to the calvarium. The infraorbital fragments can be fixed to the reconstructed osseous block of the nose without the risk of producing a saddle deformity of the nose by wire suspension of the maxilla

In 1980 the miniplate osteosynthesis developed by CHAMPY [4, 5] and MICHELET [7] has been introduced in the ENT-Department of the University of Würzburg in order to reconstruct the osseous base of the nose [2, 3, 9, 10]. Due to the stability, achieved with this osteosynthesis, normally an uncomplicated bony consolidation can be reached. Additionally, the basis for good healing of the soft-tissues is created in reconstructing the original bony contours. At first the rhinosurgical intervention with debris-clearing and sealing of the frontal skull base is performed. After this the reconstruction of the osseous base of the nose follows (Fig. 2). After restoration of the bony fronto-nasal-pillar by stable miniplate osteosynthesis, it is possible to reconstruct the lateral midface as well as perform a wire suspension of the maxilla within one operation without the risk of redislocations. The osteoplastic treatment of fractures of the medial midface pillar of the frontal skull base by miniplate osteosynthesis allows a stable medial fixation of the maxilla to the frontal bone. Thereby a bony saddle and bride nose can be avoided (Fig. 3). To avoid postoperative complications by inflammation and development of mucoceles it is very important to create a wide approach to the frontal sinus as well as to the nose [2]. An uncomplicated healing of this newly formed nasofrontal canal can be supported by the insertion of packings.

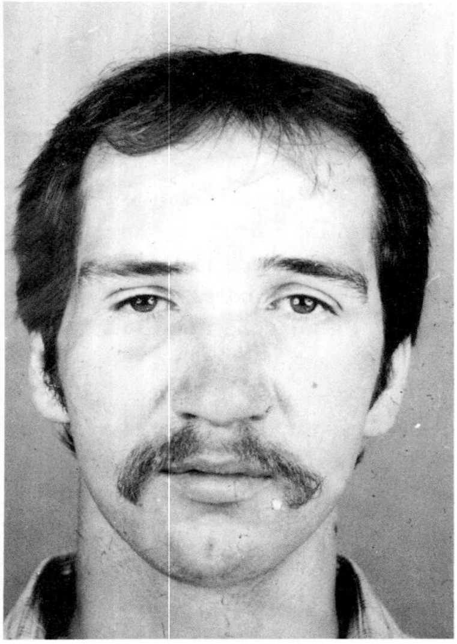

Fig. 3: Frontal appearance of a patient with former fracture of the anterior wall of the frontal sinus, Le Fort II and III fractures and fracture of the roof of the sphenoid sinus 6 weeks after the removal of the bone plates (x-ray view of the former bone plate osteosynthesis is shown in fig. 2b). The surgical approach was performed by bilateral brow incisions

Results

From 1980 to 1986 more than 100 patients with fractures of the central and lateral midface and of the frontal skull base underwent surgical treatment at the ENT-Department of the University of Würzburg using miniplate osteosynthesis. Compared with previous techniques, the results are much better when taking all aesthetical and functional aspects into account. 6 to 9 months after primary treatment, plates and screws in the neighbourhood of the upper paranasal sinuses are removed. In two cases complications could be observed, which caused a loosening of the screws and an inflammation-induced bone resorption [2]. Even in performing the osteosynthesis perfectly, it cannot be avoided that the screws contact the mucosa of the upper paranasal sinuses. Inflammation of the mucous membrane therefore causes a penetration into the bone. Periodical postoperative controls of the patients are important, first once a week and then monthly. The endoscopy of the nose and the paranasal sinuses and x-ray controls are important aids to localise defects and to avoid complications.

References

[1] Boenninghaus HG: Rhinologische Eingriffe bei der Versorgung frontobasaler Frakturen. Z Laryng Rhinol 46 (1967) 110 - 115

[2] Brunner FX, Kleine BI: Frakturen des zentralen Mittelgesichts und der Rhinobasis - operative Versorgung - postoperative Nachsorge - Komplikationsmöglichkeiten. HNO 35 (1987) 106 - 111

[3] Brunner FX, Kley W, Plinkert P: Anatomical studies and a correlative management of facial skeleton and skull base injuries with bone plate fixation. ArchORL 113 (1988) 97 - 104

[4] Champy M, Lodde JP, Muster D, Wilk A, Castelo L: Les ostéosynthèses par plaques visée miniaturesées en chirurgie faciale et cranienne. Ann chir plast 22 (1977) 261 - 264

[5] Champy M, Lodde JP, Wilk A, Grasset D: Plattenosteosynthesen bei Mittelgesichtsfrakturen und -osteotomien. Dtsch Z Mund-Kiefer-Gesichtschir 2 (1978) 26 - 29

[6] Kley W: Die Unfallchirurgie der Schädelbasis und der pneumatischen Räume. Arch HNO-Heilkd. 191 (1968) 1 - 216

[7] Michelet FX, Deymes J, Dessus B: Osteosynthesis with miniaturized screwed plates in maxillo-facial surgery. J maxillo fac surg 1 (1973) 79

[8] Richter W: Zugangswege bei Osteosynthesen des Mittel- und Obergesichtes mit extrakranieller Frontobasisrevision. Laryngol rhinol Otol 66 (1983) 260 - 265

[9] Richter W, Georgi W, Brunner FX: Die periorbitale, knöcherne Rekonstrucktion (Miniplattenosteosynthese nach Champy). HNO 30 (1983) 186 - 188

[10] Richter W, Georgi W, Brunner FX: Das Trauma des interorbitalen Raumes. Therapie. HNO 31 (1983) 303 - 310

Restoration of eye motility in orbital floor fractures

J. Esser, Ch. Mohr, D. Schettler, H. Hunz

Abstract

58 patients with orbital floor fractures were surgically treated and investigated before and 3 days, 7 days, 1 month and 6 months after surgery with regard to their eye motility (Hess-Lees screen, monocular excursion), their double vision (Harms tangent screen) and their enophthalmos (Hertel exophthalmometry). 62,5 % of the cases had no more double vision 6 months after surgery. Among these the patients in whom early surgery (within 15 days after trauma) was performed showed better results. A surgery as early as possible is thus recommended. Older patients showed significantly better results than younger patients. The measurements of bulbar excursions according the Kestenbaum principles which are technically simple to apply achieve valid results as well as haploscopic methods.

Introduction

One of the aims of therapy with orbital floor fractures is the restoration of eye motility in order to preserve binocular vision in all directions of gaze. The subject of discussion is whether and at what time a surgical orbital floor reconstruction should be performed. An immediate surgery should be declined for two main reasons: On the one hand CRIKELAIR et al. [2], PUTTERMAN et al. [18] as well as DULLEY and FELLS [3] report of a very high amount of spontaneously improved cases. Therefore it seems to be justified to wait for 10 - 14 days and in cases which changed for the better there is no more need for a surgery [4, 12]. KOMMERELL [13] explains this spontaneous improvement by means of stretching of the incarcerated orbital connective tissue [14] by normal use of the eye. On the other hand postoperative complications are described like for example sight loss due to an occlusion of the central retinal artery [1, 4, 8, 17]. These complications occur when hard implants for orbital floor plastic were used (such as bones or teflon), not when Lyodura was used [7]. Supporters of an operative therapy [1, 6, 8, 9, 11, 15, 16, 19, 20, 21] regard only an early surgery (up to 14 days after trauma) as a possibility to succeed in motility restoration, since later on scars or a Volkmann contraction of the inferior rectus muscle prevent the regaining of the motility [22].

The object of the present study is to follow the course of motility disorders of orbital floor fractures post-therapeutically in short terms and long terms by means of different complementary methods of examination and to put it in correlation to the moment of surgery, to the initial findings and to intraoperative conditions.

Patients and methods

With 58 with intraoperatively confirmed orbital floor fractures (35 zygoma and orbital floor fractures, 17 isolated orbital floor fractures, 6 mid-face fractures of the type Le Fort II/III), which were surgically treated 1986 in the Essen University Hospital, Department of Maxillo-Facial Surgery, the following examinations were carried out before surgery and also 3 days, 7 days, 1 month and 6 months after surgery:

(1) Exophthalmometry (Hertel)
(2) Haploscopic eye motility analysis (Hess-Less screen): The difference between the affected and healthy were analysed in 30 degrees elevation of gaze while in 15 degrees abduction.
(3) Determination of monocular excursion with help of Kestenbaum glasses [10]: The full extent of vertical excursion of the affected eye was analysed in comparison to the extent of excursion of the other eye.
(4) Determination of the area of binocular single vision at the Harms tangent screen: Analysed were the limits of the double vision free area in all directions of gaze.

Results

With all 58 patients a transcutaneous orbital floor reconstruction was performed, with 31/58 patients intraoperatively visible incarcerations in the fracture slit were released. In 56/58 cases an orbital floor plastic with lyodura implant was performed, in 3/58 cases an Anthony-Fisher balloon was implanted. 35/58 patients were surgically treated within the first two weeks after trauma (early surgery), 23/58 were surgically treated at a later time, whereby 5 cases were operated between the 8th and the 18the week after trauma.

Fig. 1 illustrates that postoperatively the enopthalmos decreases as well as the exophthalmos which is caused by tissue swelling and no difference between early and late surgery has been noted. Before surgery 35/58 patients had motility disorders (29 of them underfunctions) in the radius of action of the superior rectus muscle (Fig. 2). The number of patients without motility disorders increased from 29,6 % (on the 3rd day after surgery) to 57,1 % (6 months after surgery).

Some of the 25/58 patients, where no motility disorders could be found before surgery, had short-termed lasting motility differences soon after surgery (Fig. 3). On the 3rd postoperative day there were only 57,1 % without motility disorders but after 6 months however 91,7 % of the patients were without motility disorders, the rest had only minimum disorders.

The importance of the point of time of the surgery is illustrated by the fact that among all patients with preoperative motility disorders 70,6 % of those patients who had an early surgery were without motility disorders while only 45,5 % of those who had a late surgery were without motility disorders after more than one month (Fig. 4).

22/58 patients had preoperative double vision, mostly by elevation of gaze but also when looking aside and down (Fig. 5). 7 patients had double vision even in primary position so that they were forced to stay in an abnormal head positure or to wear an occlusion respectively. Shortly after surgery there is only little change for the better, but one month after surgery 30 % of the patients had no double vision and 6 months after surgery 62 % remained without double vision (Fig. 6).

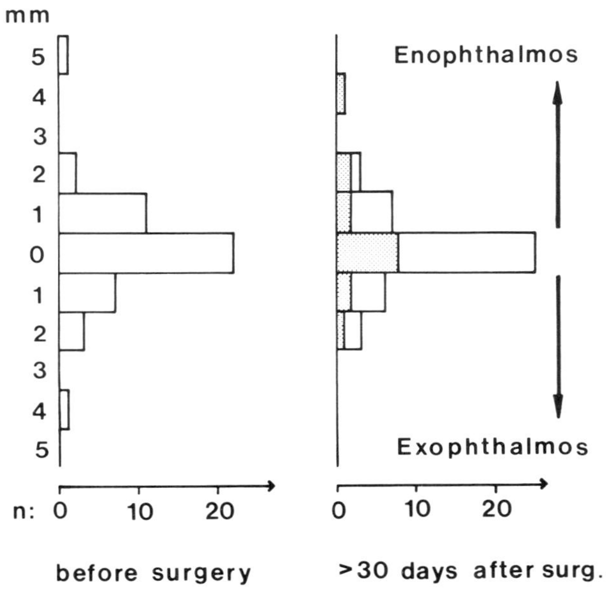

Fig. 1: Exophthalmometry after Hertel before (left) and more than 30 days after orbital floor reconstruction (right). Postoperatively there is a similar distribution of the results regarding early surgery (light) as well as late surgery (grey)

Among 36/58 patients preoperatively without double vision some suffered from a temporary double vision only shortly after surgery (Fig. 7).

The comparison of pre- and postoperative values of the Hess-Less screen as well as of the area of double vision with the results of the Kestenbaum glasses reveals that the pattern of distribution of the disorders is alike (Figs. 8 and 9).

The postoperative results do not depend on incarcerations of tissue which had been found intraoperatively (Fig. 10).

Younger patients seem to have a worse prognosis regarding the postoperative success than older ones (chi square = 6,08, $p < 0,05$, Fig. 11).

Discussion

A normalization of motility in 57,1 % of the cases and no double vision in 62,5 % of the cases which had preoperative motility disorders, by means of an orbital floor reconstruction with a lyodura plastic can be found in a similar extent in other studies. Relief from double vision is reported by GILLISSEN and OEI [8] in 311/47 cases (66 %), by FREITAG et al. [6] in 19/28 cases (68 %), by LOEWEN et al. [16] in 50/95 cases (53 %), and by HARTMANN et al. [11] in 25/37 cases (68 %).

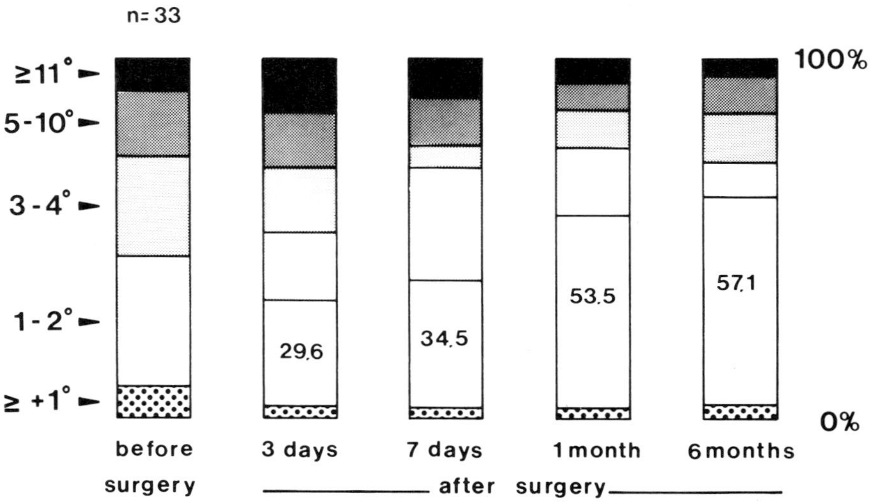

Fig. 2: Postoperative motility disorders (right columns), measured by the Hess-Lees screen with 33/58 patients, who had preoperative motility disorders (left columns, difference to the unaffected eye with 30 degrees elevation of gaze in 15 degrees abduction)

The better results of an early surgery (within the first two weeks) rather confirm the results of LOEWEN et al. [16] than those of HARTMANN et al. [11]. LOEWEN et al. [16] found a relief of double vision in 45/59 cases (69,5 %) with early surgery and 9/36 (25 %) with late surgery whereas HARTMANN et al. [11] found a relief of double vision in 15/21 cases (71 %) with early surgery and 10/16 (62,5 %) with late surgery.

In those cases in which there were no preoperative motility disorders respectively double vision, passing-bye disorders occurred because of postoperative tissue swelling, but disappeared completely in case of double vision. In 8,3 % of the cases the persisting motility disorders (Fig. 3) were only small and could be compensated by the fusion reflex. The fusion reflex explains also the better results of the double vision test in comparison to the motility test, since with haploscopic methods the possibility of fusing is disturbed. On the one hand haploscopic methods make it possible to perform a more precise objective analysis of the eye motility, on the other hand the sensation of no having double vision is the more important criterion for the patient.

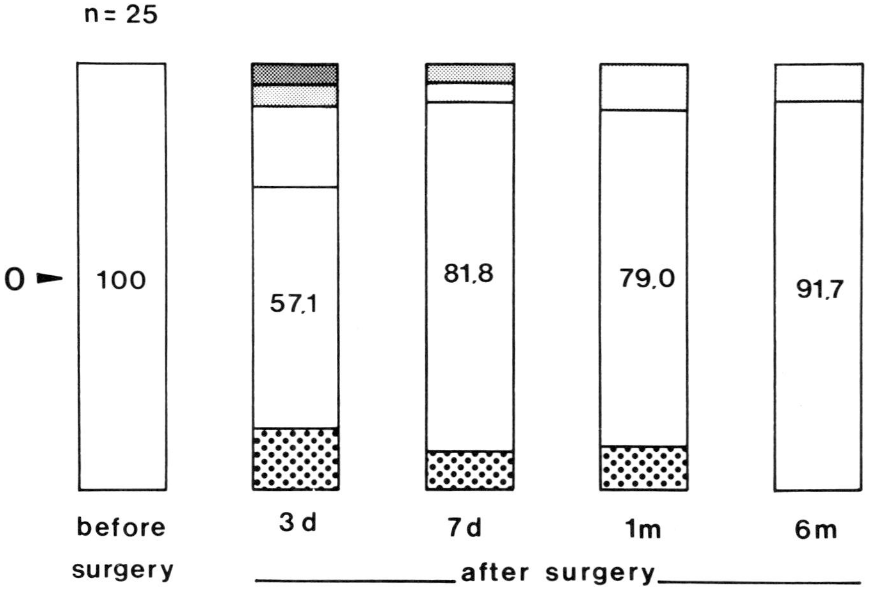

Fig. 3: Postoperative motility disorders (right columns), measured by the Hess-Lees screen with 25/58 patients who had no preoperative motility disorders. Same gradings as Fig. 2

With disorders primary on both sides a monocular measuring of motility is necessary since haploscopic methods like the Hess-Less screen base on the comparison of an affected with an nonaffected eye. A simple method are the Kestenbaum glasses, which can even be used when the patient is in a lying position. This method gives as precise results as other methods to measure the monocular excursion [5] and can be confirmed by a similar distribution pattern against the different methods and their results (Fig. 8 and 9). Intraoperatively seen tissue incarcerations seem to have no essential influence on the prognosis of the final result. This could be due to the fact that in all cases the intraoperative release of incarcerated tissue was as extensive as possible.

No definite reason can be found for the fact that the prognosis improves with the advance in years. Possibly young patients get more postoperative scars which influence the final results. Finally it should be stated that orbital floor fractures with double vision should have very early surgery, but also a later surgery may be successful. The question of a long-term success or the indication for a renewed surgery respectively cannot be answered before at least 30 days after orbital floor reconstruction. If orbital floor fractures with double vision have been proved by radiology and clinical methods they should have an early surgery as well. This should be done to avoid later onset of double vision and to release the infraorbital nerve which is incarcerated in most cases too. Furthermore the postoperatively occurring double vision is only a passing bye phenomenon.

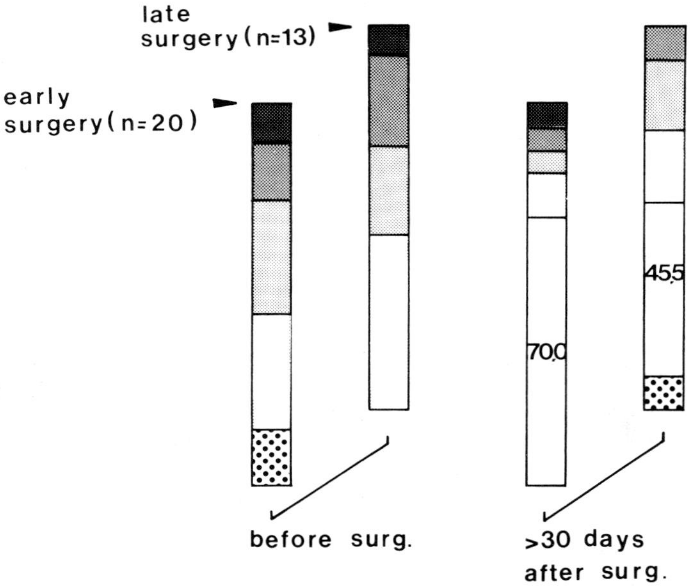

Fig. 4: Distribution of motility disorders, measured by the Hess-Less screen, preoperative (left columns) and at least one month postoperative (right columns), concerning the patients from Fig. 2 with an early surgery (1 - 14 days after trauma, front columns) and with late surgery (back columns). Same grading as in Fig. 2

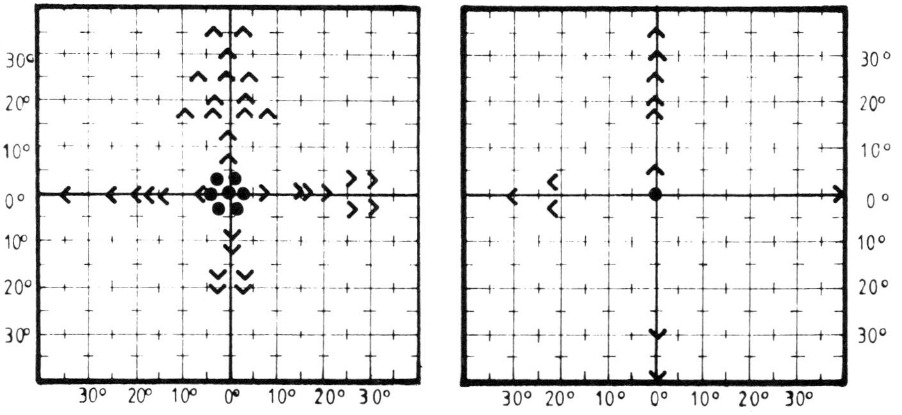

Fig. 5: Synopsis of the field of binocular single vision of all patients with double vision before (left) and 6 months after surgery (right). The pointers mark the limits where people start having double vision and the dots symbolize double vision already in primary position

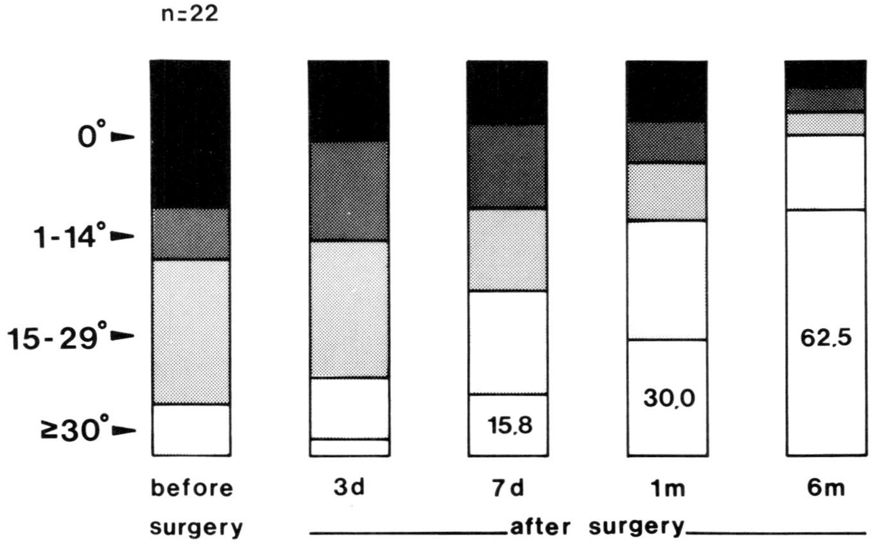

Fig. 6: Postoperative field of binocular single vision (right columns) with 22/58 patients who had preoperative double vision (left column, minimum limits of the field of binocular single vision in all directions of gaze)

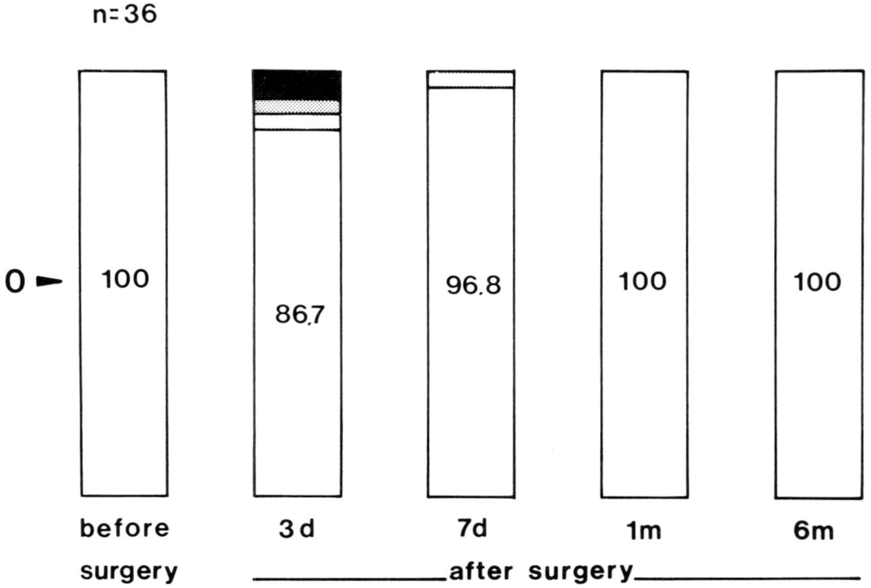

Fig. 7: Postoperative field of binocular single vision (right columns) with 36/58 patients who had no preoperative double vision (left column). Same grading as in Fig. 6

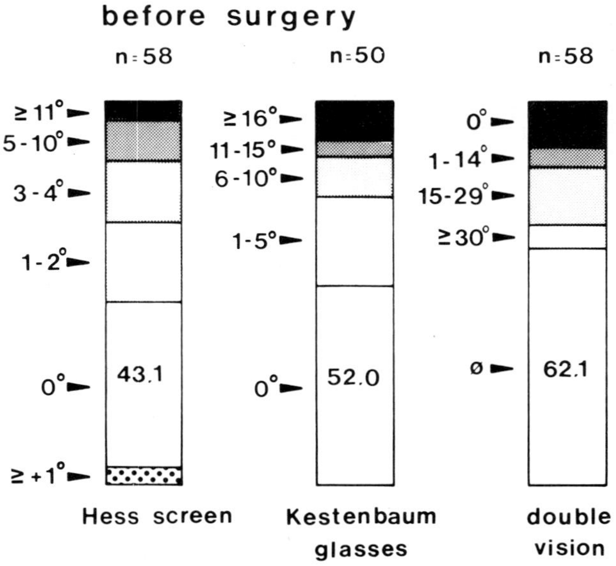

Fig. 8: Comparison of values which were found preoperatively with three different methods of eye motility examinations in all patients. the values of the Hess-Less screen method (left column, compare Figs. 2 and 3) and of measuring the field of binocular single vision (right column, compare Figs. 6 and 7) show comparable results to the Kestenbaum glasses method (medium column)

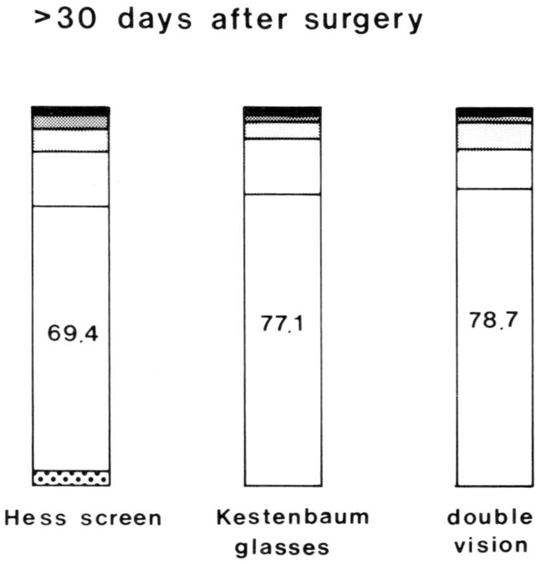

Fig. 9: Comparison of the values found at least 30 days after surgery. Arrangement as in Fig. 8

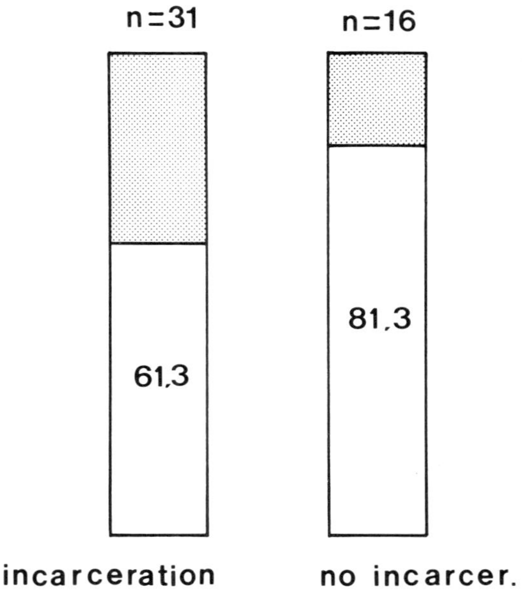

Fig. 10: Postoperative motility disorders (measured by the Hess-Less screen) of patients with (left column) and without (right column) introperatively perceptible incarceration of tissue. The white area respectively shows the patients without motility disorders in percentage (at least 30 days after surgery)

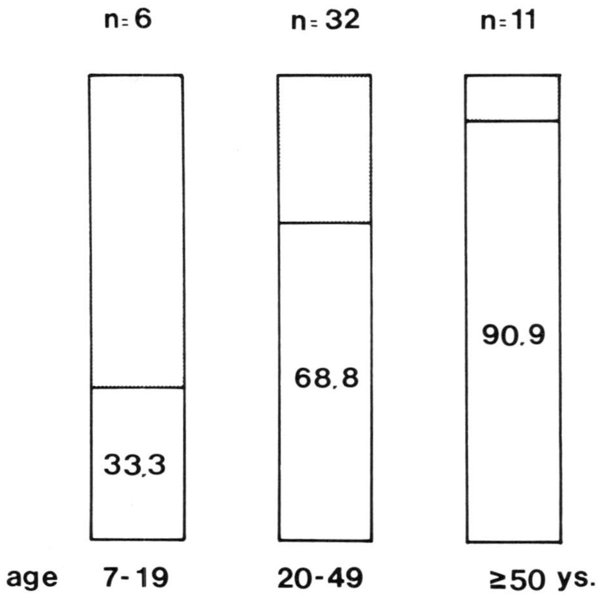

Fig. 11: Postoperative motility disorders (measured by the Hess-Less screen) according to the age of the patients when having the surgery. The white area respectively shows the patients without motility disorders in percentage (at least 30 days after surgery)

References

[1] Bleeker GM, Peeters HJF, Gillissen JPA, Oei TH, Verkerk HH: Über den Verlauf und Spätergebnisse von behandelten und unbehandelten Orbitafrakturen. Klin Mbl Augenheilk 165 (1974) 849 - 858

[2] Cricelair GF, Rein JM, Potter GD, Cosman : A critical look at the blow-out fracture. Plast Reconstr Surg 49 (1972) 347 - 379

[3] Dulley B, Fells P: Long-term follow-up of orbital blow-out fractures with and without surgery. Mod Probl Ophthal 14 (1975) 467 - 470

[4] Emery JM, Noorden von GK, Schlernitzauer DA: Orbital floor fracturs: Long term follow-up of cases with and without surgical repair. Trans Am Acad Ophthalmol Otolaryngol 75 (1971) 802 - 812

[5] Esser J, Melzer I: Comparison of monocular excursion measurements in normals and in patients with motility disorders. In: Campos (ed): International Strabismological Assiciation, Proceedings of the Fifth Meeting. Athena, Modena 1986

[6] Freitag V, Flick H, Reichenbach W: Augenmotilität nach Mittelgesichtsfrakturen mit Orbitabeteiligung (Orbitabodenrevisionen bei Mittelgesichtsfrakturen). In: Schuchardt K, Becker R (eds.): Fortschritte der Kiefer- und Gesichts-Chirurgie Band XXII. Thieme, Stuttgart 1978

[7] Fiedburg D: Blow-out Frakturen - Diagnose und Indikation zur Behandlung aus augenärztlicher Sicht. Ber Dtsch Ophthalmol Ges 78 (1981) 797 - 803

[8] Gillissen JPA, Oei TH: Follow-up of orbital fractures treated surgically. Mod Prob Ophthal 14 (1975) 471 - 473

[9] Hakelius L, Ponten B: Results of immediate and delayed surgical treatent of facial fractures with diplopia. J max-fac Surg 1 (1973) 150 - 154

[10] Haase W: Messung der maximalen Bewegungsstrecken der Bulbi. Albrecht von Graefes Arch klin exp Ophthalmol 198 (1976) 291 - 296

[11] Hartmann N, Haase W, Metz H-J: Disturbances of ocular motility and position after therapy of blow-out fractures: Late results in cases treated in the years 1968 to 1980. In: Hjorting-Hansen E (ed): Oral and maxillofacial surgery. Quintessence, Chikago-Berlin-London-Rio de Janeiro-Tokyo 1985

[12] Helveston EM: The relationship of extraocular muscle problems to orbital floor fractures: Early and late management. Trans Am Acad Opthalmol 93 (1977) 660 - 662

[13] Kommerell G: Diskussionsbemerkung. Ber Dtsch Opthalmol Ges 78 (1981) 803

[14] Koorneef L: Spatial aspects of orbital musculo-fibrous tissue in man. Swets & Zeitlinger BV, Amsterdam-Lisse 1977

[15] Lentrodt J: Zur Diagnostik und Therapei der Orbitabodenfrakturen. Dtsch Zahn-Mund-Kieferheilkd 60 (1973) 232 - 245

[16] Loewen U, Friedburg D, Westphal D: Die Bulbusmotilität bei Früh- und Spätversorgungen von Orbitabodenfrakturen. Klin Mbl Augenheilk 175 (1979) 474 - 482

[17] Nicholson MD, Guzak SV: Visual loss complicating repair of orbital floor fractures. Arch Opthalmol 86 (1971) 369 - 375

[18] Putterman AM, Stevens T, Urist MJ: Nonsurgical management of blow-out fractures in the orbital floor. Am J Ophthalmol 77 (1974) 232 - 239

[19] Rüssmann W, Friedmann G, Glanski M, Pape H-D, Riewenherm U: Okuläre Motilitätsstörungen bei Mittelgesichtsfrakturen. In: Schuchardt K, Becker R (eds): Fortschritte der Kiefer- und Gesichts-Chirurgie Band XXII Thieme, Stuttgart 1978

[20] Rüssmann W, Konen W: Operative Behandlung posttraumatischer Paresen. Orthoptik-Pleoptik 11 (1984) 59 - 67

[21] Schlöndorff G, Kaufman H: Diagnostik und Therapie der Orbitabodenfrakturen. Klin Mbl Augenheilk 162 (1973) 760 - 766

[22] Smith B: Blow-out fracture. Contribution during III. Int. symposion on periorbital surgery, New York 1980

Classification and therapy of orbital floor fractures

Ch. Milewski

Introduction

Orbital floor fractures may have poor symptoms in the beginning, but can produce severe problems later on. Since the first papers about blow out fractures (1, 6) different therapy concepts and surgical methods were recommended. Today the orbital floor fractures are integrated in the term of lateral mid-face fractures (4, 5). In the following the principles of treatment and results of surgical methods used in the ENT-Clinic of the University of Mainz are presented.

Material and Methods

Between 1978 and 1985, 265 patients with orbital floor fractures were surgically treated in the ENT-Clinic of the University of Mainz. These cases are comprised exclusively of mid-face trauma without fractures of the Le Fort Type. Diagnosis was performed clinically, radiologically and by ultrasound. An impact in anamneses and monocel or lower eye-lid haematoma and traces of blood in the nose as a possible sign of haematosinus imply a fracture of the orbital floor. By palpation discontinuities of the orbital rim are detected. Double visions and numbness or pain in the area of infra-orbital nerve are looked for. If the clinical examination leads to suspicion of an orbital floor fracture, a x-ray tomogram of the mid-face is andatory. The ultrasound diagnosis was performed by 10 mHz head to judge the discontinuities in the orbital floor. Double vision, numbness or radiological signs of fracture demand for surgical treatment.

In case of discrepancies of uncertainties in diagnosis, a preoperative endoscopic evaluation of the maxillary sinus and the orbital floor was performed. In every case an infra-orbital incision was used to optimize the surgical access to the entire orbital floor. Unaestethic eyelid swelling and scar tissue formation postoperatively was minimized by the use of a intracutaneous suturing technique. In the case of more intensive fractures, including those of the lateral mid-face, a second surgical approach through the front wall of the maxillary sinus via the vestibulum of the mouth was carried out. After the orbital hernia was properly relocated and the infra-orbital nerve fred (if required), lyophilised dura was positioned between periostium and the relocated orbital bone. Fibrin glue provided for fixation. If necessary auto- and homographs were used for reconstruction of defects of the orbital floor. When required a catheter, mainly Foley-type, was inserted into the maxillary sinus to support the reconstructed orbital floor.

Results

In 112 (42 %) cases there was only a blow out fracture with mainly a depressed medial part of the orbital floor (62), this occurred only seldom in the lateral section (6). In 44 cases there was a multiple fracture of the orbital floor.

In 153 patients (58 %), the blow out fracture was combined with a lateral mid-face fracture. 83 patients had a fracture of the rim of the bony orbit either. This was combined with a fracture of the frontal maxillary wall in 38 cases and 32 times with an additional fracture of the cheek bone.

The cause of trauma differed according to the type of fracture. In pure blow out fractures (110) the primary cause was fistfighting (39) followed by traffic accident (29) and sport and work related accidents (27). For the combined fractures (153) the primary causes were traffic accidents (42) and accidental fall (42) mainly in aged patients followed by sports and work related accidents (39).

The reconstruction of the orbital floor by lyophilisized dura was done in 186 (70 %) of our patients. Auto- and homografts of cartilage (or portions of the front wall of the maxillary sinus) were used in 30 cases of multiple fractures of the orbital floor. In 13 cases ceramics or PDS-implants were used. In 32 patients no material was needed for reconstruction. In 96 cases (36,5 %) an osteosynthesis of the orbital rim or cheek bone was requird. 88 times this was performed using wires and 8 times using miniplates. In 50 % of the patients a catheter was inserted into the maxillary sinus to support the reconstructed orbital floor.

Preoperatively 93 patients complained of numbness in the area of the infraorbital nerve. Postoperatively only 34 % of the patients showed these symptoms. In 2 patients the numbness was caused the operation itself.

Preoperatively 150 patients had double vision which was confirmed by ophthalmological examinations.

Immediately after surgical treatment 40 patients had double vision, 6 months postoperatively the number decreased to 20 patients. 9 of these 20 had only minimal double vision on extreme eye movement. The remaining 11 patients developed double vision and suffered enophthalmic problems as well. They all had had severe lateral mid-face traumata and postoperative sinking of the reconstructed orbital floor in spite of being supported by a catheter.

Discussion

A balloon catheter, in comparison with other methods like silicon-T-implants, fingerlings or ointment tamponade, has the advantage of ease of insertion and removal as well as being easy to correct intra- and postoperatively [2, 3, 7]. Besides the cosmetic disadvantage for the patients, we found the main problem with the Foley catheters to be the shape of the balloon itself. When filled, a latex balloon exhibits a round shape. Yet the sinus cavity has a completely different shape - that of an inverted pyramid [8]. When filled, the balloon reaches the orbital floor quickly, but only with a small area of contact in the middle of the orbital floor.

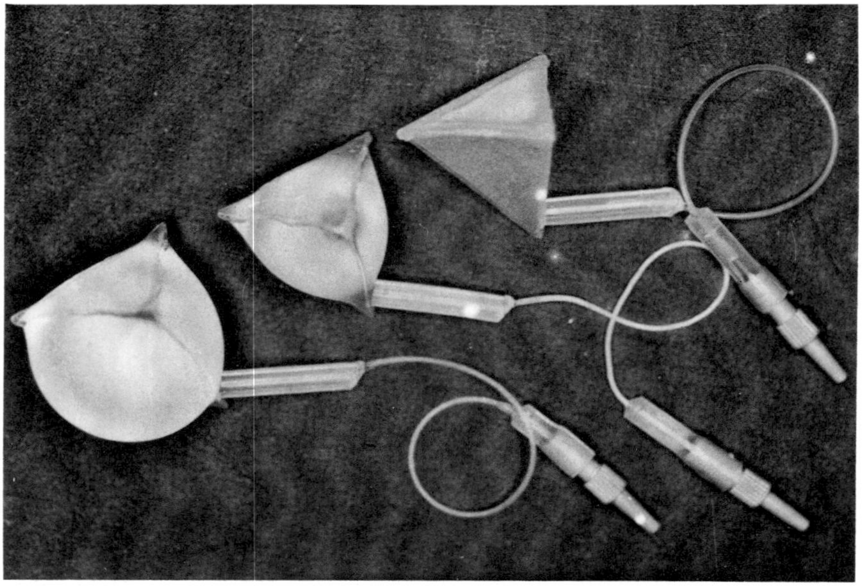

Fig. 1

In order to achieve a proper support of the peripheral areas of the orbital floor, the balloon must be inflated further, resulting in a dislocation of the middle area of the orbital floor. An exact repositioning of the entire orbital floor is thus quite difficult. And since the bulbus oculi is displaced more than the orbital fat tissue, the patient's double vision is actually increased. To cope with that problem, since 1987 we use a special low pressure silicon balloon catheter (fig. 1) (manufactured and distributed by XOMED Int.).

This balloon already has the form of an inverted pyramid, and is so constructed that even with a maximum filling volume, the superior portion of the balloon remains parallel. Yet the sides of the catheter balloon are thinner permitting an optimal fit of the antral cavity and its anatomical variations, when filled. A mixture of 1 : 10 Urografin^{R} and water used for filling the balloon, provides x-ray visibility.

1987, the catheter was used in 15 cases. In all cases the repositioning of the orbital floor was satisfactory and an endoscopic control showed healthy mucosa. No patient exhibited double vision postoperatively.

Conclusion

By adhering to the following principles a good result can be achieved in treating extended orbital floor fractures:

1. surgical treatment within the first week
2. infraorbital incision
3. examination of the entire orbital floor,
4. proper implant material
5. wire osteosynthesis
6. balloon catheter support
7. intracutaneous suturing without subcutaneous sutures,
8. preventing of edema of the eye-lid

In spite of the short frame, the special antral balloon catheter has proven to be a valuable tool in treatment of orbital fractures.

References

[1] Converse JM, Smith B: Reconstruction of the floor of the orbit by bone grafts. Arch. Ophthalmol. 44 (1950) 1 - 5

[2] Holzner K, Kränke CH, Madras H: Retension des frakturierten und reponierten Orbitabodens mit neu konzipiertem Kieferhöhlenballon. Aus: Erkrankungen der Kieferhöhle, Symposium Pfuschl, Herausg. Watzek & Mateika, Springer Verlag, 1985

[3] Masing H, Mauch P: Die Tamponade bei Trümmerbrüchen der Kieferhöhle und des Orbitabodens mit Selastic Schwamm. Vortrag auf der 51. Ver-sammlung der Vereinigten Südwestdeutschen HNO-Ärzte, Erlangen, Sept. 1969

[4] Rink B: Spätergebnisse der Behandlung lateraler Mittelgesichtsfrakturen. HNO-Praxis 11 (1986) 89 - 92

[5] Schwab W, Mang WC: Traumatologie des Mittelgesichts. HNO 34 (1986) 1 - 10

[6] Smith B, Reagan WF: Blow out fracture of the orbit: Mechanism and correction of internal orbital fracture. Am. J. Ophthalmol. 44 (1957) 733 - 737

[7] Weidauer H, Alexandridis E: Zur Dignostik und Therapie der medianen Blow-out Fraktur. Laryngologie, Rhinologie, Otologie Band 64 (1985) 567 - 570

[8] Zuckerkandl E: Normale und pathologische Anatomie der Nasenhöhle und ihre pneumatischen Anhänge. Wilhelm Braunmüller, Wien 1882

Functional results achieved by the surgical management of blow-out fractures

H. Iro, D. Horst

Summary

Sixtyfive blow-out fractures of different degrees of severity were reviewed retrospectively. Within the first 2 weeks following the injury the fractures were treated surgically via the transorbital route. The impaired sensitivity of the infraorbitalnerve, which was present in 26 patients prior to surgery, had either disappeared or substantially improved after surgery in all patients. In 49 patients (74 %) diplopia existed preoperatively. Six months after surgical management diplopia was either no longer verifiable or found to have greatly improved in 44 patients (90 %). In 5 instances, diplopia resisted treatment.

Considering the functional results obtained by non-surgical treatment of pure blow-out fracture, we feel that early exploration of the orbital floor is justified in the event of blow-out fractures.

Introduction

Fractures of the orbital floor may occur as blow-out fractures proper with intact intraorbital rim or as orbital floor fractures resulting from a complex "middle-third" fracture. As to the causal mechanism underlying an isolated blow-out fracture, two theories are put forwards: The theory of bone transmission and that of increased orbital pressure increase [1].

The incarceration of orbital tissue in the blow-out fracture and the resulting restriction of eyeball motility [2], the displacement of orbital contents into the maxillary sinus as well as enlargement of the orbit (wide orbit syndrome [3]) lead to enophthalmus and diplopia which is very distressing to the patient.

For the prevention of sequelae difficult to correct later on, orbital floor fractures should be treated early and expertly. However, the indication for surgery in the case of pure blow-out fractures is still debatable. The opinions of the authors range from "never resort to surgery" to "surgery is always a must". We advocate early surgical treatment of blow-out fractures and thus agree with SALLAND et al. (1984).

In the following a report is presented on our functional results obtained by the surgical management of pure blow-out fractures.

Material, Method and Results

Within the last 5 years a total of 65 pure blow-out fractures of different extent were surgically treated by us (Table I). Table II indicates the pre-operative diagnosis when a blow-out fracture is suspected. With suspected orbital floor fracture, the indication for surgery was established on the basis of the following prerequisites:

1) Clear evidence of the fracture and of orbital tissue displaced into the maxillary sinus (confirmed radiographically or by antroscopy of the maxillary sinus).
2) Enophthalmus
3) Diplopia when looking straight ahead or in the customary field of vision

Surgery was instituted within the first 2 weeks following injury.

Table I

Blow-out fracture n = 65	
- Fracture without displacement of orbital tissue	n = 9
- Comminuted fracture without displacement of orbital tissue	n = 2
- Comminuted fracture with displacement into the maxillary sinus	n = 48
- Comminuted fracture with bony defect and displacement of	
- orbital tissue into the maxillary sinus	n = 6

The transorbital approach via an infraorbital incision was used in all 65 cases. In 11 patients additional fenestration of the maxillary sinus in the lower meatus of the nose was required for the placement of an antral balloon. As in this case major comminuted fractures of the orbital floor were involved, additional stabilisation from the direction of the maxillary sinus appeared reasonable and necessary. The detailed intervention after visualization of the blow-out fracture and, if required, repositioning of the orbital tissue is shown in table III and IV. In 20 patients (30 %) enophthalmus was present before surgery. This was detected in only 4 patients (6 %) six months after surgery.

Table II

Pre-operative diagnosis on suspected blow-out fracture
- Clinical examination
- Radiological exploration
  - survey (large film) of paranasal sinuses
  - if necessary, conventional of computed tomography
- Antroscopy of the maxillary sinus
- Ophthalmologic examination

Impairment of sensitivity detected preoperatively in 26 patients (40 %) and involving the infra-orbital nerve, had completely subsided in 21 patients 6 months after surgery, and noticeably improved in the remaining 5. Immediately after the trauma, 38 patients (57 %) had developed diplopia. In another 11 patients (17 %) diplopia developed within 10 days of the accident. As a result, diplopia was present in 49 out of 65 (74 %) pure blow-out fractures verified radiological. Six months after surgery, diplopia was no longer found to exist in 27 cases, in 17 patients diplopia had subsided considerably and was only detectable at extreme lines of sight. In 5 patients (7 %) surgical intervention failed to allay diplopia. However, in no case was surgery found to worsen the original ophthalmological findings prior to surgery.

Compared with the pre-operative findings, early surgery managed to eliminate diplopia either completely or to mitigate it considerably in 90 % of cases.

Discussion

Important criteria for success in treating pure orbital floor fractures are both the functional (diplopia) and aesthetic (enophthalmus) disorders. Therapy-resistant enophthalmos is likely to lead to social isolation due to reactive psychic alterations. Whereas hypo-aesthesia in the area of distribution of infra-orbital nerve is generally well-tolerated by patients, persistent diplopia, especially in the main lines of vision, is felt to be very distressing. BUTTERBEAN et al. (1974) who expect a high percentage of diplopia cases to regress spontaneously, definitely suggest allowing 4 to 6 months to elapse before undertaking surgical repair. Based on this publication, however, diplopia still persisted after six months in 25 %of patients, and enophthalmus was seen in as many as 65 % of patients 6 months after injury. According to a retrospective study by EMERY et al. (1971) conservative treatment of blow-out fractures revealed long-term diplopia in 60 % of cases.

Table III

Materials used in lining the orbital floor

- Lyophilized dura	n = 42
- plus xenogenous cartilage	n = 2
- plus antral balloon	n = 10
- plus silicone foil	n = 6

Late revision of the orbital floor in cases of persistent diplopia or enophthalmus is frequently aggravated by cicatricial entrapment of the orbital tissue in the fracture gap. Therefore, late surgical intervention yields much poorer results than an early exploration of the orbital floor [6].

Table IV

Materials used in lining the orbital floor

- xenogenous cartilage only	n = 1
- antral balloon only	n = 1
- xenogenous cartilage with antral balloon	n = 1
- silicone foil only	n = 2

SALLAND et al. (1984) favour surgical treatment of blow-out fractures within the first days of injury, an approach with which they have obtained very good functional results. Two months after surgery, diplopia was only seen in 11 % of patients. Similar results are reported by GRAY and associated (1985) with a postoperative diplopia rate of 9 %. The retrospective study of our patients also revealed persistent diplopia in just on 10 % of cases. The 6 % incidence of therapy-resistant enophthalmos in our patients is also relatively low. Of course, a comparison between patients with orbital floor fractures of different severity and extent cannot be accepted without reservation. Nevertheless, in the light of our experience, we agree with the two last-named authors that proper and early exploration of the orbital floor, i.e. within the first 2 weeks of the injury, is the method of choice in the case of pure blow-out fractures. Only in this manner can difficult to correct functional after-effects and aesthetic late sequelae be prevented.

References

[1] Austermann K-H: Untersuchungen zum Entstehungsmechanismus der blow-out Frakturen. Dtsch. Z. Mund. Kiefer-Gesichts-Chir. 3 (1979) 220 - 223

[2] Bumm P, de Decker W: Erfahrung in der Traumatologie der Periorbita. Arch Otorhinolaryngol. 235 (1982) 399 - 402

[3] de Decker W, Bumm P, Haase L, Koorneef L, Mühlendyck H: Rundtischgespräch über blow-out Frakturen. Fortschr. Ophthalmol. 79 (1982) 174 - 178

[4] Emery JM, von Noorden GK: Orbital floor fractures: longterm follow-up cases with and without surgical repair. Trans. Amer. Acad. Ophthal. Otolaryng. 75 (1971) 802 - 812

[5] Gray LN, Kalimuthu B, Jayaram B, Lewis N, Sohaey M: A retrospective study of treatment of orbital floor fractures with the maxillary sinus approach. Brit. J. Plast. Surg. (1985) 113 - 115

[6] Herzau V: Über Symptome, Behandlung und Verlauf der isolierten Orbitabodenfraktur. Albrecht v. Graefes Arch. klin. exp. Ohthal. 196 (1975) 145 - 151

[7] Puttermann AM, Stevens T, Urist MJ: Nonsurgical management of blow-out fractures of the orbital floor. Am. J. Ophtal. 77 (1974) 232

[8] Salland T, Hammerstein W, Lentrodt J: Zur Indikation der primären chirurgischen Intervention bei Orbitabodenfrakturen. In: Plastische und wiederherstellende Maßnahmen bei Unfallverletzungen. Jungbluth KH, Mommsen U (Hrsg.) Springer-Verlag (1984) 49 - 56

Transethmoidal decompression of the optic nerve in the case of craniocerebral trauma

H. Kolenda, M. Schröder, H. Mühlendyck, B. Rama, E. Markakis

Abstract

Over a period of ten years 39 patients who suffered an optic nerve compression after a craniocerebral trauma underwent transethmoidal decompression surgery. The operation has been performed bilaterally on 5 patients.

50 % of patients involved suffered a blunt head or brain injury, the others a brain compression or contusion. On the side of optic nerve compression we found specific signs and symptoms such as negative or sluggish direct light reaction of the pupil, wound on the lateral side of the eyebrow, bleeding from the nose, eyelid hematoma, maximum number of skull fractures and intracranial hematomas.

The coincidence of radiological and intraoperative findings was only 67 %. The ophthalmological findings such as lack of direct pupil reaction with preserved consensual light-reaction or progressive loss of vision after a corresponding traumatic incident are our guideline for performing transethmoidal decompression of the optic nerve.

In comparison with the results of conservative therapy as published in the literature our operative results were good or acceptable in about 20 % or more of the cases.

Introduction

According to different statistics (5, 6, 11, 14) a lesion of the optic nerve is to be expected in 0,35 to 3,6 % of all patients suffering a craniocerebral trauma.

As former surgical treatment of an optic nerve compression by a craniotomy and transfrontal osteoclastic decompression proved to be dangerous in cases of severe brain injuries and ineffective compared to conservative treatment, the transethmoidal surgical approach to the optic canal was proposed in 1961 (8). This technique allows the remove of up to 75 % of the bony canal. Operating under local anesthesia, return of pupils light-reaction or return of visual function may direct the extent of the decompression (2, 8, 13). A disadvantage is the inability to decompress the optic nerve at its entry to the canal

Nethertheless excellent success was reported by SUGITA (13) and FUKADO (3) with a great number of patients. European findings were with smaller number of patients and their results remained poorer (1, 4, 12).

Since 1976, we performed decompression of the optic nerve on 37 patients with craniocerebral trauma by the transethmoidal approach. The diagnostic procedure was carried out in close cooperation between neurosurgeons and ophthalmologists, while the operation was performed by the otolaryngologists.

Results

Pattern of injuries

Age distribution showed 60 % of the patients to be in the groups of the second and third decade, most of them being between 15 and 25 years of age (Fig. 1).

Road traffic accidents were the most common reason for optic nerve injury (60 %) followed by occupational accidents (16 %). A polytrauma was frequent (40 %).

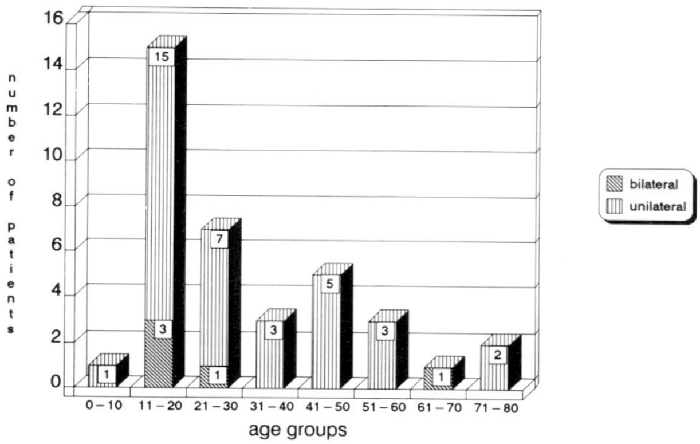

Fig. 1: Age distribution of patients, male = 32, female = 5

More than half of the patients suffered a blunt head trauma or a brain concussion only (Fig. 2). The rest of them had brain contusion, in 5 cases combined with considerable space-occupying intracerebral hemorrhage. Additionally, we found extracerebral hematomas in 5 patients. Thirteen patients had to undergo a neurosurgical intervention, mainly an evacuation of hematomas.

Brain contusion was localized mainly in the frontal lobe (75 % of the total), the rest in the temporoparietal region. They were located always on the same side as the optic nerve compression, like the extracerebral hematomas, with one exception: a seven year old girl, in whom the primary contusion side and all visible injuries were seen contralaterally, because the main fracture line crossed the other optic canal. Fractures of the orbit were seen most frequently, followed by fractures of the skull base (Fig. 3). Fractures of the facial skull outside the bony canal of the optic nerve were found in 84 % of the cases. These fractures influenced exclusively or predominant by the side of optic nerve compression. Visible bruises or injuries of the face and galea were found as well, always on the side of the optic nerve compression except in the one case mentioned above. They proved to be more frequent supra- as infraorbital, the majority situated in the fronto - temporal border.

Leading and misdirecting symptoms

Two thirds of the patients showed the triad of symtomatology reported by FUKADO (2) with "loss or sluggishness of the direct light reaction of the pupil on the affected side, a wound on the lateral side of the eyebrow and bleeding from the nose".

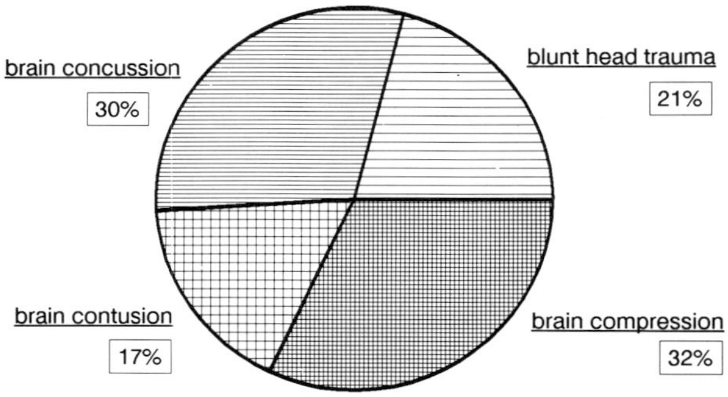

Fig. 2: Brain trauma (n = 37): light = 51%, severe = 49 %

In 90 % we also found an ipsilateral eyelid hematoma. It might either be a hint or distract from diagnosis if the hematoma is extensive. Besides an eyelid hematoma a contusion of the ocular bulb makes diagnosis more difficult (Tab. I). A hyposphagma was found in 65 % of the eyes concerned. In such a case only a sensitive investigation according to other bleedings inside the ocular bulb or effects of contusion to the iris or fundus of the bulb may lead to the diagnosis (7). Other factors impeding correct diagnosis were lack of cooperation with nearly half of the patients, posttraumatic space-occupying complications (compressio cerebri) in one third of the total, or a primary traumatic injury of the oculomotor nerve. We diagnosed this injury in five patients ipsilateral to the optic nerve compression.

A simultaneous lesion of the oculomotor nerve delayed the diagnosis for about ten hours. The average delay between traumatic insult and diagnosis was 35 hours. Unexpectedly, this interval was about twenty hours longer with conscious, cooperative patients as with unconscious patients after a severe brain injury.

We relate it to the more frequent primary defect of pupils' reaction and to more intensive primary care with patients after a severe brain damage. While only 20 % of the latter showed secondary compression of the optic nerve, 55 % of the primary conscious patients came to an amaurosis by secondary compression.

Pathogenetic factors

Comparison between preoperative radiological and intraoperative findings showed a concordance of only 67 % (Fig. 4). This might be due to the fact that during operation procedure the lateral part of the optic canal is invisible and consequently a fracture in that area shown by x-ray is not verifiable. Additionally, compression inside the canal is difficult to demonstrate through the transethmoidal approach.

In five cases an indication for the decompression of the nerve was seen although we had no pathological findings by plain x-rays or computerized tomography. In two of these cases operative findings were inconspicuous too.

Operative decompression results

As three patients died during the first two weeks after traumatic insult, the success of the transethmoidal operative decompression could be pursued on 38 decompressed optic nerves only (Tab. II).

Table II: Postoperative visus and visual field

Nearly complete restitution (80 - 100 % of pretraum. stage)	16 %
Restitution to about 50 % of pretraumatic stage	21 %
Restricted visual function	16 %
	53 %
Persisting amaurosis	37 %
Deterioration	10 %
	47 %

In 37 % we succeeded in turning out a good or sufficient visual function. All of these cases showed restitution of pupillary reaction up to the forth day. In up to 16 % of cases the postoperative visual function remained at recognition of hand movement or gleam of light. In those cases where a fracture and compression of the optic canal had been proved by radiodiagnostic means, restitution of visual function occurred to a maximum of 50 % only.

Bilateral optic nerve compression

With regard to the five patients being decompressed bilaterally, we found them all suffering from polytrauma and severe central fractures of the facial skull. All of them had fractures of Le Fort II and Le Fort III type, three had fragmentation fractures of the facial skull.

These five patients could be divided into two groups.

In the first one with two patients after a blunt craniocerebral trauma a limited direct reaction of the pupils was seen on both sides. Ophthalmoscopy showed streaky hemorrhages on both sides and blurredness of the papillas in the other patient. After operative treatment by maxillary surgery, loss of the pupillary reaction developed and remained unchanged in spite of decompressive procedure carried out on the second or third day. Intraoperative findings were inconspicuous. Retrospectively the explanation in one of the cases was a lesion of the chiasmatic region. In the other case a bilateral occlusion of the ateria centralis retinae was diagnosed.

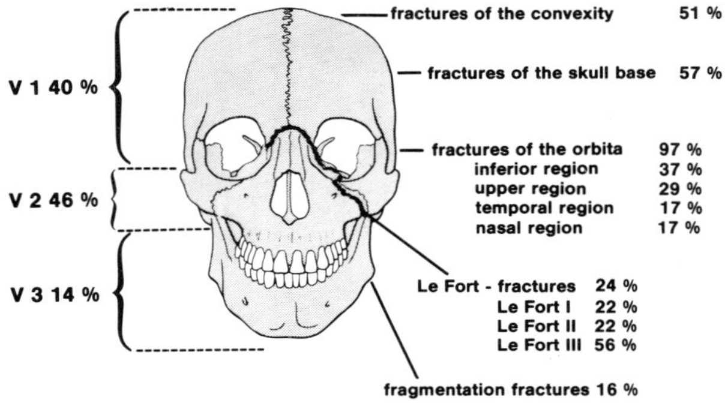

Fig. 3: Fractures of the skull in the case of traumatic optic nerve compression (n = 37). The percentages on the left side of the figure demonstrate the relative quantity of skull fractures according to the trigeminal nerve areas

The three patients in the second group suffered a severe craniocerebral trauma and because of loss of pupils' light reaction, decompression was performed during the first twelve hours after excluding brain compression as a reason for this. Intraoperatively fragmentation fractures of the ethmoidal structures and the optic canal were seen.

One of these patients died after three days, one kept half of his visual capacity and field in one of his eyes, the other a limited visual capacity in the upper nasal visual field.

Complications

In the 42 operations that we performed, one purulent secondary infection developed in the operation site five years afterwards and two after-bleedings. One of the after-bleeding might have been responsible for a postoperative deterioration of visual capacity.

Discussion

Comparing our results with extensive statistics in literature (6, 9, 10, 14) referred to the results of conservative therapy, we see an improvement in 40 to 75 % of the patients. Nearly complete restitution of visual function or restitution to about 50 % of pretraumatic stage, were seen after conservative treatment at an average of about 15 to 20 % of cases, while we achieved the same results with 37 % of our patients.

For this reason, transethmoidal optic nerve decompression should be performed, if after ophthalmological investigation and supporting radiodiagnostic evidence an optic nerve compression is suspected.

It has to be emphasised that on the one hand we perform a thorough radiological procedure, if we suspect an optic nerve compression, but on the other hand concerning the relevance for the indication of operative proceeding the characteristic ophthalmological findings are of greater relevance to us:

- lack of direct pupillary reaction and preserved consensual light - reaction and inconspicuous eyes fundus or
- progressive loss of vision after a craniocerebral trauma.

As other authors we think that decompression of the optic nerve should be performed as quick as possible, although we were not able to prove that with significant statistics.

Conclusions

A typical pattern of injuries to the orbita with an awake or unconscious patient has to be dealt with closely meshed controls of direct and consensual light reaction of the pupils, even if a considerable eyelid hematoma is hindering the diagnosis.

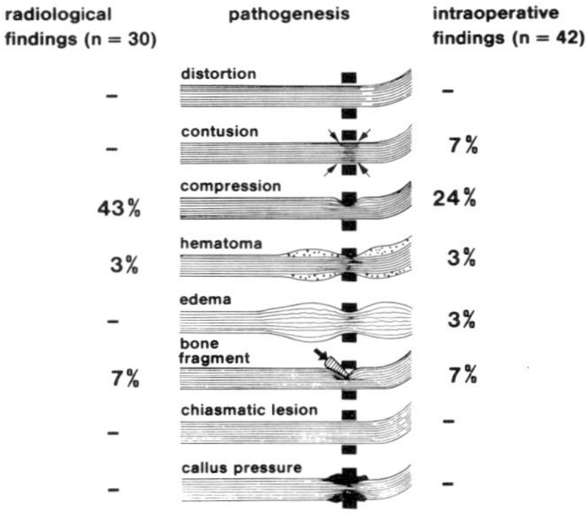

Fig. 4: Radiological and introperative findings of pathogenetic factors leading to an optic nerve lesion in sequence of their frequency from above to below; modified according to HAGER [4]

In the case of severe bilateral middle face fractures of a Le Fort II or Le Fort III type, we advice a conservative approach consisting of external fixation without mobilisation of the fractures, as majority among plastic surgeons in the USA concluded in 1984 (15), since a secondary amaurosis might be induced as in two of our patients.

Eyelid haematoma	90%
Hyposphagma (eyeball contusion)	65%
Lack of patient's cooperation	47%
Brain compression	32%
Oculomotor nerve lesion	14%
Light reaction bilaterally absent	14%

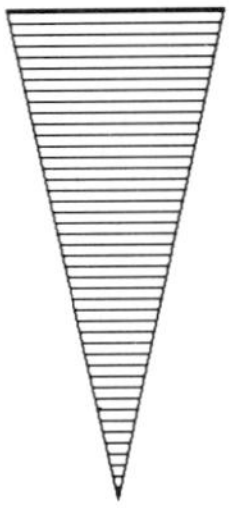

Tab. I: Results of transethmoidal optic nerve decompression (n = 38)

We propose to perform a detailed layered computerized tomography of the orbita immediately, if a light - resistant pupil after a craniocerebral trauma does not find its explanation by brain compression during computertomographic procedure.

References

[1] Behrens-Baumann W, Chilla R: Zur medikamentösen und chirurgischen Therapie der traumatischen Optikuskompression. Fortschr Ophthalmol 81 (1984) 87 -89

[2] Fukado Y: Results in 400 cases of surgical decompression of the optic nerve. Mod Probl Ophthal 14 (1975) 474 - 481

[3] Fukado Y: Microsurgical transethmoidal optic nerve decompression: experience in 700 cases. In Samii M, Jannetta PJ (eds): The cranial nerves. Springer-Verlag, Berlin-Heidberg-New York 1981

[4] Hager G, Gerhardt HJ, Maruniak M: Indikationen und Ergebnisse operativer Freilegung traumatisch geschädigter Sehnerven. Klin Monatsbl Augenheilkd 167 (1975) 515 - 526

[5] Hughes B: Verletzungen der Hirnnerven. In Kessel FK, Guttmann L, Maurer G (eds): Neuro-Traumatologie mit Einschluß der Grenzgebiete, Vol I. Urban und Schwarzenberg, München-Berlin-Wien 1969

[6] Landolt E: Zur Opticusschädigung bei Schädeltrauma. Acta Neurochir 4 (1956) 128 - 142

[7] Mühlendyck H, Leithäuser D: Diagnostic problems in cases with blow-out fractures and motility disturbances of other origin. Proc 3rd Int Symp on Orbital Disorders, Amsterdam (1977) 229 - 239

[8] Niho S, Yasuda K, Sato T et al.: Decompression of the optic canal by the transethmoidal route. Am J Ophthalmol 51 (1961) 659 - 665

[9] Otradovec J: Das Gesichtsfeld bei indirekten Sehnervenverletzungen. Klin Monatsbl Augenheilkd 153 (1968) 485 - 495

[10] Scheschy H, Benedikt O: Optikusatrophie durch indirekte Traumen. Klin Monatsbl Augenheilkd 161 (1972) 309 - 315

[11] Schmaltz B, Schürmann K: Traumatische Optikusschäden. Klin Monatsbl Augenheilkd 159 (1971) 33 - 51

[12] Siegl H: Zur Dekompression des Nervus opticus. Laryngol Rhinol Otol 64 (1985) 118 - 129

[13] Sugita S, Sugita Y, Jamada J et al.: Die Sehstörung nach Schädeltrauma und ihre operative Behandlung. Klin Monatsbl Augenheilk 147 (1965) 720 - 730

[14] Turner JWA: Indirect injuries of the optic nerve. Brain 66 (1943) 140 - 151

[15] Weymuller EA: Blindness and Le Fort III fractures. Ann Otol Rhinol Laryngol 93 (1984) 2 - 5

AUTHOR'S INDEX

Author's Index

SUBJECT INDEX

Subject Index